New Image-Enhanced Endoscopy

NBI/BLI Atlas

| Supervisor | Hisao Tajiri |

Editors	Mototsugu Kato
	Shinji Tanaka
	Yutaka Saito
	Manabu Muto

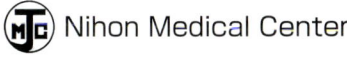
Nihon Medical Center

New Image-Enhanced Endoscopy
NBI/BLI Atlas

Supervisor　Hisao Tajiri

Editors　　　Mototsugu Kato

　　　　　　Shinji Tanaka

　　　　　　Yutaka Saito

　　　　　　Manabu Muto

Copyright © 2014 by Nihon Medical Center, Inc.
1-64 Kanda-jinbo-cho, Chiyoda-ku, Tokyo 101-0051, Japan

All rights reserved.
Any reproduction or other unauthorized use of the material or images herein is prohibited without the prior permission of the publisher.

Japanese edition published in Tokyo in 2013 by Nihon Medical Center, Inc.
English Translation　Atsushi Chiba

ISBN: 978-4-88875-274-9

New Image-Enhanced Endoscopy
NBI/BLI Atlas
新しい画像強調内視鏡システム　NBI/BLI アトラス〔英語版〕

2014年11月1日　第1版1刷発行

監　修　田尻　久雄
編　集　加藤　元嗣／田中　信治／斎藤　豊／武藤　学
発行者　増永　和也
発行所　株式会社日本メディカルセンター
　　　　東京都千代田区神田神保町1-64（神保町協和ビル）
　　　　〒101-0051　TEL 03(3291)3901㈹
印刷所　三報社印刷株式会社

ISBN978-4-88875-274-9
©2014　乱丁・落丁は，お取り替えいたします．

本書に掲載された著作物の複写・転載およびデータベースへの取り込みに関する許諾権は日本メディカルセンターが保有しています．

|JCOPY| <㈳出版者著作権管理機構　委託出版物>
本書の無断複写は著作権法上での例外を除き禁じられています．複写される場合は，そのつど事前に，㈳出版者著作権管理機構（電話 03-3513-6969，FAX03-3513-6979，e-mail：info@jcopy.or.jp）の許諾を得てください．

■ Supervisor

Hisao Tajiri — Professor, Department of Gastroenterology and Hepatology/Department of Endoscopy, The Jikei University School of Medicine

■ Editors

Mototsugu Kato — Clinical Professor, Division of Endoscopy, Hokkaido University Hospital

Shinji Tanaka — Professor, Department of Endoscopy, Hiroshima University Hospital

Yutaka Saito — Director, Endoscopy Center/Gastrointestinal Endoscopy Division, National Cancer Center Hospital

Manabu Muto — Professor, Department of Therapeutic Oncology, Graduate School of Medicine, Kyoto University

■ Authors (in order of appearance)

Kazuhiro Gono	R & D Planning Division, Olympus Medical Systems Corp.
Masayuki Kuramoto	Medical Systems R & D Center, R & D Management Headquarters, Fujifilm Corp.
Masahiro Kubo	Medical Systems R & D Center, R & D Management Headquarters, Fujifilm Corp.
Shuko Morita	Assistant Professor, Department of Gastroenterology and Hepatology, Graduate School of Medicine, Kyoto University
Tomomasa Hayashi	Assistant Professor, Department of Therapeutic Oncology, Graduate School of Medicine, Kyoto University
Manabu Muto	Professor, Department of Therapeutic Oncology, Graduate School of Medicine, Kyoto University
Yuichi Shimizu	Associate Professor, Department of Gastroenterology, Hokkaido University Graduate School of Medicine
Kenro Kawada	Assistant Professor, Department of Esophageal and General Surgery, Tokyo Medical and Dental University
Tatsuyuki Kawano	Professor, Department of Esophageal and General Surgery, Tokyo Medical and Dental University
Akira Dobashi	Assistant Professor, Department of Endoscopy, The Jikei University School of Medicine
Kenichi Goda	Assistant Professor, Department of Endoscopy, The Jikei University School of Medicine
Hisao Tajiri	Professor, Department of Gastroenterology and Hepatology/Department of Endoscopy, The Jikei University School of Medicine
Miwako Arima	Deputy Director, Department of Gastroenterology, Head of Department of Endoscopy, Saitama Cancer Center
Mika Tsunomiya	Chief, Department of Gastroenterology, Saitama Cancer Center
Takako Yoshii	Chief, Department of Gastroenterology, Saitama Cancer Center
Fumiko Yamamoto	Department of Gastroenterology and Hepatology, Nagoya University Graduate School of Medicine
Ryoji Miyahara	Assistant Professor, Department of Gastroenterology and Hepatology, Nagoya University Graduate School of Medicine
Hidemi Goto	Professor, Department of Gastroenterology and Hepatology, Nagoya University Graduate School of Medicine
Seiichiro Abe	Endoscopy Division, National Cancer Center Hospital
Shigetaka Yoshinaga	Endoscopy Division, National Cancer Center Hospital
Ryoji Kushima	Chief, Pathology and Clinical Laboratory Division, National Cancer Center Hospital
Satoshi Mochizuki	Department of Gastroenterology, University of Tokyo Hospital
Mitsuhiro Fujishiro	Associate Professor, Director of the Department of Endoscopy and Endoscopic Surgery, University of Tokyo Hospital
Kazuhiko Koike	Professor, Department of Gastroenterology, University of Tokyo Hospital
Mototsugu Kato	Clinical Professor, Division of Endoscopy, Hokkaido University Hospital
Shoko Ono	Assistant Professor, Division of Endoscopy, Hokkaido University Hospital
Nobuaki Yagi	Professor, Department of Gastroenterology, Murakami Memorial Hospital, Asahi University (Visiting professor, Department of Molecular Gastroenterology and Hepatology, Graduate School of Medical Science, Kyoto Prefectural University of Medicine)
Shigeto Yoshida	Clinical Lecturer, Department of Endoscopy, Hiroshima University Hospital
Kazuyoshi Yagi	Director, Department of Internal Medicine, Niigata Prefectural Yoshida Hospital
Yujiro Nozawa	Chief, Department of Internal Medicine, Niigata Prefectural Yoshida Hospital
Atsuo Nakamura	Director, Department of Internal Medicine, Niigata Prefectural Yoshida Hospital
Noriya Uedo	Vice-Director, Department of Gastrointestinal Oncology, Endoscopic Training and Learning Center, Osaka Medical Center for Cancer and Cardiovascular Diseases
Shinya Kodashima	Assistant Professor, Department of Gastroenterology, The University of Tokyo Hospital
Azumi Suzuki	Department of Gastroenterology, Kyoto Second Red Cross Hospital
Kenjiro Yasuda	Deputy Hospital Director, Department of Gastroenterology, Kyoto Second Red Cross Hospital
Shunsuke Kamba	Department of Gastroenterology and Hepatology, Department of Endoscopy, The Jikei University School of Medicine
Kazuki Sumiyama	Department of Endoscopy, The Jikei University School of Medicine
Yoji Takeuchi	Deputy Director, Gastrointestinal Oncology, Osaka Medical Center for Cancer and Cardiovascular Diseases
Yasuhiko Tomita	Senior Director, Department of Pathology, Osaka Medical Center for Cancer and Cardiovascular Diseases
Yoshimasa Miura	Assistant Professor, Endoscopy Center, Jichi Medical University
Hironori Yamamoto	Professor, Endoscopy Center, Jichi Medical University
Takashi Kawai	Professor, Endoscopy Center, Tokyo Medical University Hospital
Hiroaki Sawai	Department of Gastroenterology, Hyogo Cancer Center

Hiroyuki Ono	Deputy Hospital Director, Director of Endoscopy Division, Shizuoka Cancer Center
Kayoko Matsushima	Research Associate, Department of Gastroenterology and Hepatology, Nagasaki University
Hajime Isomoto	Associate Professor, Department of Gastroenterology and Hepatology/Department of Endoscopy, Nagasaki University Hospital
Ken Onita	Lecturer, Department of Gastroenterology and Hepatology, Nagasaki University Hospital
Saburo Shikuwa	Director, Sankokai Miyazaki Hospital
Shin Ichihara	Chief, Department of Pathology, Hokkaido P. W. F. A. C Sapporo-Kosei General Hospital
Shinji Tanaka	Professor, Department of Endoscopy, Hiroshima University Hospital
Naohisa Yoshida	Lecturer, Department of Molecular Gastroenterology and Hepatology, Graduate School of Medical Science, Kyoto Prefectural University of Medicine
Yuji Naito	Associate Professor, Department of Molecular Gastroenterology and Hepatology, Graduate School of Medical Science, Kyoto Prefectural University of Medicine
Yoshito Itoh	Professor, Department of Molecular Gastroenterology and Hepatology, Graduate School of Medical Science, Kyoto Prefectural University of Medicine
Shoichi Saito	Lecturer, Department of Endoscopy, The Jikei University School of Medicine
Masahiro Ikegami	Professor, Department of Pathology, The Jikei University School of Medicine
Daisuke Ide	Department of Gastroenterology and Hepatology/Department of Endoscopy, The Jikei University School of Medicine
Yoshikazu Hayashi	Research Associate, Division of Gastroenterology, Department of Medicine, Jichi Medical University School of Medicine
Noriyoshi Fukushima	Professor, Department of Pathology, Jichi Medical University School of Medicine
Takeshi Yamashina	Department of Gastrointestinal Oncology, Osaka Medical Center for Cancer and Cardiovascular Diseases
Taku Sakamoto	Endoscopy Division, National Cancer Center Hospital
Takeshi Nakajima	Endoscopy Division, National Cancer Center Hospital
Takahisa Matsuda	Chief, Endoscopy Division, National Cancer Center Hospital
Yutaka Saito	Director, Endoscopy Center/Gastrointestinal Endoscopy Division, National Cancer Center Hospital
Takuji Kawamura	Chief, Department of Gastroenterology, Kyoto Second Red Cross Hospital
Akira Yokoyama	Department of Clinical Oncology, Kyoto University Graduate School of Medicine
Takahiro Horimatsu	Department of Clinical Oncology, Kyoto University Graduate School of Medicine
Toshio Uraoka	Medical director, Department of Gastroenterology, National Hospital Organization Tokyo Medical Center
Naohisa Yahagi	Professor, Division of Research and Development for Minimally Invasive Treatment, Cancer Center, Keio University
Motoya Tominaga	Research Associate, Division of Gastroenterology and Hematology/Oncology, Department of Medicine, Asahikawa Medical University
Mikihiro Fujiya	Associate Professor, Division of Gastroenterology and Hematology/Oncology, Department of Medicine, Asahikawa Medical University
Yutaka Kohgo	Professor, Division of Gastroenterology and Hematology/Oncology, Department of Medicine, Asahikawa Medical University
Kinichi Hotta	Chief, Division of Endoscopy, Shizuoka Cancer Center
Kenichiro Imai	Deputy Chief, Division of Endoscopy, Shizuoka Cancer Center
Yuichiro Yamaguchi	Division of Endoscopy, Shizuoka Cancer Center
Yoshiki Wada	Research Associate, Digestive Disease Center, Showa University Northern Yokohama Hospital (presently Assistant Professor, Department of Endoscopy, Tokyo Medical and Dental University Hospital)
Shin-ei Kudo	Professor, Director of the Digestive Disease Center, Showa University Northern Yokohama Hospital
Masashi Misawa	Digestive Disease Center, Showa University Northern Yokohama Hospital
Hiroshi Kawano	Clinical Director, Department of Gastroenterology, St. Mary's Hospital
Osamu Tsuruta	Professor, Department of Medicine, Division of Gastroenterology, Kurume University School of Medicine/Department of Endoscopy, Digestive Disease Center, Kurume University Hospital
Shozo Osera	Department of Gastroenterology, Endoscopy Division, National Cancer Center Hospital East
Hiroaki Ikematsu	Department of Gastroenterology, Endoscopy Division, National Cancer Center Hospital East
Tatsushi Shingai	Department of Surgery, Osaka Medical Center for Cancer and Cardiovascular Diseases
Takashi Hisabe	Lecturer, Department of Gastroenterology, Fukuoka University Chikushi Hospital
Santa Hattori	Gastrointestinal Center, Sano Hospital
Yasushi Sano	Director, Gastrointestinal Center, Sano Hospital
Chiko Sato	Endoscopy Division, National Cancer Center Hospital
Nana Hayashi	Department of Endoscopy and Medicine, Hiroshima University Hospital
Daiki Nemoto	Department of Coloproctology, Aizu Medical Center, Fukushima Medical University
Shungo Endo	Professor, Department of Coloproctology, Aizu Medical Center, Fukushima Medical University
Kazutomo Togashi	Professor, Department of Coloproctology, Aizu Medical Center, Fukushima Medical University
Shin Haruyama	Endoscopy Center/Gastrointestinal Endoscopy Division, National Cancer Center Hospital
Yasushi Iwao	Professor, Center for Preventive Medicine, Keio University Hospital

Preface

The history of endoscopy over the past three decades has been marked by steady and rapid progress in endoscopic treatment, as arisen from the development of the video endoscope in 1983, leading to rapid advances in the subsequent years. The 1980s were characterized by improvements in endoscopic treatment of early gastrointestinal cancers using EMR, while in the 1990s, previous concepts of diagnosis and treatment of gastric diseases were overturned when the association between *H. pylori* and diseases of the gastrointestinal tract was verified. In the 2000s, the rapid dissemination of ESD has led to further advances in endoscopic treatment, while the introduction of the HDTV endoscope to the market in 2002, together with more recent innovations such as image-enhanced endoscopy (IEE) and magnifying endoscopy, has provided the basis for new diagnostic study. Now, thanks to the introduction of high-resolution endoscopes and magnifying endoscopes with NBI (Narrow Band Imaging), which provide clear and accurate observation of the microstructures and microvascular architectures on the mucosal surfaces, the grade of tissue atypism can be estimated with endoscopy. Soon we will enter a new era of endoscopic diagnosis, an era of what we can call "endoscopic pathology" in pretherapeutic examinations.

These minute diagnostics have triggered a quantum leap in traditional endoscopic diagnosis. Supported by the achievements of prospective multicenter studies, these developments have had a profound impact on gastrointestinal endoscopists and cancer researchers around the world. As a result, it has been propagated worldwide and made a significant contribution to actual cancer treatments, as well as to clinical studies.

Since the summer of 2012, two systems have been released which are designed to obtain images with even higher definition easily than before. They are the EVIS LUCERA ELITE system with built-in NBI from Olympus Medical Systems Corporation and the LASEREO laser endoscopy system from Fujifilm Corporation featuring another new method called BLI (Blue Laser Imaging). This book was written in order to give you an idea of what the endoscopic images obtained with the new systems look like, explain how to incorporate IEE in endoscopic diagnosis and provide tips on observation using the new IEE techniques. Drawing on a comprehensive collection of case images as ATLAS sourced from hospitals that have already introduced these new systems, this book will guide you step by step through the diagnostic process, enabling you to observe minute changes in the endoscopic images and compare those observations with the explanations given by the authors. We are confident that this book will serve as a leading reference with high quality for a wide range of people, from young physicians aiming at becoming endoscopy specialists to doctors who are already acting as specialists or trainers, providing them with the knowledge they need to understand the new image-enhanced endoscopy and the guidance they need to take advantage of.

We hope that the material included in this book will give our readers the confidence to take on the challenge of pioneering the use of second-generation NBI, which has surmounted the problems associated with conventional NBI and/or BLI in routine procedures, and to perform evaluations and studies in order to establish more sophisticated diagnostics and advance new functional studies.

Finally, we would like to express our gratitude to the many doctors who contributed to this book even though they were very busy. We would also like to express gratitude to Ms. Setsuko Kurozoe at Nihon Medical Center for her work in the editing of this book.

October 2013   Hisao Tajiri
President, Japan Gastroenterological Endoscopy Society
Professor, Department of Gastroenterology and Hepatology/
Department of Endoscopy, The Jikei University School of Medicine, Tokyo, Japan

Abbreviations

Japanese classifications

DM	distal margin
EGJ	esophagogastric junction
EP	tumor confined to the epithelium
HM0	no involvement of the horizontal margin
INFa	expanding growth with a distinct border from the surrounding tissue
INFb	intermediate pattern between INFa and INFc
INFc	infiltrative growth with no distinct border with the surrounding tissue
int	intermediate type
LPM	tumor confined to the lamina propria mucosae
ly0/1/2	no/ minimal/ moderate lymphatic invasion
MM	tumor confined to the muscularis mucosae
por	poorly differentiated adenocarcinoma
Ra	rectum above the peritoneal reflection
Rb	lower rectum
RM	radial margin
SCJ	squamocolumnar junction
sig	signet-ring cell carcinoma
SM	tumor confined to the submucosa
tub1	well differentiated tubular adenocarcinoma
tub2	moderately differentiated tubular adenocarcinoma
UL	ulcer/ ulcer scar
v0/1/2	no/ minimal/ moderate venous invasion
VM0	no involvement of the vertical margin
p (prefix)	pathological classification (ex. pDM0; pathologically no involvement of the distal margin, pPM0; pathologically no involvement of the proximal margin)

Others

AVA	avascular area
BLI	Blue LASER Imaging
CO	crypt opening
CP	capillary pattern
EMR	endoscopic mucosal resection
ESD	endoscopic submucosal dissection
FICE	Flexible spectral Imaging Color Enhancement
IPCL	intraepithelial papillary capillary loop
LBC	light blue crest
LEL	lymphoepithelial lesion
LST	laterally spreading tumor
MCE	marginal crypt epithelium
NBI	Narrow Band Imaging
SECN	subepithelial capillary network
WLI	white light imaging
WOS	white opaque substance
WZ	white zone

CONTENTS

Principles of NBI and BLI

NBI (Narrow Band Imaging) ·············· Olympus Medical Systems Corp. 12
BLI (Blue Laser Imaging) ·· Fujifilm Corp. 16

Oropharynx and Hypopharynx

● **General Theory** : How to Observe These Regions with NBI or BLI
Tips on NBI Observation ·················· Morita, S., Hayashi, T., Muto, M. 24
Tips on BLI Observation ·· Shimizu, Y. 26

● **Case Atlas**

Case 1	NBI	Inflammatory pharyngeal lesion	Morita, S., Muto, M.	30
Case 2	BLI	Hypopharyngeal papilloma	Kawada, K., Kawano, T.	32
Case 3	NBI	Pharyngeal melanosis	Dobashi, A., Goda, K., Tajiri, H.	34
Case 4	BLI	Pharyngeal melanosis	Shimizu, Y.	36
Case 5	NBI	Oropharyngeal superficial carcinoma (0 – Ⅱa)	Morita, S., Hayashi, T., Muto, M.	38
Case 6	BLI	Oropharyngeal superficial carcinoma (0 – Ⅱb)	Kawada, K., Kawano, T.	40
Case 7	NBI	Hypopharyngeal superficial carcinoma (0 – Ⅱb)	Morita, S., Muto, M.	42
Case 8	BLI	Hypopharyngeal superficial carcinoma (0 – Ⅱa + Ⅱb)	Shimizu, Y.	44

Esophagus

● **General Theory** : How to Observe This Region with NBI or BLI
Tips on NBI Observation ··············· Goda, K., Dobashi, A., Tajiri, H. 48
Tips on BLI Observation ·············· Arima, M., Tsunomiya, M., Yoshii, T. 56

● **Case Atlas**

Case	Mode	Title	Authors	Page
Case 9	NBI	Glycogenic acanthosis (GA)	Morita, S., Muto, M.	62
Case 10	BLI	Esophageal papilloma	Arima, M.	64
Case 11	NBI	NERD	Dobashi, A., Goda, K., Tajiri, H.	66
Case 12	BLI	NERD	Yamamoto, F., Miyahara, R., Goto, H.	68
Case 13	NBI	GERD	Goda, K., Dobashi, A., Tajiri, H.	70
Case 14	BLI	GERD	Yamamoto, F., Miyahara, R., Goto, H.	72
Case 15	NBI	Type 0–I superficial esophageal carcinoma	Morita, S., Muto, M.	74
Case 16	BLI	Type 0–I s superficial esophageal carcinoma	Arima, M.	76
Case 17	BLI	Type 0–II a superficial esophageal carcinoma	Kawada, K., Kawano, T.	78
Case 18	BLI	Type 0–II b superficial esophageal carcinoma	Arima, M.	80
Case 19	NBI BLI	Type 0–II c superficial esophageal cancer	Abe, S., Yoshinaga, S., Kushima, R.	82
Case 20	NBI BLI	Type 0–II c superficial esophageal cancer	Abe, S., Yoshinaga, S., Kushima, R.	84
Case 21	BLI	Type 0–II c superficial esophageal carcinoma	Yamamoto, F., Miyahara, R., Goto, H.	86
Case 22	NBI	Barrett's esophagus	Goda, K., Dobashi, A., Tajiri, H.	88
Case 23	BLI	Barrett's esophagus	Yamamoto, F., Miyahara, R., Goto, H.	90
Case 24	NBI	Barrett's esophageal adenocarcinoma	Goda, K., Dobashi, A., Tajiri, H.	92
Case 25	BLI	Barrett's esophageal adenocarcinoma	Arima, M.	94

Stomach and Duodenum

● **General Theory**: How to Observe These Regions with NBI or BLI

Tips on NBI Observation ················ Mochizuki, S., Fujishiro, M., Koike, K. 98
Tips on BLI Observation ················ Kato, M., Ono, S., Yagi, N., Yoshida, S. 104

● **Case Atlas**

[Stomach]

| Case 26 | NBI | Chronic gastritis | Yagi, K., Nozawa, Y., Nakamura, A. | 110 |

Case 27	BLI	Chronic gastritis	Uedo, N. 112
Case 28	NBI	Gastric adenoma	Kodashima, S. 114
Case 29	BLI	Gastric adenoma	Yoshida, S. 116
Case 30	NBI	Differential diagnosis of adenoma and gastric carcinoma	Suzuki, A., Yasuda, K. 118
Case 31	BLI	Differential diagnosis of erosion and early gastric carcinoma	Ono, S. 120
Case 32	NBI	Diagnosis of extent of early gastric cancer	Morita, S., Muto, M. 122
Case 33	BLI	Diagnosis of extent of early gastric carcinoma	Yoshida, S. 124
Case 34	BLI	Diagnosis of extent of early gastric carcinoma	Yagi, N. 126
Case 35	NBI	Type 0 – IIc differentiated early gastric carcinoma	Kamba, S., Sumiyama, K., Tajiri, H. 128
Case 36	NBI	Diagnosis of histological type of early gastric carcinoma	Mochizuki, S., Fujishiro, M., Koike, K. 130
Case 37	BLI	Diagnosis of histological type of early gastric carcinoma	Takeuchi, Y., Uedo, N., Tomita, Y. 132
Case 38	BLI	Diagnosis of histological type of early gastric carcinoma	Miura, Y., Yamamoto, H. 134
Case 39	NBI	Transnasal endoscopic observation of early gastric carcinoma	Kawai, T. 136
Case 40	NBI	Early carcinoma in gastric remnant	Sawai, H., Ono, H. 138
Case 41	NBI	MALT lymphoma	Matsushima, K., Isomoto, H., Onita, K., Shikuwa, S. 140
Case 42	BLI	MALT lymphoma	Ono, S. 142

[Duodenum]

Case 43	NBI	Duodenal adenoma	Dobashi, A., Goda, K., Tajiri, H. 144
Case 44	BLI	Duodenal adenoma	Yoshida, S. 146
Case 45	NBI	Duodenal carcinoma	Dobashi, A., Goda, K., Tajiri, H. 148
Case 46	BLI	Duodenal carcinoma	Yagi, N. 150
Case 47	BLI	Duodenal carcinoma	Ono, S. 152

Featured Article

· Pathological correlative approach to magnified images   Ichihara, S. 154

Colon and Rectum

- **General Theory**: How to Observe These Regions with NBI or BLI

  NBI Observation—Basic Principles and Operation Tips ················· Tanaka, S. 158

  Tips on BLI Observation ························· Yoshida, N., Naito, Y., Ito, Y. 168

- **Case Atlas**

Case 48	NBI	Hyperplastic polyp	Saito, S., Ikegami, M., Tajiri, H.	174
Case 49	NBI	SSA/P (sessile serrated adenoma/polyp)	Ide, D., Saito, S., Ikegami, M.	176
Case 50	BLI	SSA/P (sessile serrated adenoma/polyp)	Hayashi, Y., Yamamoto, H., Fukushima, N.	178
Case 51	BLI	SSA/P (sessile serrated adenoma/polyp)	Takeuchi, Y., Yamashina, T., Tomita, Y.	180
Case 52	NBI	Protruding serrated adenoma	Sakamoto, T., Nakajima, T., Matsuda, T., Saito, Y.	182
Case 53	NBI	Elevated tubular adenoma	Kawamura, T., Yasuda, K.	184
Case 54	NBI	Superficial tubular adenoma	Yokoyama, A., Horimatsu, T.	186
Case 55	NBI	Tubulovillous adenoma	Uraoka, T., Yahagi, N.	188
Case 56	BLI	Villous adenoma	Tominaga, M., Fujiya, M., Kohgo, Y.	190
Case 57	NBI	Protruding M carcinoma	Hotta, K., Imai, K., Yamaguchi, Y.	192
Case 58	NBI	Slightly elevated M carcinoma	Imai, K., Hotta, K., Yamaguchi, Y.	194
Case 59	NBI	Slightly depressed M carcinoma	Wada, Y., Kudo, S., Misawa, M.	196
Case 60	NBI	Elevated SM carcinoma	Kawano, H., Tsuruta, O.	198
Case 61	NBI	Slightly depressed SM carcinoma	Osera, S., Ikematsu, H.	200
Case 62	BLI	Composite (Ⅱa+Ⅱc) SM carcinoma	Takeuchi, Y., Shingai, T., Tomita, Y.	202
Case 63	BLI	Composite (Ⅱa+Ⅱc) SM carcinoma	Hisabe, T.	204
Case 64	NBI	Composite (Ⅱa+Ⅱc) SM carcinoma	Hattori, S., Sano, Y.	206
Case 65	NBI	Composite (Ⅰs+Ⅱc) SM carcinoma	Sato, C., Matsuda, T., Saito, Y.	208
Case 66	NBI	LST-G, homogeneous type	Misawa, M., Wada, Y., Kudo, S.	210

Case 67	BLI	LST-G, nodular mixed type	Yoshida, N., Yagi, N., Naito, Y.	212
Case 68	NBI	LST-NG, pseudo-depressed type	Hayashi, N., Tanaka, S.	214
Case 69	BLI	LST-NG, pseudo-depressed type	Nemoto, D., Endo, S., Togashi, K.	216
Case 70	NBI BLI	LST-NG, pseudo-depressed type	Haruyama, S., Saito, Y., Kushima, R.	218
Case 71	NBI	LST-NG, pseudo-depressed type	Hayashi, N., Tanaka, S.	222
Case 72	BLI	LST-NG, pseudo-depressed type	Yoshida, N., Yagi, N., Naito, Y.	224
Case 73	BLI	Ulcerative colitis	Tominaga, M., Fujiya, M., Kohgo, Y.	226
Case 74	NBI	Tumor associated with inflammatory colon diseases (carcinoma/dysplasia)	Uraoka, T., Iwao, Y.	228

Featured Articles

· Magnifications in Near Focus electronic zoom observation
  of the LUCERA ELITE system　　　　　　　　　　　Tanaka, S., Hayashi, N.　230

· Importance of structure enhancement in NBI magnifying observation
　　　　　　　　　　　　　　　　　　　　　　　　　Tanaka, S., Hayashi, N.　232

Cover
　①② Hattori, S., et al. (p. 206, 207)
　③ Yoshida, N., et al. (p. 212)
　④ Goda, K., et al. (p. 53)
　⑤ Kato, M., et al. (p. 106)

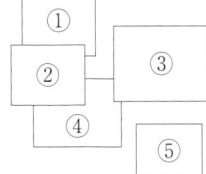

Principles of NBI and BLI

See page 4 for explanation of abbreviations.

Principles of NBI and BLI

Olympus Medical Systems Corporation

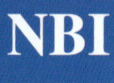 NBI (Narrow Band Imaging)

Introduction

In May 2006, Olympus introduced the EVIS LUCERA SPECTRUM, a next-generation endoscopy system incorporating the NBI (Narrow Band Imaging) function. NBI is an image enhancement technology that improves the contrast of the microvascular structure and fine mucosal patterns in the mucosal surface layer[1,2]. It is classified as "image-enhanced endoscopy, optical digital technology, narrow band technique" because it is implemented by optimizing the observation light and signal processing[3]. Since its introduction in Japan, NBI has been adopted by many medical facilities and clinical studies have been performed for a variety of diseases. With its establishment as a legitimate diagnostic tool, NBI was added as "narrow-band light enhancement" in the fiscal year 2012 amendment of the Japanese Medical Expenses Reimbursement System. It was also awarded the Prime Minister's Prize at the 2011 National Commendation for Invention and Innovation for its originality as an industrial product and its contribution to the medicine. To give you a better understanding of NBI, we will summarize its principles here, as well as offer a few tips on how to use it in endoscopic observation.

I. Targets enhanced by NBI

The standard technique used in endoscopic observation is white light imaging (WLI), which displays natural mucosal colors on the monitor. In some cases, endoscopists focus on specific areas of interest such as the microvascular structure or fine patterns in the mucosal surface layer. To support observation and diagnosis, these targets have been enhanced by digital image processing techniques such as color enhancement and structure enhancement. Although these techniques can enhance colors and structures while maintaining relatively accurate WLI color reproduction so that the image appears natural to the observer, their enhancement effects are limited by the inherent characteristics of digital image processing. A better solution was needed, and in the late 1990 s, Olympus began developing a new technique to perform enhancement using light. Since this technique achieves its effects by manipulating light wavelengths, which means the color, using it means discarding the natural color reproduction available with WLI. However, in doing so, this technique is able to achieve enhancement effects that are virtually impossible to obtain with digital image processing. In other words, this function specializes in enhancing the contrast of targets such as vessels or patterns, rather than accurately reproducing colors. This means that NBI findings should be understood as changes in contrast rather than changes in color.

Contrast can be defined as the ratio of brightness between the background and the

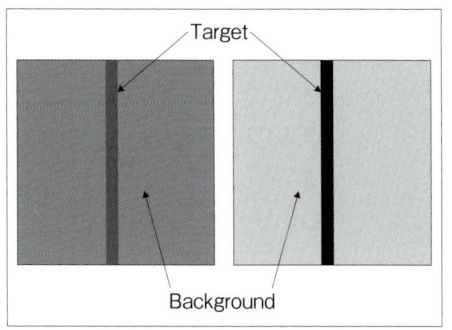

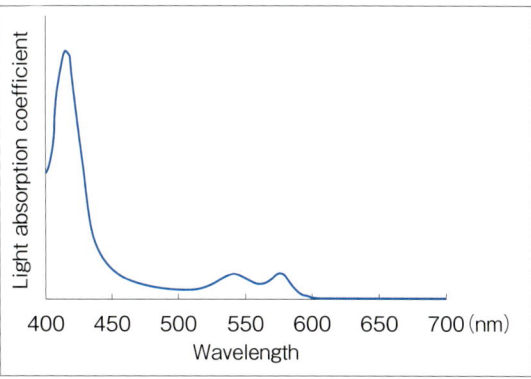

Fig. 1 Contrast

Fig. 2 Characteristics of Hemoglobin

target that the endoscopist is focusing on. If the target is blood vessels, the contrast represents the ratio of brightness between the vessels and the surrounding mucosa.

II. Principles

Enhancing the contrast means changing the brightness of the target so that it stands out from the background. Specifically, the target is made darker, while the background is made brighter as shown in **Fig. 1** or vice versa. If the endoscopist wants to observe the vessels, the contrast can be enhanced by darkening the vessels and brightening the surrounding mucosa. So how is this achieved? How bright or how dark something appears depends on how much of the incident light is returned to the endoscope. The amount of light returned from the vessels is determined by how much light is absorbed by the hemoglobin inside the vessels. Absorption of light means the conversion of the energy of the incident light into heat.

Since light, like sound, travels in waves, different types of light have different wavelengths. Changing the wavelength significantly alters the characteristics of the light. A human being can perceive light with wavelengths from 400 nm to 700 nm. When the light wavelength changes, we perceive it as a change in color—for example, light with a wavelength of 400 nm light appears blue, 550 nm is green, and 700 nm is red. In addition, when an object absorbs light of a specific wavelength, we see that object as being of a specific color. For instance, an apple looks red because the pigment in its skin absorbs the blue and green light, while the unabsorbed red light is reflected toward our eyes.

Hemoglobin primarily absorbs light energy with wavelengths of 415 and 540 nm—that is, blue light and green light (**Fig. 2**). Normal white light (as used in WLI) is composed of the three primary colors—red, green and blue (RGB). However, the blue light contains multiple wavelengths ranging from 400 to 500 nm, and the green light also contains multiple wavelengths around 550 nm. This is too broad a spectrum to enable significant absorption by the hemoglobin. Instead, the illumination light has to be filtered and converted into focused two narrow-band beams of 415 nm and 540 nm. When this narrow-band illumination is used, the hemoglobin will absorb more of the light incident on the vessels, making the vascular regions appear much darker. This dramatically enhances the contrast between the vascular regions and the background mucosa.

III. How NBI enhances images

Fig. 3 shows the blood vessels on the underside of the tongue. NBI renders the

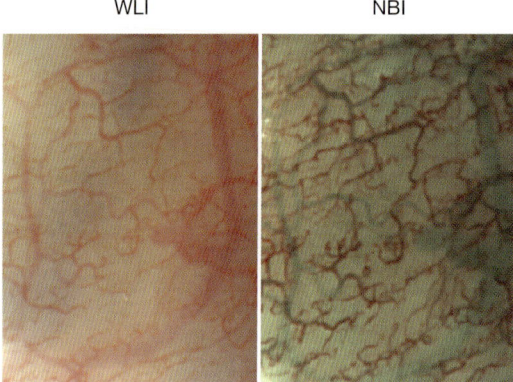

Fig. 3   Images of the Mucosa on the Underside of the Tongue

capillaries in the surface layer in brown, while the vessels in the deeper layers are shown in cyan. The way it works with an actual endoscopy system is quite simple. The NBI and WLI modes can be switched over by pressing a switch on the scope control section. When the scope switch is pressed, the filter that converts WLI light into narrow-band wavelengths of 415 and 540 nm is engaged in the light path. Then, the RGB rotary filter intermittently irradiates the mucosa with RGB-sequential narrow-band beams. At the 415 nm irradiation timing, a monochrome image corresponding to the capillary structure on the mucosal surface layer is generated, while at the 540 nm irradiation timing, a monochrome image corresponding to the vascular structure in the deep layer is generated. The video processor synthesizes the final color image from the two monochrome images (**Fig. 3**). The synthesis is executed by applying the 415 nm monochrome image signal to the B and G input terminals of the monitor and applying the 540 nm monochrome image signal to the R input terminal of the monitor. At first glance, it may appear as if this method—which is specific to NBI—destroys the color balance, but it is the only way to effectively achieve the vascular contrast enhancement effect.

IV. Evolution of NBI

Initially, the biggest problem hampering the effectiveness of NBI was its brightness. Since the narrow-band components are extracted from WLI using optical filters, the energy, or brightness, of the illumination light is reduced, resulting in a corresponding reduction in image brightness. This reduced brightness has been especially problematic in gastric observation. In October 2012, Olympus Medical Systems Corp. introduced the EVIS LUCERA ELITE system, which incorporates improved NBI technology (**Fig. 4**) that effectively resolves problem of NBI brightness.

To improve the brightness, Olympus modified the system so that the 415 nm narrow-band beam is irradiated twice. The result is a significant improvement in image clarity that makes it possible to now use NBI in the stomach as well. **Fig. 5** shows a comparison between the old and new versions of NBI using a stomach model. Assuming that the NBI technology used in the EVIS LUCERA SPECTRUM system can be considered the first generation of NBI, that used in the EVIS LUCERA ELITE system can be regarded as the second generation of NBI.

Conclusion

As described above, NBI works by exploiting the wavelength selectivity of the

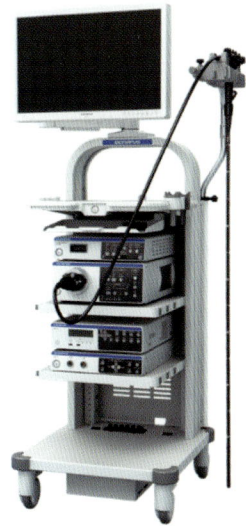

Fig. 4 EVIS LUCERA ELITE

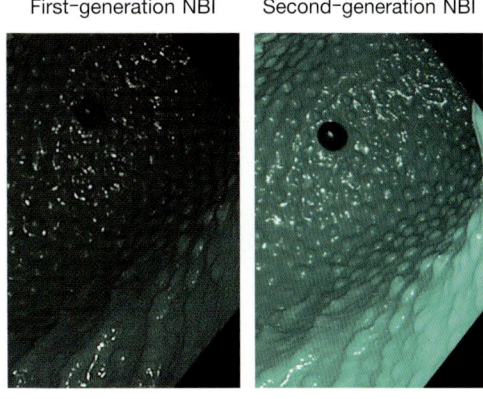

Fig. 5 Improvement of NBI Brightness

absorption characteristics of hemoglobin. As for NBI's clinical efficacy, you can read the numerous reports contributed to this book by many doctors. When developing NBI, we soon became convinced that the ability to control light characteristics would prove of enormous benefit to medicine. Now, having solved the brightness problem with the development of second-generation NBI, we are more certain of its potential than ever. In the future, we hope to build on the possibilities inherent in this light control technology, both by improving NBI still further and by developing innovative new functions.

References
1) Gono, K., Yamazaki, K., Doguchi, N. et al. : Endoscopic Observation of Tissue by Narrowband Illumination. Opt. Rev. 2003 ; 10 : 211-215
2) Gono, K., Obi, T., Yamaguchi, M. et al. : Appearance of enhanced tissue features in narrowband endoscopic imaging. J. Biomed. Opt. 2004 ; 9 : 568-577
3) Niwa, H., Tajiri, H. : Proposal of new classification of endoscopic observation method (in Japanese, title translated). Rinsho Shokaki Naika (Clinical Gastroenterology), 2008 ; 23 (1) : 137-141

(Gono, K.)

Principles of NBI and BLI

Fujifilm Corporation

BLI (Blue Laser Imaging)

Introduction

Previous Fujifilm endoscopy systems used FICE (Flexible spectral Imaging Color Enhancement), which enhances images by extracting spectral images at the desired wavelengths by applying signal processing to the white light generally used by endoscopes. However, because the ability of conventional white light illumination to image microvessels in the mucosal surface layer in high contrast is limited, a more effective way to achieve this was felt to be of critical importance.

In our new-generation endoscopy system called LASEREO, introduced in September 2012, we incorporated laser illumination technology that combines two types of laser light with a phosphor and unique image processing technology. The result is BLI (Blue Laser Imaging), a powerful new technique for observing images and enhancing the information considered important for cancer diagnoses, specifically changes in the microvessels in the mucosal surface layer and in the mucosal surface structure[1]. Here we will discuss the outline, principles and performance of the system, as well as highlight to consider the future potential of laser endoscopy.

I. System outline and features

The LASEREO is the first gastroenterological endoscopy system to use laser light as illumination. It is equipped with a narrow-band light observation function that takes advantage of the characteristics of laser light, as well as a white light observation function. Other features include lower power consumption and heat generation than xenon light sources. The system is composed of the VP-4450HD processor, the LL-4450 laser light source and four laser-dedicated scope models (as of April 2013).

1. Features of the LL-4450 laser light source

The LL-4450 incorporates laser diodes with two wavelengths. Illuminations suitable for white light observation and narrow-band light observation can be obtained by varying the light intensity ratio between two lasers.

One of the two lasers—the white light mode laser (450 nm laser)—provides white light with a wide spectral width, which is suitable for normal observation. In this mode, the phosphor emits the light, irradiating a mixture of laser light and fluorescence (**Fig. 1**). As the intensity of the light emitted from the phosphor varies depending on the intensity of the laser light, the amount of white light irradiation can be controlled by adjusting the light emission intensity of the laser. The other laser—the BLI laser (410 nm laser)—is used for narrow-band light observation, obtaining high-contrast information on the microvessels and slight mucosal surface irregularities in the mucosal surface layer and on the vessels in the deep layer. This is achieved by

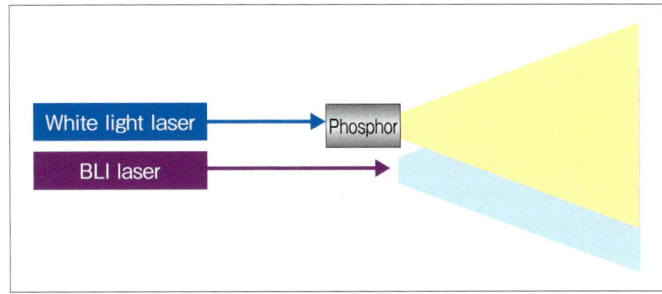

Fig. 1   Concept of Laser Illumination

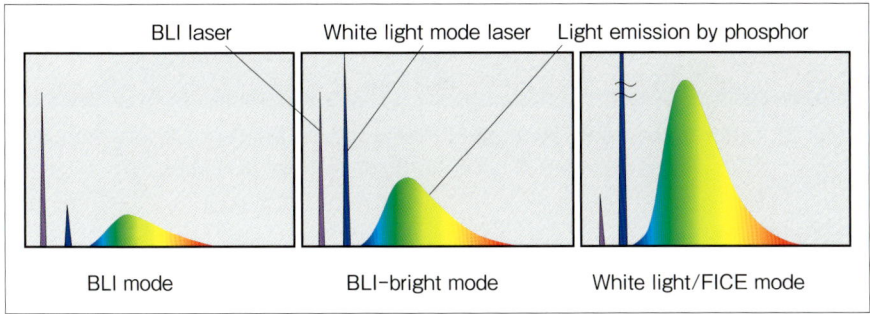

Fig. 2   Illumination Spectrum of Each Observation Mode

exploiting the properties of narrow-band light such as short wavelength and narrow spectral width. The wavelength bandwidths of the lasers are no more than 2 nm. The product specifications define wider wavelength ranges (400-420 nm and 440-460 nm), considering individual differences in the central wavelengths of lasers, but the actual variances are less than a few nanometers. Deviations of 5 nm or more are extremely rare.

In endoscopic observation, the illumination system has to enable brightness adjustment across a wide dynamic range from the far view to close-up view, while maintaining a constant color temperature. This means that extremely precise control is necessary in order to ensure that the ratio of light intensity between the two lasers remains constant. The LL-4450 combines several kinds of generally used laser modulation drive systems to achieve high-precision control in the wide brightness adjustment range.

2. Illumination patterns and observation modes

The LASEREO provides three patterns of illumination with different spectral distributions (**Fig. 2**). These are used in different combinations to obtain four different observation modes.

FICE is available with the illumination pattern for white light observation. The newly developed BLI function for narrow-band light observation generates images with improved mucosa-vessel contrast by irradiating an appropriate balance of narrow-band short-wavelength light and white light, then applying special image processing to the narrow-band signal obtained with the narrow-band, short-wavelength light and the broad-band signal obtained with the white light (**Fig. 3**).

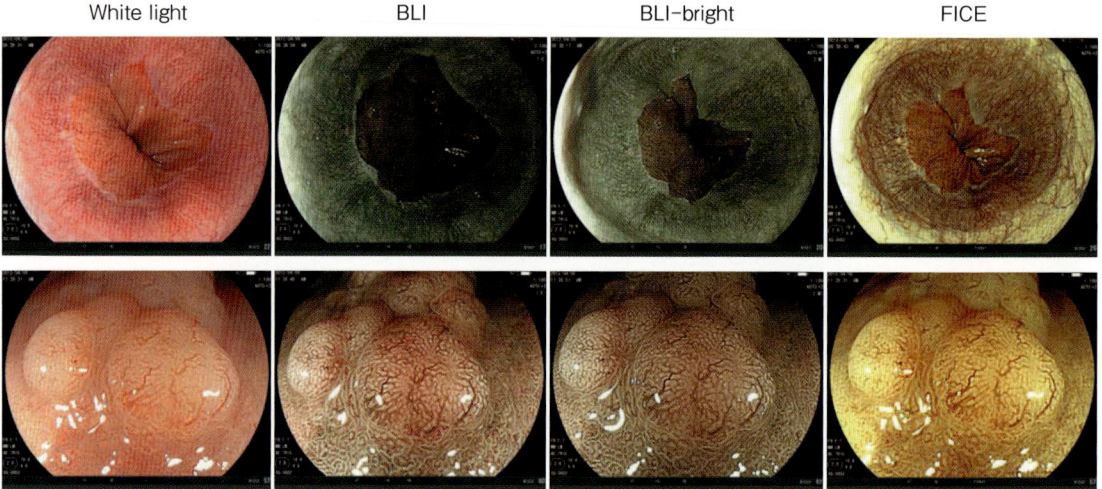

Fig. 3 Differences between Images Produced in Different Observation Modes
(Images courtesy of Kyoto Prefectural University of Medicine)

■ Ⅱ. BLI function

1. Principles of BLI

BLI is an endoscopic imaging technique that makes it possible to distinguish between the superficial microvessels and deep blood vessels based on the light absorption characteristics of the hemoglobin and the light scattering characteristics of the mucosa.

Short-wavelength light easily penetrates the mucosa without scattering, and in turn is easily absorbed by the vessels. As a result, the superficial microvessels are imaged in high contrast. Long-wavelength light, on the other hand, scatters easily when it hits the mucosa and is poorly absorbed by the vessels, so superficial microvessels are imaged in low contrast with blurred contours due to the scattering, while deep blood vessels are imaged in high contrast.

Together, these two types of image make it possible to view and clearly distinguish the superficial microvessels and deep blood vessels (**Fig. 4**).

2. Setting the narrow-band light observation modes

The LASEREO provides two narrow-band light observation modes.

・**BLI mode**：This mode increases the ratio of the BLI laser light in order to maximize the contrast between the superficial microvessels. It is designed primarily for close-up to magnifying observation.

・**BLI-bright mode**：This mode employs a balance of BLI laser light and white light mode laser light to improve both image brightness and vessel image contrast. It is designed mainly for middle/far view to close-up observation.

Proper switching between these two narrow-band light observation modes lets you observe images with high brightness and high vessel imaging contrast from the middle/far view to the close-up/magnifying observation.

3. Structure enhancement

The targets of endoscopic examinations are highly variable, from a far view of a lesion a few centimeters in size to a magnified view of a microvessel a mere 10 μm across. In magnifying observation, treatment policy is determined by observing not only the

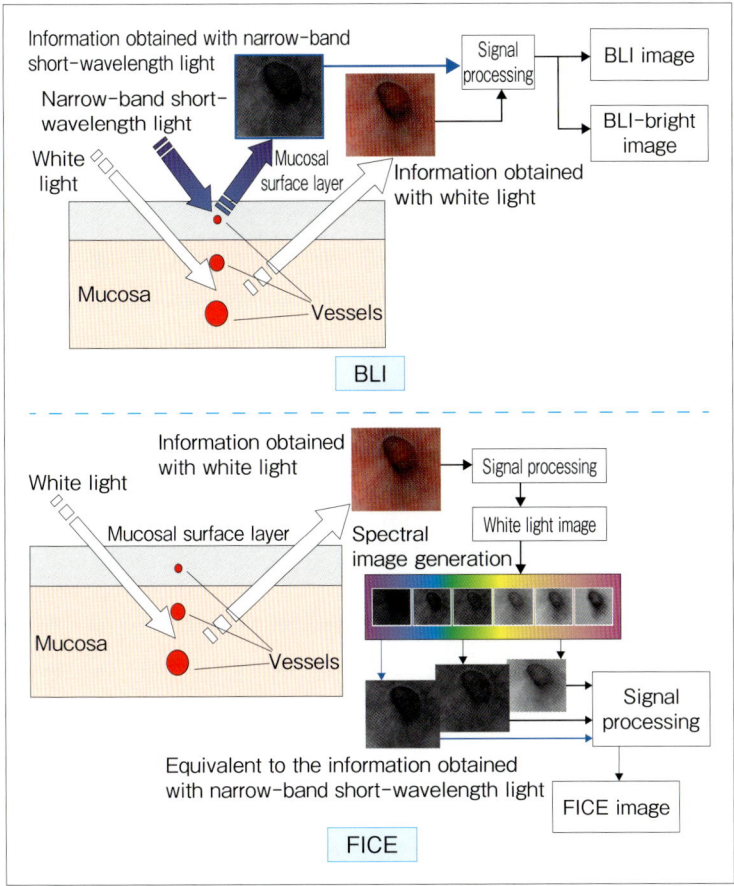

Fig. 4 BLI/FICE Processing Flow

microvessels, but also the mucosal surface structures. To handle the requirements of various observation conditions and targets, the structure enhancement of BLI has two enhancement modes that use different frequency bands (**Fig. 5**). A-mode is designed to enhance lower frequencies than B-mode and is suitable for enhancing slightly broader areas and structures. B-mode is designed to enhance thin lines, making it suitable for observing microvessels.

4. Color enhancement

The type of mucosal epithelium and the density of vessels in the gastrointestinal tract differ depending on the location. Reproduced color tones are also greatly variable. To make lesions in various locations such as the pharynx, esophagus, stomach and colon more easily distinguishable, the BLI mode provides three color tones. The BLI-bright mode also provides a no color enhancement option with color tone close to white light observation (**Fig. 5**).

5. Difference between BLI and FICE

The FICE function improves the mucosa-vessel contrast by generating a narrow-band image created by applying signal processing to the white light image and reconstructing the result as an RGB image. The BLI function, on the other hand, enhances the mucosa-vessel contrast by irradiating high-intensity narrow-band

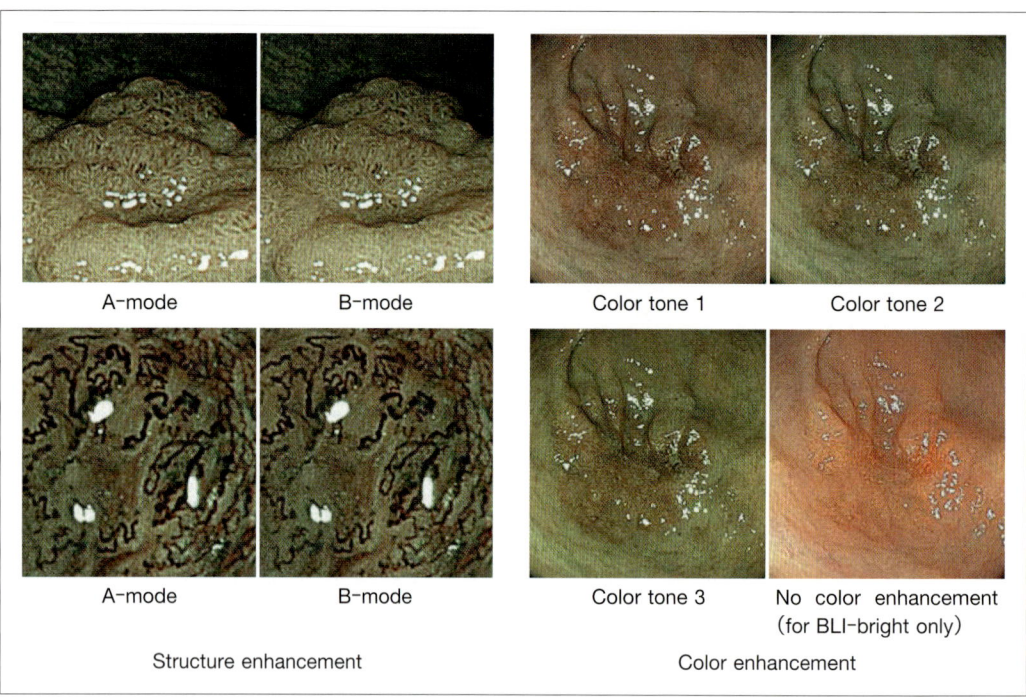

Fig. 5 Differences between the Structure Enhancement and Color Enhancement Modes
(Images courtesy of the National Cancer Center Hospital East)

Table   Characteristics of Each Observation Mode

Mode	Purpose	Laser intensity White light mode laser	Laser intensity BLI laser	Characteristics
White light	White light imaging	High	Low	Equivalent color tone to previous systems (xenon light sources).
FICE	Color enhancement	Same as WLI mode		Fine color tone changes are enhanced by spectral image processing. Enhancement of the color difference between the mucosa and vessels can improve vessel visibility. Brightness is equivalent to white light images and far view observation is possible.
BLI	Vascular/mucosal surface structure observation	Low	High	An image suitable for enhancing the superficial microvessels is generated by increasing the short-wavelength component from the laser to increase the contrast produced by the hemoglobin. Suitable for close-up/magnifying observation.
BLI-bright	Vascular/mucosal surface structure observation	Medium	High	The white light component is increased slightly compared to the BLI mode to generate an image bright enough for middle/far-view observation with vessel/surface structure imaging performance equivalent to the BLI mode.

short-wavelength light, and then enhancing the resulting narrow-band image (**Fig. 4** and **Table**).

The FICE, BLI and BLI-bright modes all enable narrow-band light observation. However, the brightness and degree of vessel contrast enhancement vary as outlined below.

Image brightness
　　　Low⟵──────────────⟶High
　　　BLI＜BLI-bright＜FICE≈White light observation
Vessel-mucosa contrast
　　　High⟵──────────────⟶Low
　　　BLI＞BLI-bright＞FICE＞White light observation

Conclusion

The LASEREO gastrointestinal endoscopy system uses lasers as its illumination light source and incorporates BLI, a function for narrow-band light observation that displays mucosa and vessels in high contrast by taking advantage of the high-intensity, narrow-band properties of the lasers. A BLI-bright mode is also provided ; by varying the intensities of the BLI and white light mode lasers, this mode enables bright narrow-band light observation at relatively far views.

Laser technology offers enormous potential. Using lasers with different wavelengths from those used with the LASEREO will make it possible to implement new diagnostic functions. In the future, technologies for visualizing a large variety of biological and functional changes in cancers can be expected to provide the basis for developing endoscopy systems that facilitate early detection of cancerous lesions and support more detailed treatment policy.

Reference
1) Yoshida, N., Hisabe, T., Inada, Y. et al. : The ability of a novel blue laser imaging system for the diagnosis of invasion depth of colorectal neoplasms. J. Gastroenterol. 2013 Mar [Epub ahead of print]

(Kuramoto, M., Kubo, M.)

Oropharynx and Hypopharynx

See page 4 for explanation of abbreviations.

Oropharynx and Hypopharynx

General Theory : How to Observe These Regions with NBI or BLI

Tips on NBI Observation

I. Light source settings

1. Structure enhancement
   By enhancing fine patterns and contours, NBI makes it possible to increase the sharpness of an endoscopic image. There are two types of enhancement available (Types A and B) and the level of enhancement can be selected from 9 steps (Steps 0 to 8). Type A can enhance relatively large targets, while type B can be used for more precise enhancement of smaller targets. In upper gastrointestinal endoscopy, the most frequently used mode is <u>Type B, Step 8</u>.
2. Color enhancement
   With the EVIS LUCERA ELITE, minute changes in mucosal color tone are enhanced to generate clear images with high contrast. The color enhancement level can be selected from 3 steps, but the most suitable enhancement level is selected automatically when the endoscope is connected to the light source. Step 1 or 2 is usually selected in the upper gastrointestinal endoscopy.

II. Actual observation

To remove saliva and mucus before pharyngeal anesthesia, the patient drinks a glass of water. As observation is difficult during endoscope withdrawal because of attached saliva/mucus or mucosal erythema/bleeding due to contact with the scope, it is preferable to perform observation when the endoscope is being inserted. NBI is recommended because it can discover oropharyngeal and hypopharyngeal tumors more easily than WLI[1]. If it is difficult to observe a location in the oropharyngeal or hypopharyngeal region, take advantage of the movement induced by the patient speaking or breathing. Using a sedative can reduce the pharyngeal reflex, but makes it more difficult to take advantage of speaking during observation. When observing a location that tends to present blind spots such as the pyriform sinus or epiglottic vallecula, attaching the distal attachment to the endoscope may facilitate observations.

III. Presence diagnosis

The findings to be noted for identifying a pharyngeal tumor are identical to those in the esophagus, the inside of which is composed of squamous epithelium. They include slight color changes including erythema and fading, loss of normal vascular shadows and slight surface irregularities. However, these findings are hard to distinguish with WLI because the pharynx tends to cause reflexes and has many natural surface irregularities (**Fig. 1**). When NBI is used, there are two typical findings suggesting a pharyngeal tumor—a well-demarcated brownish area and a proliferation of atypical vessels presenting vasodilation, tortuosity, irregular diameters and/or irregular shapes in a well-demarcated brownish area. These findings are usually easier to

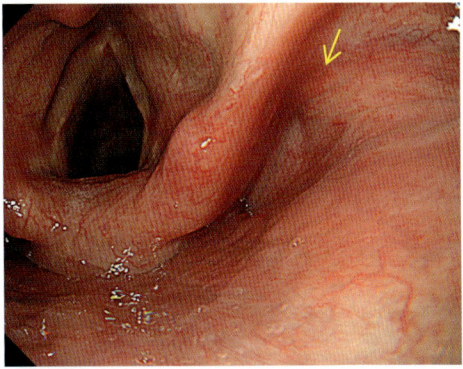

Fig. 1 WLI Non-Magnifying Observation
An erythematous flat lesion where normal vessels cannot be seen is observed in the right pyriform sinus (indicated by the arrow). This lesion is very difficult to distinguish.

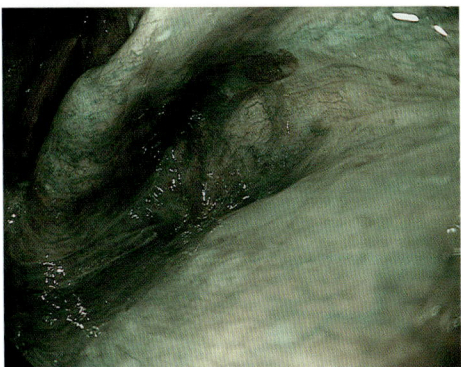

Fig. 2 NBI Non-Magnifying Observation
With the NBI image, a well-demarcated brownish area in the right pyriform sinus can be easily discerned.

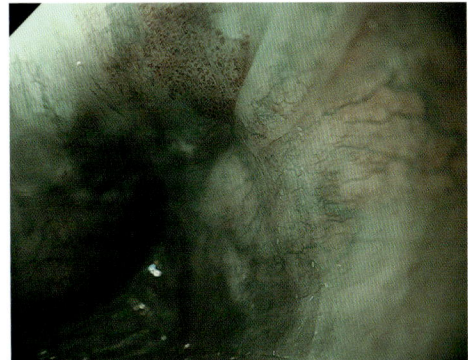

Fig. 3 NBI Magnifying Observation
Magnifying observation shows an increase of atypical vessels inside the brownish area.

(Figs. 2 and 3 were obtained in NBI mode, with structure enhancement B8 and color mode 2.)

discern with NBI than WLI.

A brownish area likely indicates the presence of a pharyngeal tumor (**Fig. 2**). If the boundary of the brownish area is well demarcated and contains atypical vessels, the likelihood of pharyngeal tumor is even greater (**Fig. 3**).

IV. Invasion depth diagnosis

With an esophageal superficial carcinoma, invasion depth diagnosis is based on the intrapapillary capillary loop (IPCL) pattern classification proposed by Arima, Inoue et al.[2,3] However, this depth diagnosis is intended for the esophagus and is not always applicable to the pharynx even though both are composed of squamous epithelium. For now, it is safe to say that a lesion with few surface irregularities will probably only invade within the epithelium, while a lesion with noticeable surface irregularities is likely to invade beneath the epithelium.

References
1) Muto, M., Minashi, K., Yano, T. et al. : Early detection of superficial squamous cell carcinoma in the head and neck region and esophagus by narrow band imaging : a multicenter randomized controlled trial. J. Clin. Oncol 2010 ; 28 : 1566-1572
2) Inoue, H., Honda, T., Nagai K. et al. : Ultra-high magnification endoscopic observation of carcinoma in situ of the esophagus. Dig Endosc 1997 ; 9 : 16-18
3) Arima, M., Tada, S., Arima, H. et al. : Evaluation of microvascular patterns of superficial esophageal cancers by magnifying endoscopy. Esophagus 2005 ; 2 : 191-197

(Morita, S., Hayashi, T., Muto, M.)

Oropharynx and Hypopharynx

General Theory : How to Observe These Regions with NBI or BLI

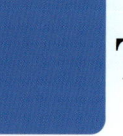

Tips on BLI Observation

■ Introduction

The growing sophistication of endoscopic diagnosis techniques has led to increased detection of early laryngopharyngeal cancers, improving the chances of a benign prognosis even with minimally invasive treatments such as ESD (endoscopic submucosal dissection)[1)-5)]. However, as detailed observation of the laryngopharyngeal regions takes time and causes discomfort to the patient, narrowing down the risk group would greatly enhance the efficiency of early cancer screening.

■ I. Endoscopic observation in the laryngopharyngeal region

Background studies of a large number of early laryngopharyngeal cancer cases indicate that the risk group is males aged 55 years or older[3),4)]. The following observation method is considered the most appropriate for this group.

Since the pharyngeal reflex produces a major obstruction in the pharyngeal region, the pharynx should be anesthetized using Xylocaine® Viscous, and Xylocaine Spray should also be used whenever possible. It helps to have the patient say, "Ahh," while spraying. The recommended patient position during observation is the so-called "sniffing position," in which the patient stays in the left lateral position, while pushing out their face and sticking out their chin. In this position, the space between the tongue base and palatine arch is expanded, making it possible to avoid contact with the tongue base and the pharyngeal wall, preventing the pharyngeal reflex and facilitating observation.

Laryngopharyngeal observation is performed with the endoscope in the BLI-bright mode from the time it is inserted (recommended setup : B8, C1). The region that should be observed first is the area from the posterior wall of the oropharynx to the posterior wall of the hypopharynx (**Figs. 1, 2**). As saliva in the oral cavity can interfere with observation, be sure to suction the saliva whenever possible. The saliva in the oral cavity is highly viscous and relatively easy to suction. Also wash the region frequently using the endoscope's irrigation valve. Never attempt to feed water from the biopsy port as this will cause aspiration. Since many early laryngopharyngeal cancers are accompanied with vascular proliferation, the findings to be noted are the vasodilation or proliferation of capillaries (IPCLs), well-demarcated brownish areas, and interruption of surrounding vessels. Slough on erosion is another important finding.

Next, observe the region from the pyriform sinuses to the larynx. As the left pyriform sinus often looks closed due to the effect of gravity, start observation from the right pyriform sinus. Observe the region that is as close as possible to the esophagus entrance by suctioning saliva whenever possible (**Fig. 3**). As the advantage of the BLI-

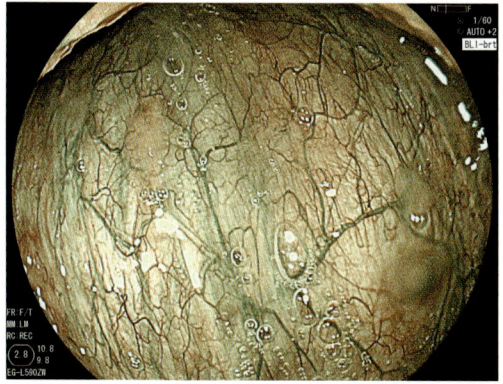

Fig. 1 Posterior Wall of Oropharynx
(Figs. 1 to 11 were obtained in BLI-bright mode, with structure enhancement B8, color enhancement C1.)

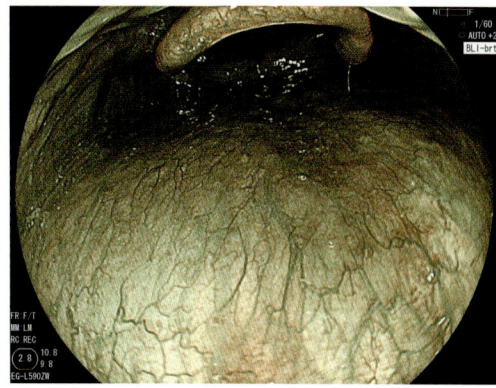

Fig. 2 Posterior Wall of Hypopharynx

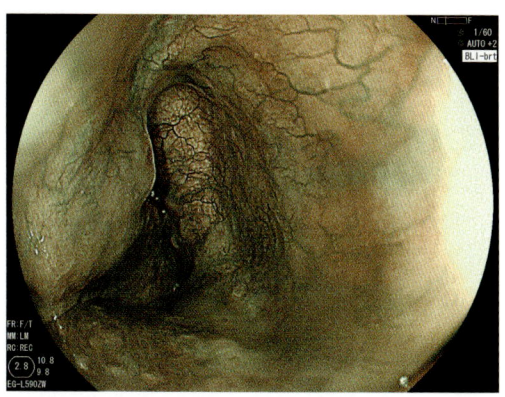

Fig. 3 Right Pyriform Sinus

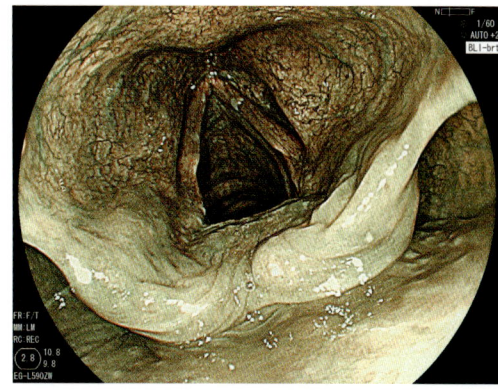

Fig. 4 Pharynx

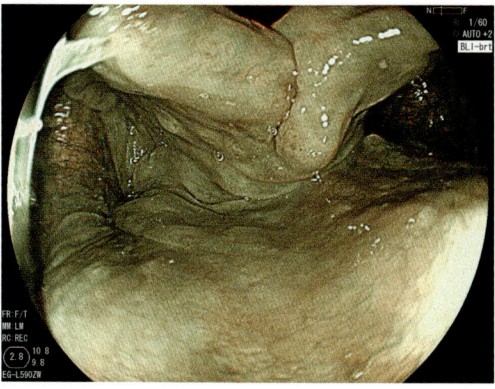

Fig. 5 Postcricoid Area and Posterior Wall of Hypopharynx

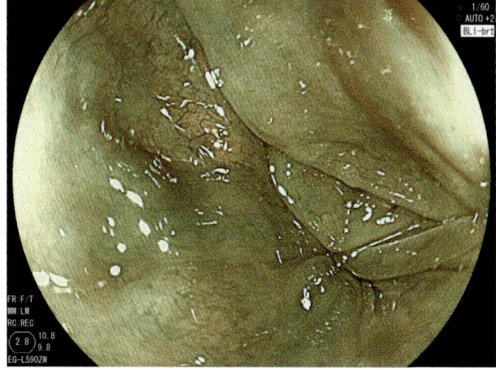

Fig. 6 Left Pyriform Sinus

bright mode is its effectiveness in the absence of brightness, be sure to observe not only the supraglottic region, but also observe the subglottic region (as a far view) whenever possible during laryngeal observation (**Fig. 4**). The postcricoid area is the hardest region to observe, but the field of view can be enlarged slightly by utilizing the motions produced by breathing or by reflexive action. You can also ask the patient to

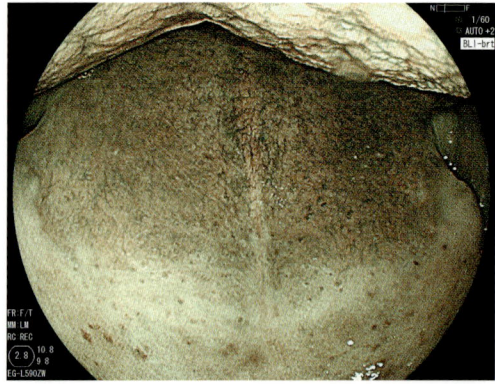

Fig. 7　Hard Palate and Soft Palate

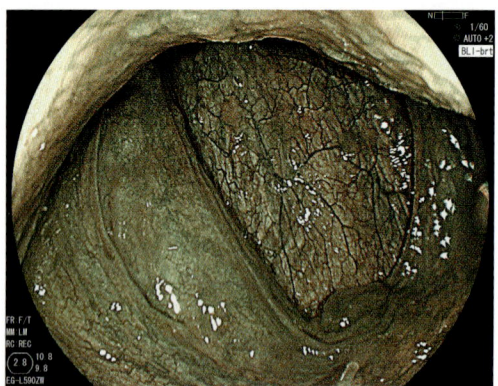

Fig. 8　Palatine Arch

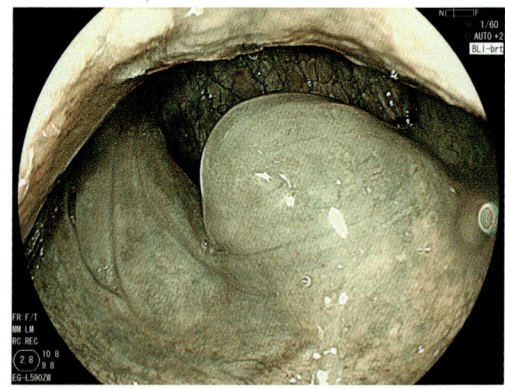

Fig. 9　Uvula

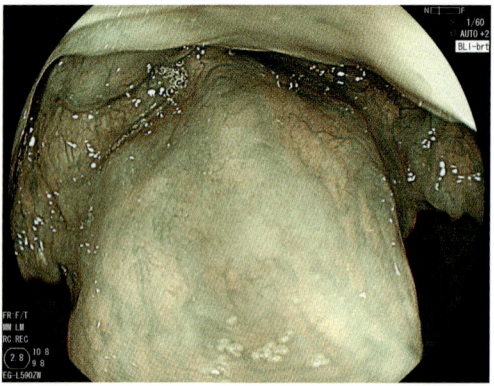

Fig. 10　Lingual Surface of Epiglottis

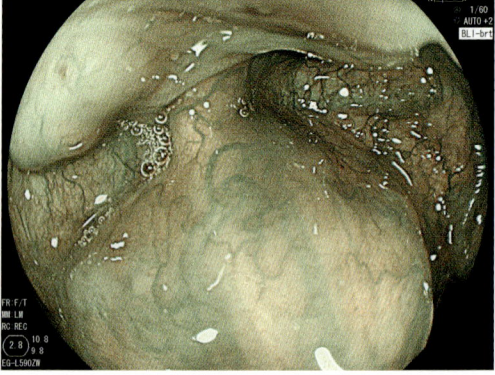

Fig. 11　Epiglottic Vallecula

say something or to attempt exhalation against a closed airway (Valsalva maneuver) (**Fig. 5**). Finally, observe the left pyriform sinus while pushing the endoscope against it to expand (**Fig. 6**), and then enter the esophagus. Since the pyriform sinus is necessarily observed in close-up view, the brightness of the BLI-bright mode may sometimes seem excessive. In this case, switch to the BLI mode and use the low magnification as required.

II. Endoscopic observation of high-risk group

Patients with a history of esophageal squamous cell carcinoma complications, patients found to be chronic drinkers who have an alcohol flush reaction, and patients found to be heavy drinkers/smokers should be assigned to the high risk group. With these patients, it is recommended to perform the following observations in addition to the laryngopharyngeal observations described above.

Before (afterward is also fine) observing the posterior wall of the pharynx, observe the region from the hard palate to the soft palate (**Fig. 7**), and then observe the palatine arches, tonsils and uvula (**Figs. 8, 9**). The uvula should be observed all the way to the tip. If the uvula tilts to the left due to gravity, hindering palatine arch observation, push the endoscope to expand the space.

Next, advance the endoscope to the back of the epiglottis and observe its lingual surface (**Fig. 10**). This region is normally invisible unless you deliberately look for it, but it is also a common site for cancer. When observing it, push down the epiglottis with the endoscope and observe as far as the epiglottic vallecula (**Fig. 11**). Although observation in the tangential direction is difficult, try to observe the base of the tongue as far back as possible. If it is determined that detailed observation of the base of the tongue is necessary, you will have to perform retroflexed observation using a transnasal endoscope. In observation of the vicinity of the lingual surface of the epiglottis, the pharyngeal reflex is easily induced due to the contact of the endoscope with the base of the tongue. To avoid this, you should wait until near the end of the laryngopharyngeal observation to observe this region, or do it while withdrawing the endoscope.

References

1) Muto, M., Nakane, M., Katada, C. et al. : Squamous cell carcinoma in situ at oropharyngeal and hypopharyngeal mucosal sites. Cancer 2004 ; 101 : 1375-1381
2) Shimizu, Y., Yamamoto, J., Kato, M. et al. : Endoscopic submucosal dissection for treatment of early stage hypopharyngeal carcinoma. Gastrointest. Endosc 2006 ; 64 : 255-259
3) Iizuka, T., Kikuchi, D., Hoteya, S. et al. : Endoscopic submucosal dissection for treatment of mesopharyngeal or hypopharyngeal carcinomas. Endoscopy 2009 ; 41 : 113-117
4) Muto, M., Satake, H., Yano, T. et al. : Long-term outcome of transoral organ-preserving pharyngeal endoscopic resection for superficial pharyngeal cancer. Gastrointest Endosc 2011 ; 74 : 477-484
5) Shimizu, Y., Yoshida, T., Kato, M., et al. : Long-term outcome after endoscopic resection in patients with hypopharyngeal carcinoma invading the subepithelium : a case series. Endoscopy 2009 ; 41 : 374-376

(Shimizu, Y.)

Case 1 Inflammatory pharyngeal lesion

Male in 50s　*Purpose* Screening　*Location* Right pyriform sinus

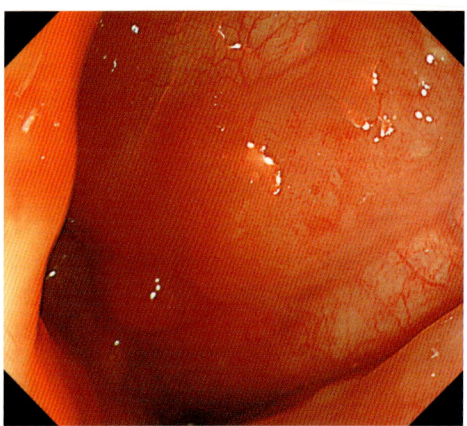

WLI low-magnification observation : A reddish elevated lesion with unclear demarcation and a diameter of about 3 mm is observed on the right pyriform sinus. The elevation is not sharp but rather gentle.

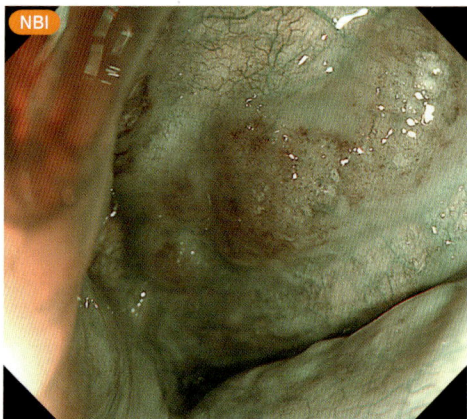

NBI low-magnification observation : This is an elevated lesion with a not very clearly demarcated brownish area. Multiple similar lesions are found in the surrounding area. White coat is attached to each lesion.

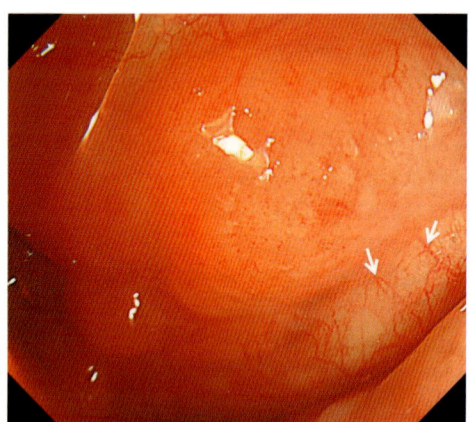

WLI high-magnification observation : Linear normal vessels (white arrows) are observed around the elevation. Dotted vessels can be seen on the elevation, while normal vessels have disappeared. As the thickness of the dotted vessels is identical to the surrounding normal vessels, it can be assumed that they are not dilated. In addition, as the vessel density is not high, the possibility that the lesion is an epithelial tumor should be considered as negative.

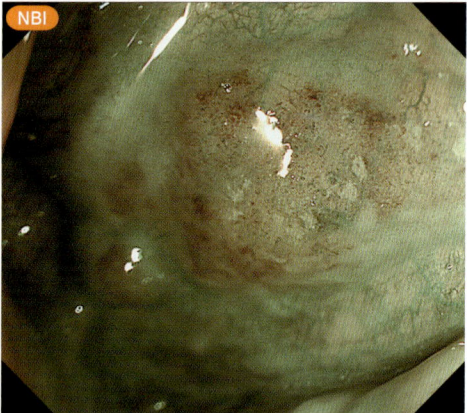

NBI high-magnification observation : Vessels that are difficult to observe with WLI can be observed easily and clearly with NBI.

Endoscope : GIF-H260Z (Olympus)　　Light source : EVIS LUCERA ELITE (Olympus)
NBI setup : Structure enhancement B8, color mode 2

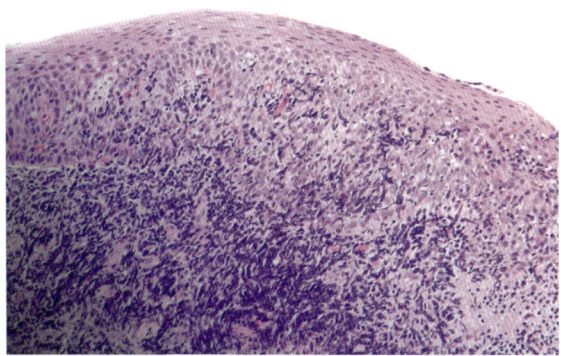

Histopathological image : Biopsy leads to a diagnosis of lymphoid inflammation.

Comment

WLI non-magnifying observation finds an elevation that appears to be a uncleary demarcated submucosal tumor with a diameter of about 3 mm on the right pyriform sinus. A slightly elevated lesion is also observed with NBI non-magnifying observation. It has a brownish area, but its demarcation is unclear.

Neither WLI nor NBI magnifying observation finds atypical vessels with morphological abnormalities such as dilation, bending or tortuosity accompanying the elevation.

▶**Observation tips** A finding like this case is often observed on the hypopharynx. Multiple inflammations of this kind are observed in many cases. Diagnosis is possible because the brownish area is uncleary demarcated and is not accompanied with mucosal irregularities or atypical vessels.

(Morita, S., Muto, M.)

Case 2　Hypopharyngeal papilloma

Male in 30s　**Purpose** Observation of anomaly found in health check
Location Left pyriform sinus of hypopharynx　**Macroscopic type** 0-Ⅰp

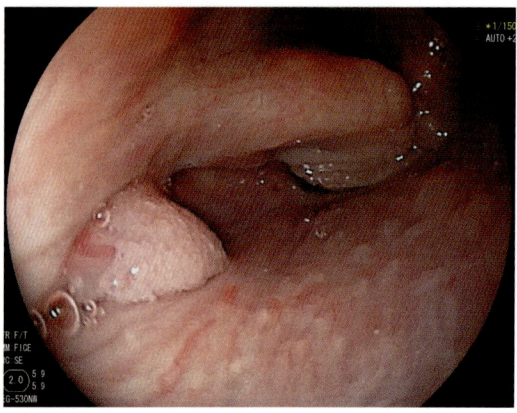

Transnasal endoscope：A whitish protruding lesion is observed on the left pyriform sinus of the hypopharynx. A grainy structure is observed on the surface.

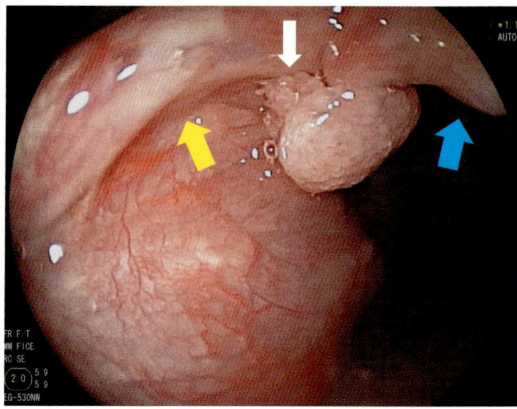

Transnasal endoscopy (with larynx expanded with the Valsalva maneuver)：The lesion looks as if it is hanging down toward the posterior wall from the intersection of the left aryepiglottic fold (blue arrow) and pharyngoepiglottic fold (yellow arrow). A small protrusion (white arrow) that looks like a sea anemone can be seen on the outer side of the protrusion.

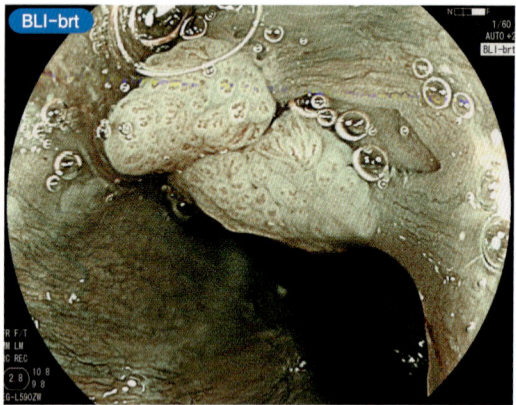

Magnifying endoscope (BLI-bright)：The lesion consists of a whitish protrusion with a papillary structure and a long, thin stem. It is divided into two parts.

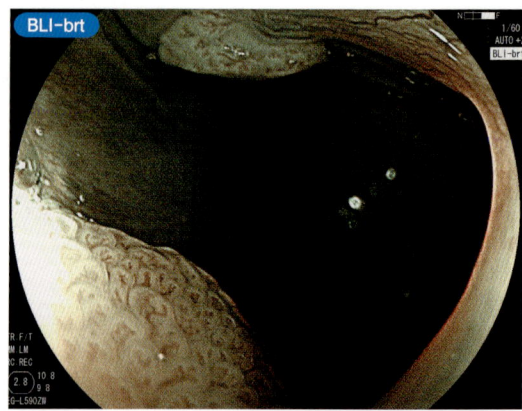

Magnifying endoscope (BLI-bright)：When the endoscope is inserted between the two parts, it is found that what seemed to be a single lesion is actually two lesions with bases some distance apart.

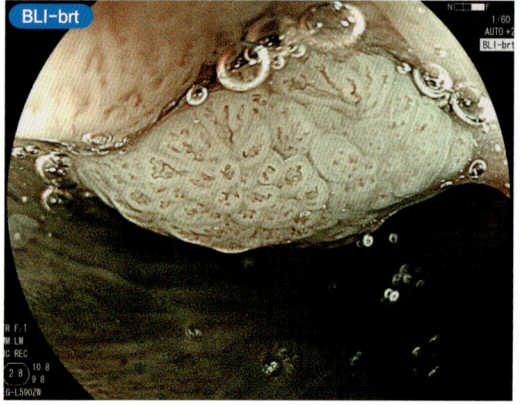

Magnifying endoscope (BLI-bright)：Feeding vessels are arranged in an orderly manner on the center of each papilla,

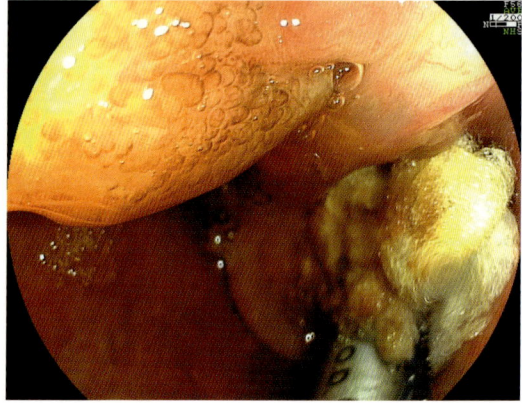

Intraoperative magnifying endoscopy (iodine stained)：The lesions are stained with iodine.

> Endoscope: EG-530NW transnasal endoscope (Fujifilm),
> EG-L590ZW/EG-590ZW magnifying endoscopes (Fujifilm)   Light source: LASEREO (Fujifilm)
> BLI setup: Structure enhancement A6, color enhancement C1

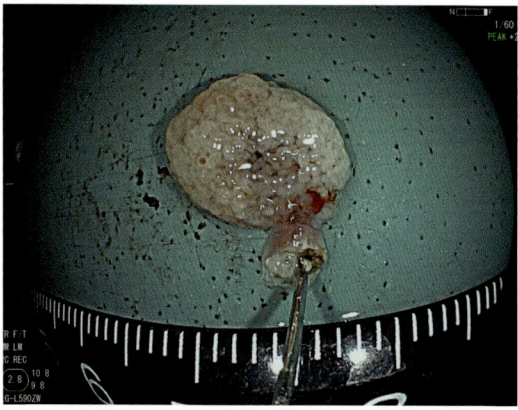

Resected specimen (main lesion): This lesion is a papillary protrusion with a thin stem and a diameter of 10 mm.

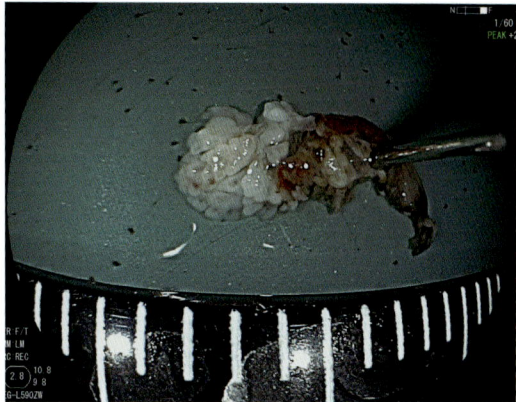

Resected specimen (secondary lesion): This has a diameter of 5 mm and a structure like a sea anemone.

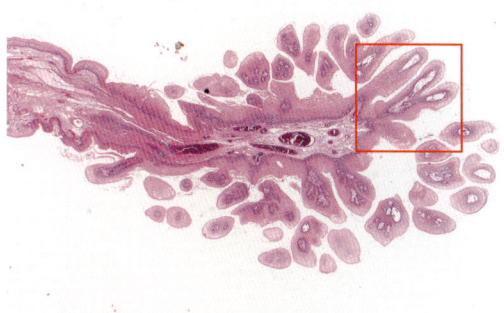

Pathology (low magnification): A large vessel is observed on the center of the stem. The vessel is branched on the periphery.

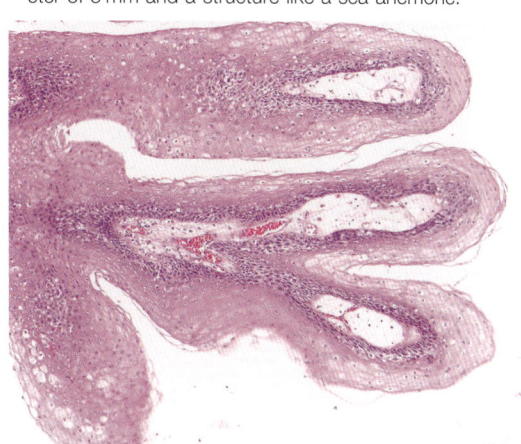

Pathology (high magnification): Magnified image of the part enclosed in the red square. Papillary growth of stratified squamous epithelia is observed around the core composed of vascular connective tissues.

Comment

A papilloma is a benign epithelial tumor. It is a projecting lesion with a whitish color tone and is either lobulated and sessile or pedunculated. It looks like a sea anemone, mulberry fruit or polyp. Some papillomas are distinguishable at a glance because of the papillary structure on the superficial layer, and some are flat and hardly distinguishable from white superficial carcinoma or glycogenic acanthosis (GA). They are soft when pinched by forceps. Pedunculated papillomas float in the saliva and move well. They can be stained with iodine.

▶ **Observation tips** The posterior wall and postcricoid area of the hypopharynx are usually bounded, so it is not unusual for the position of the lesion to be clarified using the Valsalva maneuver or through direct visualization of the larynx under general anesthesia. A pedunculated papilloma is soft and easily movable so it should be observed in a well-stretched condition. When it is observed with BLI magnifying observation, it is also characterized by the presence of relatively well-arranged feeding vessels in each papilla. Images in the laryngopharyngeal region should be taken quickly by taking care to minimize the pharyngeal reflex as much as possible.

(Kawada, K., Kawano, T.)

Case 3 Pharyngeal melanosis

Female in 60s | Purpose | Detailed examination of hypopharynx | Location | Posterior wall of hypopharynx

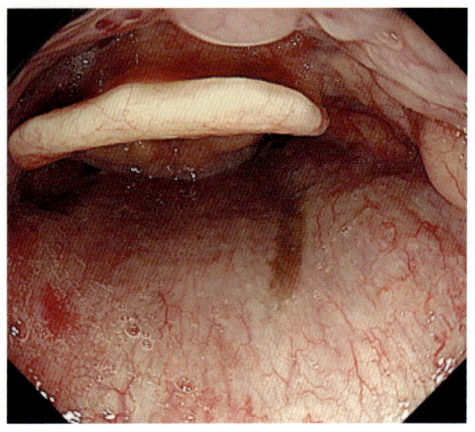

WLI observation : A flat, well-demarcated brownish lesion with a size of 6×2 mm is observed on the right posterior wall of the hypopharynx.

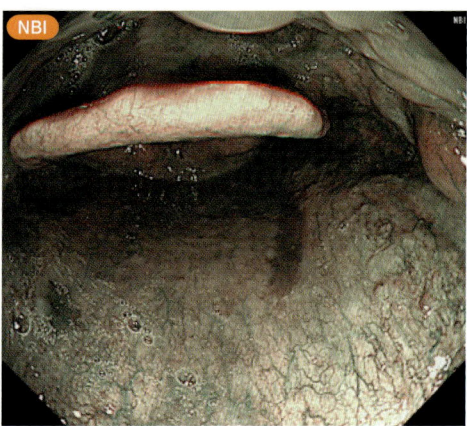

NBI non-magnifying observation : The lesion showed a well-demarcated brownish area.

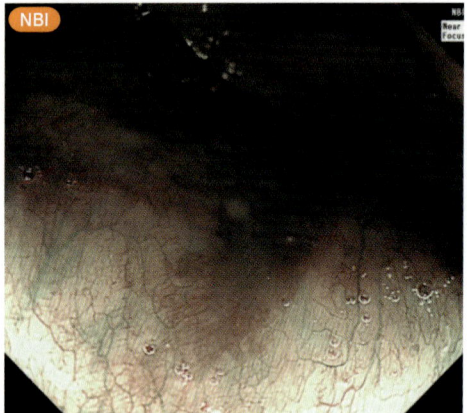

NBI magnifying observation (lesion periphery : Near Focus) : No abnormal microvessels are observed in the brownish area compared to the surrounding normal mucosa.

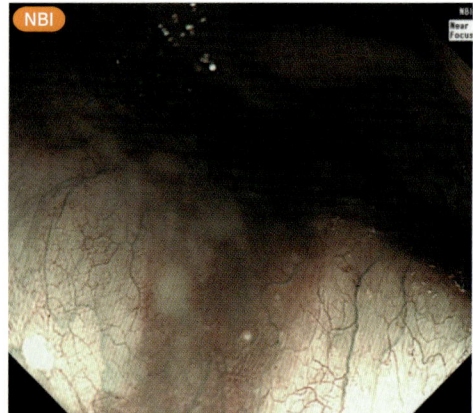

NBI magnifying observation (legion center : Near Focus) : Relatively thick green vessels are observed in the brownish area. These are similar to the normal microvessels in the surrounding area. No abnormal microvessels are observed in the superficial layer.

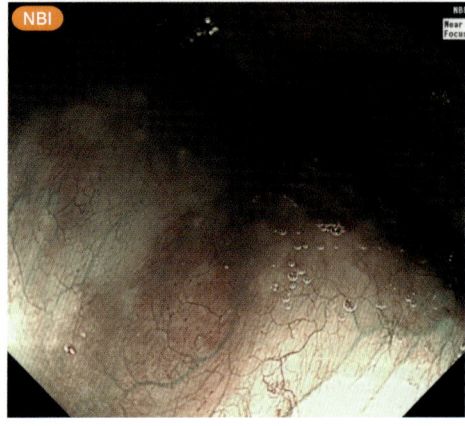

On the distal side of the lesion, no abnormal microvessels are observed in the superficial layer of the brownish area.

Endoscope : GIF-HQ290 (Olympus)　Light source : EVIS LUCERA ELITE (Olympus)
NBI setup : Structure enhancement of A7, color mode 1

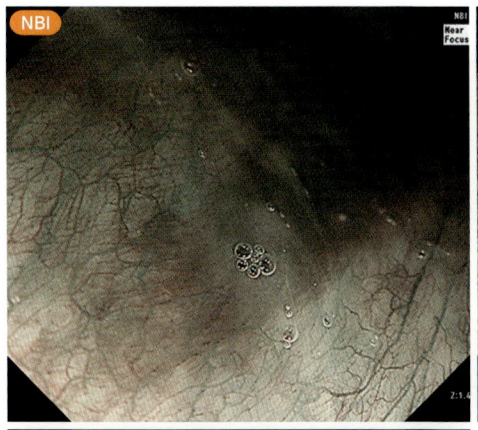

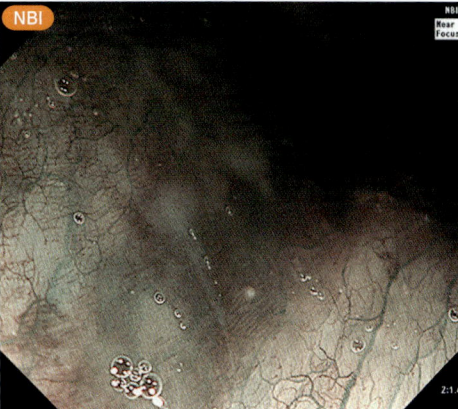

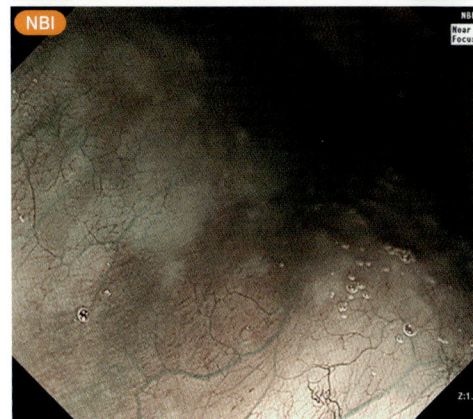

NBI magnifying observation (Near Focus＋1.4× Electronic Zoom, proximal side of lesion) : Subepithelial greenish vessels are observed in the brownish areas on the proximal side, the center and the distal side of the lesion. No obvious anomalies appear to be associated with the superficial vessels.

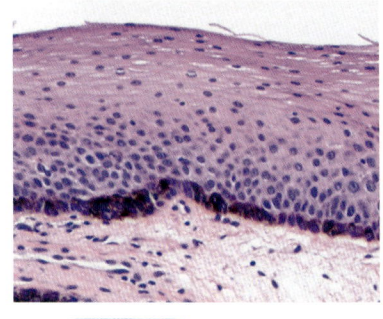

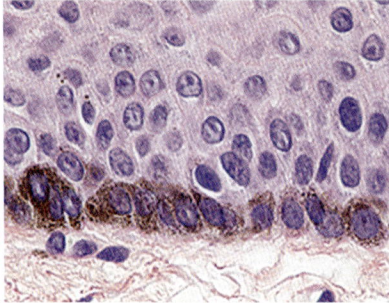

Biopsy specimens
Left : Low magnification, HE stained
Right : High magnification, HE stained
As deposition of brownish pigment granules is observed with the epithelial basal cells, the lesion is histologically confirmed as a melanosis.

Comment

Many superficial squamous cell carcinomas on the pharynx and esophagus present well-demarcated brownish areas when they are observed with NBI. Since the melanosis is also imaged as a brownish area by NBI, differentiation from superficial squamous cell carcinoma is necessary. Differentiation is usually possible by switching to WLI and observing the pigmentation.

▶Observation tips Malignant melanoma is one of the differentiation targets of the melanosis. Its WLI image is characterized by a deep color tone and accompanied by an elevation presenting a growing tendency. As melanosis often accompanies a squamous cell carcinoma, observing changes in IPCLs with NBI magnifying observation will facilitate more reliable diagnosis.

(Dobashi, A., Goda, K., Tajiri, H.)

35

Case 4　Pharyngeal melanosis

Male in 70s　|Purpose|　Screening after esophageal carcinoma ESD　|Location|　Posterior wall of oropharynx

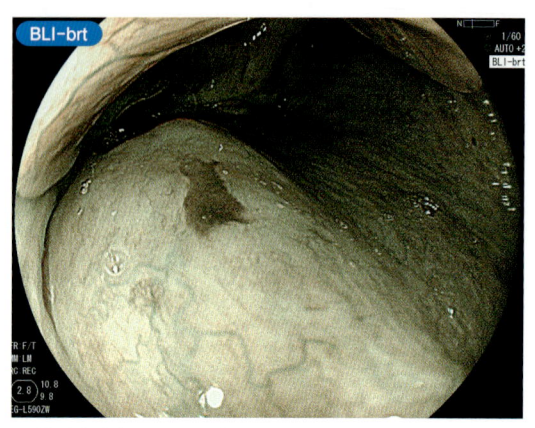

BLI-bright mode image：A brownish area is observed on the posterior wall of the oropharynx.

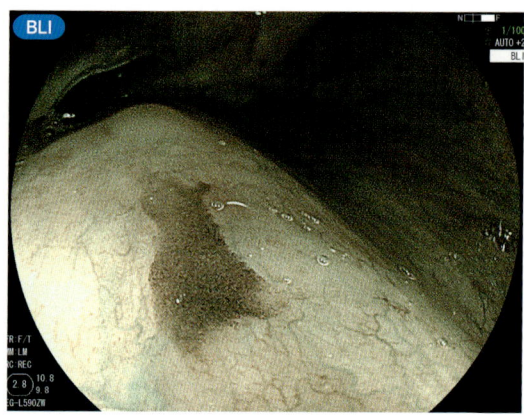

BLI mode image：The vascular construction cannot be confirmed with low magnification.

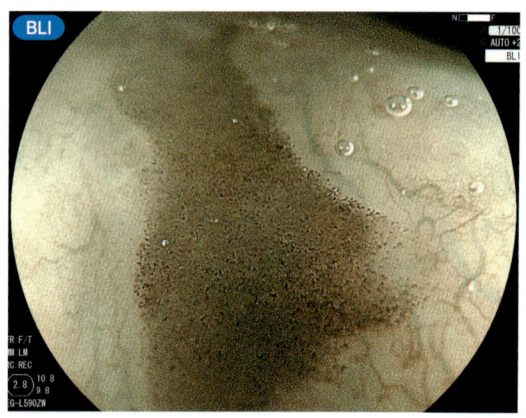

BLI mode image：Granular pigmentation is observed with high magnification.

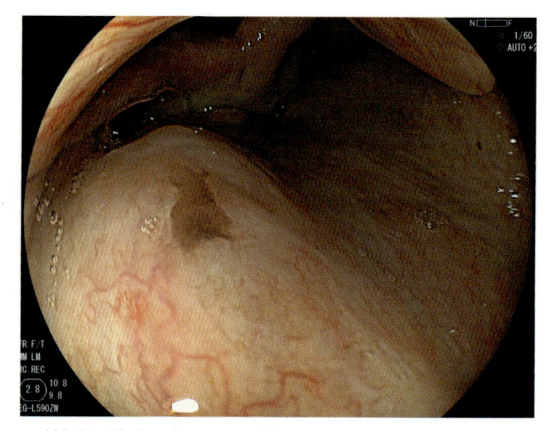

White-light image：Blackish pigmentation is recognized.

Endoscope : EG-590ZW (Fujifilm)　　Light source : LASEREO (Fujifilm)
BLI setup : Structure enhancement B8, color enhancement C1

Comment

The causes and pathological significance of pharyngeal melanosis are unknown. However, as it is often detected in chronic drinkers with ALDH2 hetero-deficiency, it is believed that it could potentially serve as a biomarker for pharyngeal carcinoma. In pharyngeal observation using BLI, melanosis catches the eye as a well-demarcated brownish area, but the IPCL structure cannot be confirmed. But differentiation is easy by checking for the blackish color tone observed in the white-light observation. As the possibility of melanosis becoming malignant is considered low, a biopsy is not usually performed.

▶**Observation tips** The findings in the BLI image could be mistaken for a type 0-Ⅱb early carcinoma. However, it is not possible to make such a mistake in white-light observation.

(Shimizu, Y.)

Case 5 Oropharyngeal superficial carcinoma (0-Ⅱa)

Male in 70s　**Purpose**　Further evaluation of pharyngeal lesion
Location　Oropharynx (epiglottic vallecula, tongue base)　**Macroscopic type** 0-Ⅱa

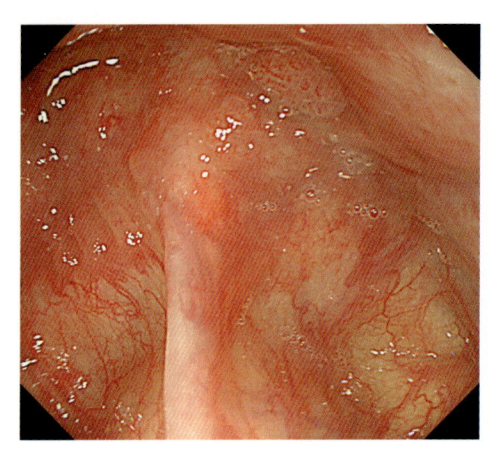

WLI non-magnifying observation : A well-demarcated, erythematous, flat elevated lesion is recognized on the tongue base side of the epiglottic vallecula. No normal vessels are observed in the lesion, which is accompanied by irregular minor elevations.

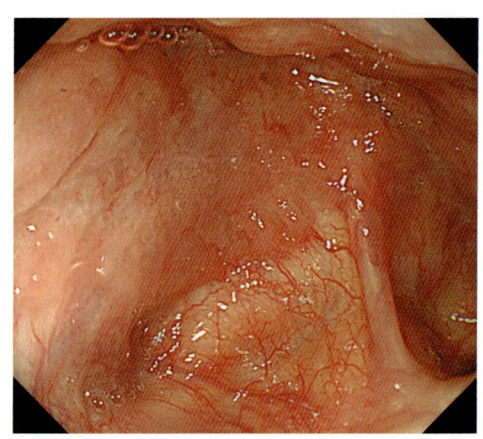

WLI non-magnifying observation : The lesion is also extended toward the left.

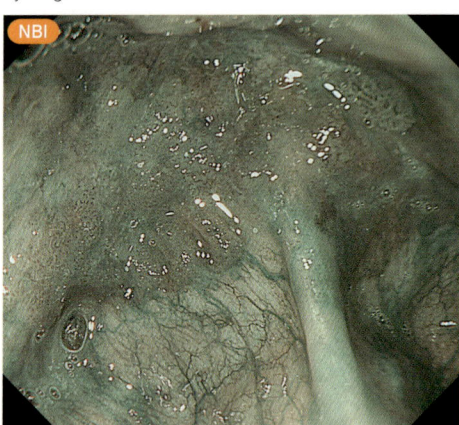

NBI non-magnifying observation : The lesion is recognized as a well-demarcated brownish area.

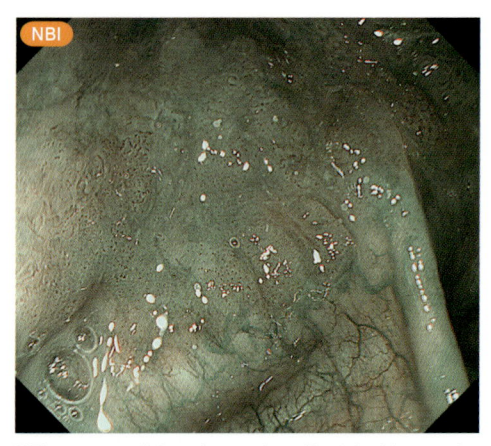

NBI non-magnifying observation : The left side can also be recognized as a well-demarcated brownish area.

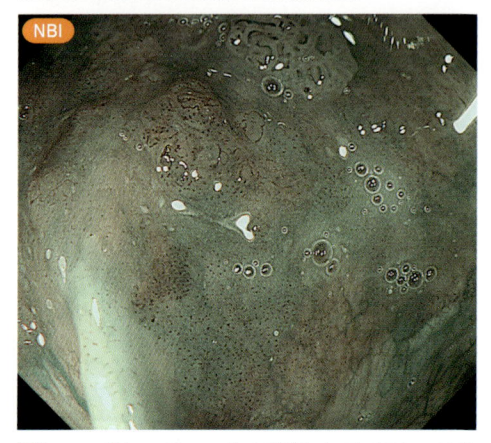

NBI magnifying observation : Dilated atypical vessels accompanied with morphological abnormalities such as tortuosity or stretching are growing in irregularly arranged minor elevations.

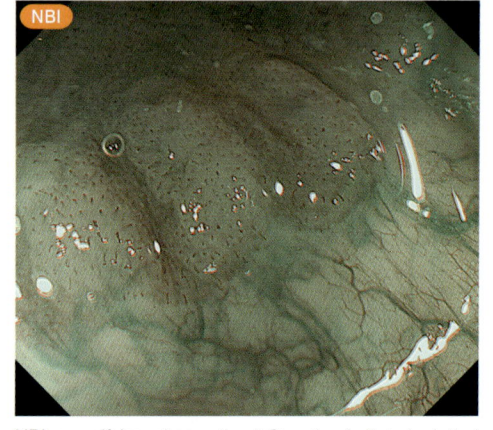

NBI magnifying observation : Growth of dilated, dotted atypical vessels is observed.

Endoscope : GIF-H260Z ; Only in the case of iodine stained image (★)—GIF-HQ290 (Olympus)
Light source : EVIS LUCERA ELITE (Olympus)　　NBI setup : Structure enhancement B8, color mode 2

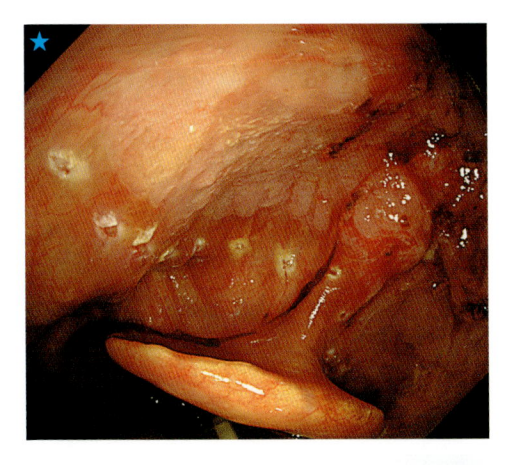

Iodine-stained non-magnifying observation (day of procedure) : When iodine is sprayed, the lesion stands out as a well-demarcated, unstained area.

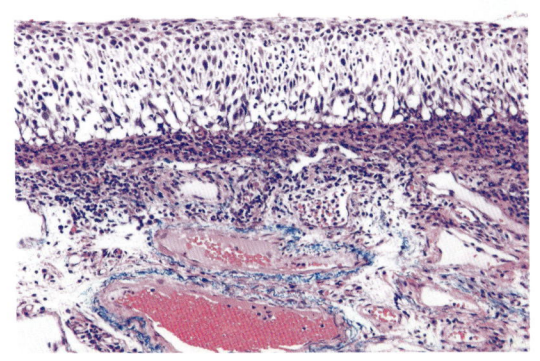

Histopathological image : A squamous cell carcinoma localized in the epithelium is recognized without surface irregularities where dilated dotted atypical vessels are observed.

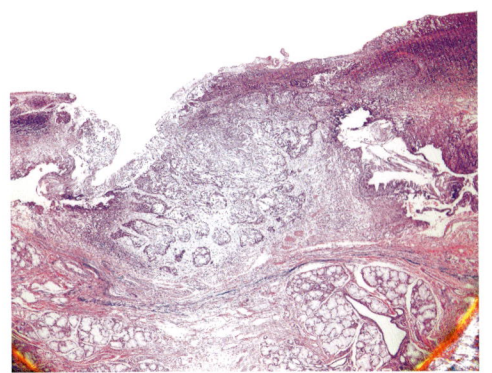

Histopathological image : The irregular minor elevation is an invasive carcinoma.

Comment

This is an elevated lesion in the area from the epiglottic vallecula to the tongue base. It is flat with a low elevation. The macroscopic type appears to be 0-Ⅱa. Nodular irregular protrusions are observed in the lesion, which is accompanied by a 0-Ⅰ lesion. Since the lesion appears as a well-demarcated brownish area with atypical vascularization, it can be diagnosed as an epithelial tumor. Although, unlike the esophagus, invasion depth diagnosis based on vascular morphology has not yet been established for the pharyngeal region, it can be said that most lesions with few surface irregularities, but with dotted vessels, remain within the epithelium. On the other hand, lesions with noticeable surface irregularities, vascular morphological abnormalities such as bending, tortuosity or stretching and/or dilated atypical vessels tend to be more invasive, penetrating to the sub-epithelial layer or deeper. In this case, also, the nodular protrusions form an invasive carcinoma.

▶**Observation tips** Carcinoma occurs often in the epiglottic vallecula region, but endoscopists sometimes hesitate to observe this region for fear that contact with the endoscope will induce the cough reflex. However, the risk of a strong reflex is not so high if the observation target is the tongue base side of the epiglottis. Observation can be facilitated by using the distal attachment.

(Morita, S., Hayashi, T., Muto, M.)

Case 6 Oropharyngeal superficial carcinoma (0-Ⅱb)

Male in 60s *Purpose* Oral cavity/laryngopharyngeal screening before esophageal superficial carcinoma operat｜
Location Posterior wall of oropharynx *Macroscopic type* 0-Ⅱb

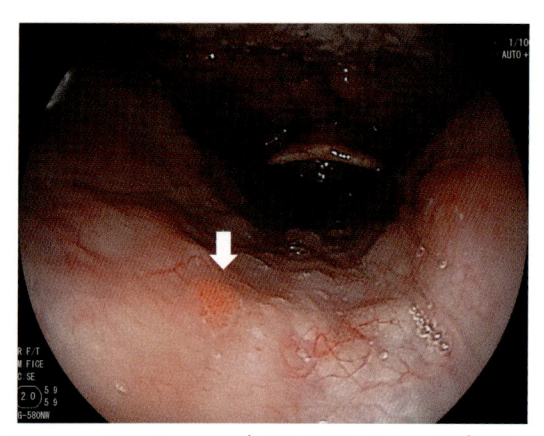

Transnasal endoscope (white-light observation): Localized erythema (arrow) is observed on the posterior wall of the oropharynx.

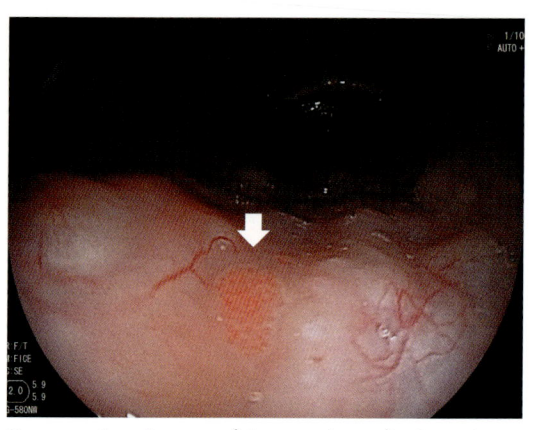

Transnasal endoscope (close-up image): Dotted vessels (arrow) can be observed, though not clearly, in the erythema.

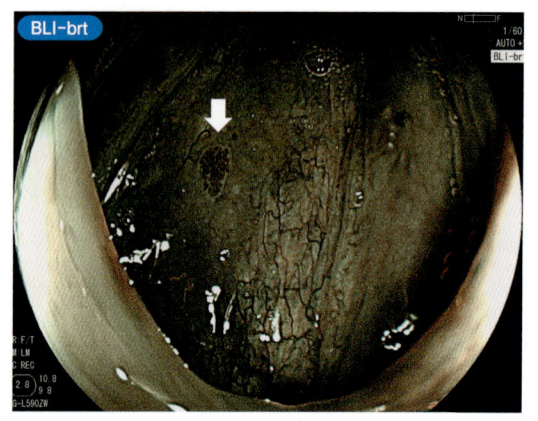

Magnifying endoscope (BLI-bright, far view): Clear brownish area (arrow) is observed on the posterior wall of the oropharynx.

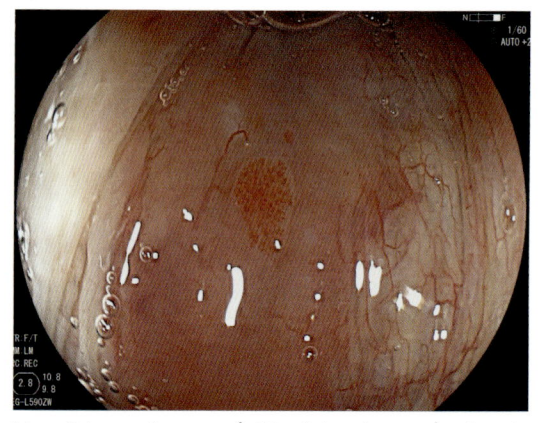

Magnifying endoscope (white-light, close-up): A well-demarcated, localized erythema is observed.

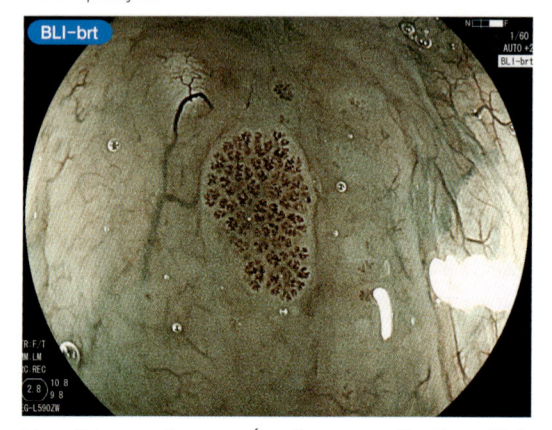

Magnifying endoscope (medium magnification, BLI-bright): Dotted B1 vessels are recognized clearly. Demarcation from the surrounding area is also clear.

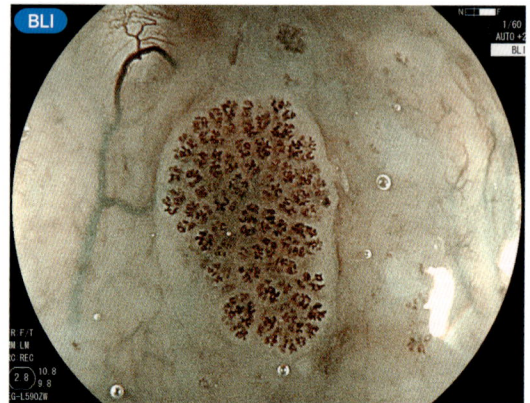

Magnifying endoscope (high magnification, BLI): The presence of B1 vessels, the intervascular background coloration and the interruption of normal vessels in the surrounding area leads to recognition of the lesion as a squamous cell carcinoma.

Scope：EG-580NW transnasal endoscope（Fujifilm）, EG-L590ZW magnifying endoscope（Fujifilm）
Light source：LASEREO（Fujifilm）　BLI setup：Structure enhancement A6, color enhancement C1

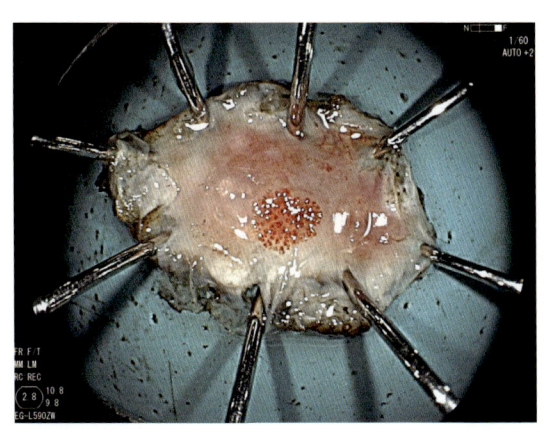

Resected specimen：The size of the part with vascularization is about 2 mm.

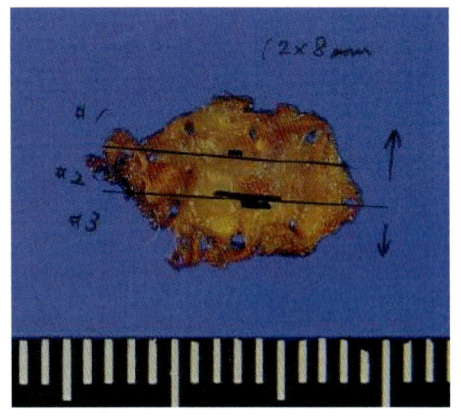

Mapping：The carcinoma extends over an area larger than the part with vascularization. The lesion size is 5×4 mm.

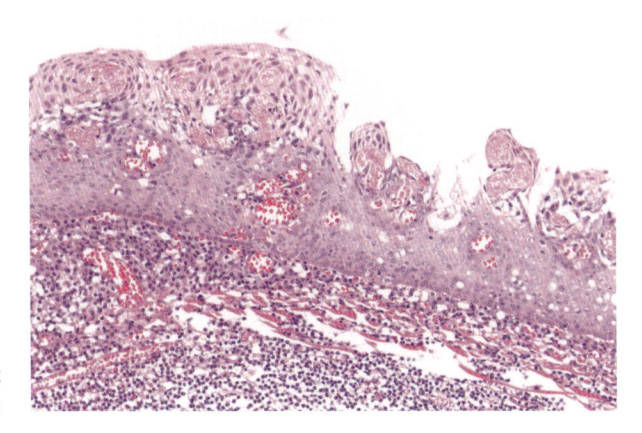

Microscopic pathology：Squamous cell carcinoma.

Comment

Advances in image-enhanced endoscopy and magnifying endoscopy, together with the clarification of the clinical characteristics of squamous cell carcinoma have made it possible to find microcarcinomas of a few millimeters in size — such as the present specimen — in the pharyngeal region. The characteristics include clear demarcation, atypical vessels with dilation, tortuosity, irregular diameters and irregular shapes, and a brownish area in the background. However, as differentiation from an inflammation, atypical epithelium or lymphoid follicles may be difficult, it is a good idea to always perform a biopsy before treatment. The treatment of such a microlesion can sometimes be completed with biopsy only. As the lesion will not progress quickly, there is no need to hurry the treatment.

▶**Observation tips** With white-light observation, both the background and carcinoma are red so it is difficult to tell them apart. However, diagnosis can be facilitated by using BLI to enhance the difference and magnifying endoscopy to visualize the superficial vessels and the color tone of intervascular background mucosa. The judgment criteria are whether or not the vessels can be seen through on the background of vascularization and whether the demarcation with the surrounding area is clear.

(Kawada, K., Kawano, T.)

Case 7 Hypopharyngeal superficial carcinoma (0-Ⅱb)

Male in 60s |Purpose| Screening |Location| Posterior wall of oro-hypopharynx |Macroscopic type| 0-Ⅱb

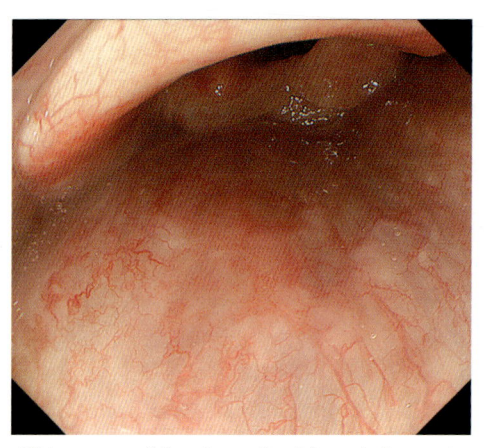

WLI non-magnifying observation: A poorly demarcated erythema in which normal vessels cannot be seen through is recognized on the posterior wall of the oro-hypopharynx. The lesion is a flat lesion without surface irregularities.

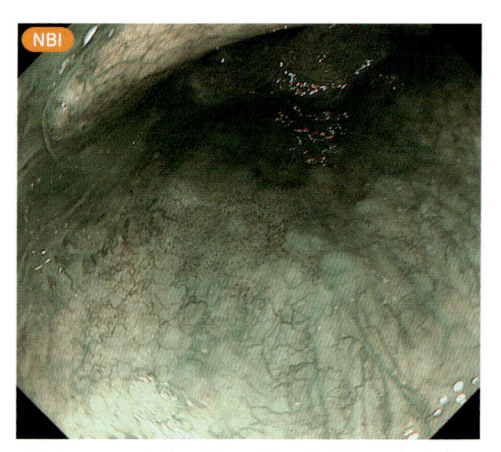

NBI non-magnifying observation: NBI allows the lesion to be recognized as a brownish area.

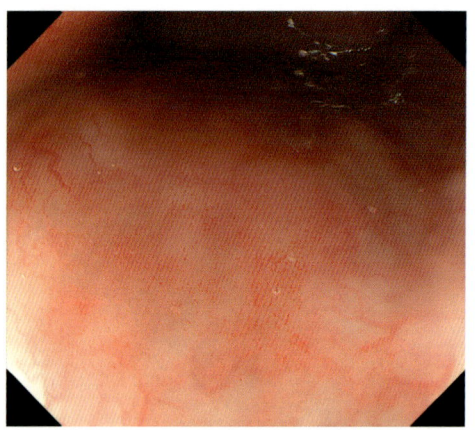

WLI low-magnification observation: No norrmal vessels are observed inside the lesion. Instead, growth of dilated, dotted atypical vessels are observed.

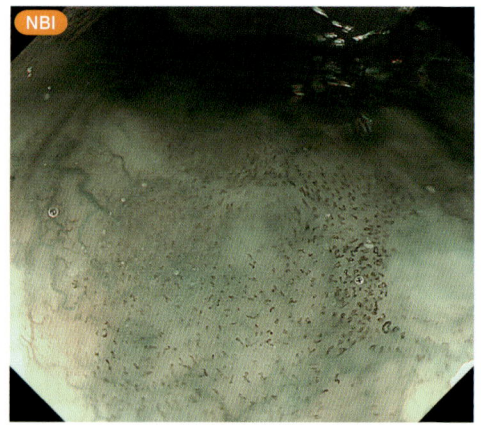

NBI low-magnification observation: NBI shows the growth of dotted atypical vessels more clearly than WLI.

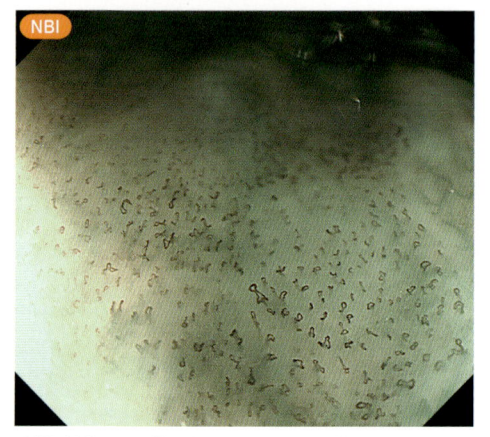

NBI high-magnification observation: When the magnification is increased, it can be confirmed that the atypical vessels that looked like dots actually consist of dilated vessels forming loops on the mucosal surface layer.

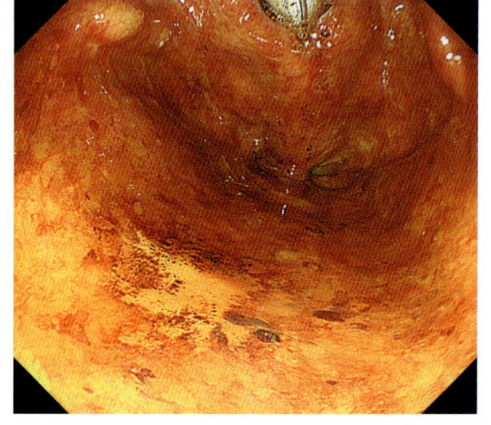

Iodine-stained non-magnifying observation (day of procedure): When iodine is sprayed, the lesion remains unstained, making it more visible.

Scope：GIF-H260Z（Olympus） Light source：EVIS LUCERA ELITE（Olympus）
NBI setup：Structure enhancement B8, color mode 2

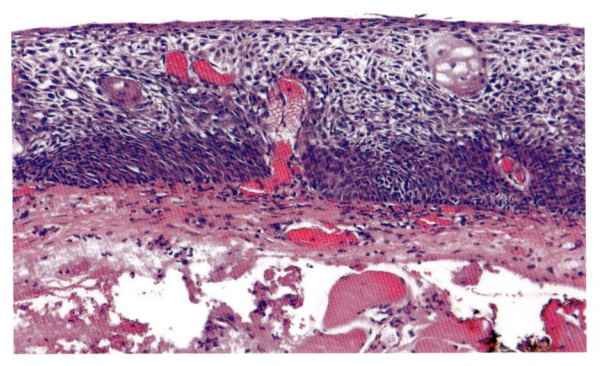

Histopathological image：A squamous cell carcinoma localized within the epithelium is recognized.
Squamous cell carcinoma, Tis, ly0, v0, pHM0, pVM0, 0-Ⅱb, 11mm

Comment

This is a case of superficial carcinoma on the posterior wall of the oro-hypopharynx. The absence of surface irregularities suggests that the macroscopic type of the lesion is Ⅱb. The findings that are hard to detect with WLI, such as slight color tone changes, disappearance of normal vessels and atypical vascularization can be observed easily with NBI. A lesion can be diagnosed as an epithelial tumor if a well-demarcated brownish area and atypical vascularization are observed with NBI. Assessment of whether the tumor is a high-grade dysplasia to SCC for which treatment is indicated or a low-grade dysplasia for which follow-up observation may be recommended is based on the grade of vessel atypism, degree of vascularization and clarity of demarcation. In case you are unsure of the diagnosis, perform a biopsy or an endoscopic follow-up in 1 to 3 months.

▶**Observation tips** A lesion can be diagnosed as an epithelial tumor if a well-demarcated brownish area and atypical vascularization are observed with NBI.

(Morita, S., Muto, M.)

Case 8 **Hypopharyngeal superficial carcinoma（0-Ⅱa+Ⅱb）**

Male in 60s　Purpose Screening after esophageal carcinoma ESD　Location Posterior wall of hypopharynx
Macroscopic type 0-Ⅱa+Ⅱb

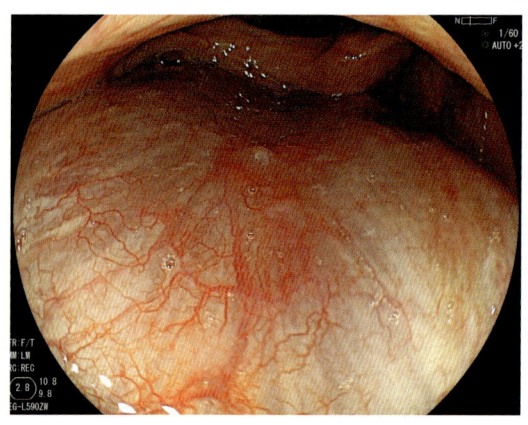

White-light image：Far view shows slight erythema on the posterior wall of the hypopharynx.

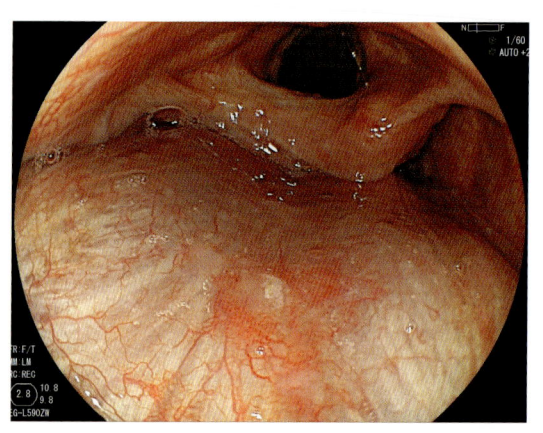

White-light image：Near view shows a 0-Ⅱa+Ⅱb type erythematous lesion accompanied by slough.

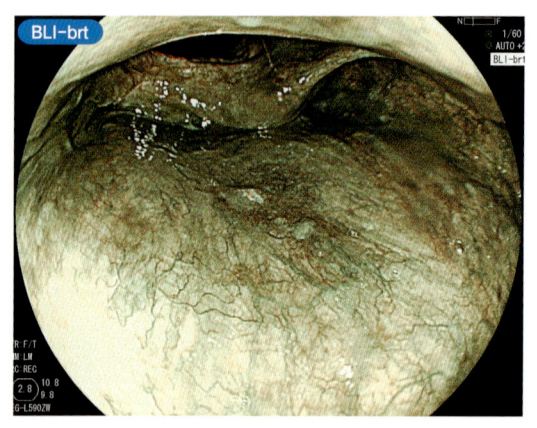

BLI-bright mode image：Far view shows an obscure brownish area on the posterior wall of the hypopharynx.

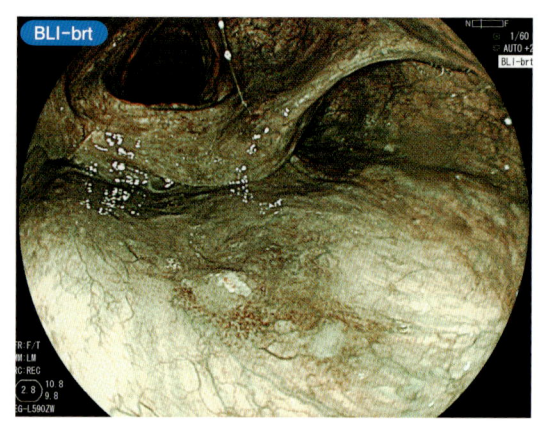

BLI-bright mode image：Near view shows the brownish area clearly.

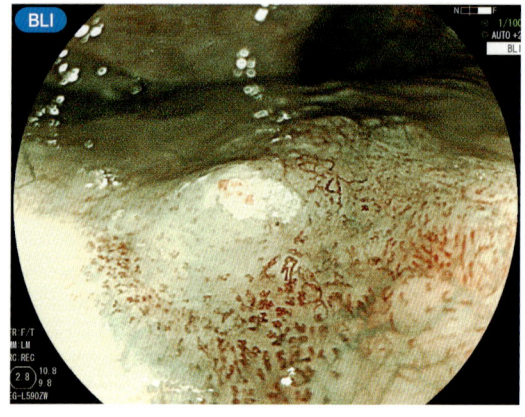

BLI mode image：Low magnification presents irregular dilation of the IPCLs.

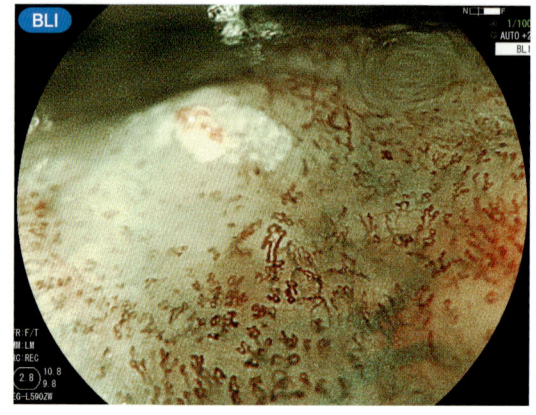

BLI mode image：High magnification shows type B2 vessels partially.

Scope：EG-590ZW（Fujifilm）　Light source：LASEREO（Fujifilm）
BLI setup：Structure enhancement B8, color enhancement C1

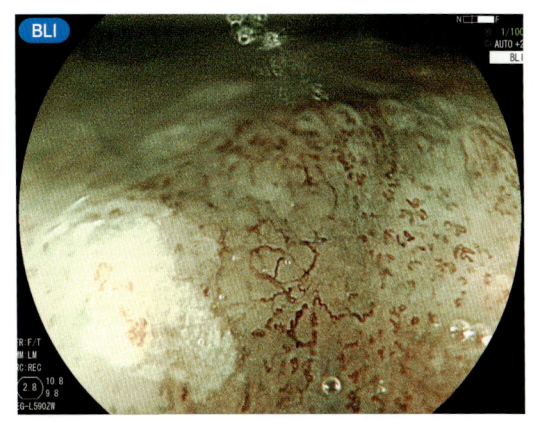

BLI mode image：High magnification shows avascular areas, middle, partially.

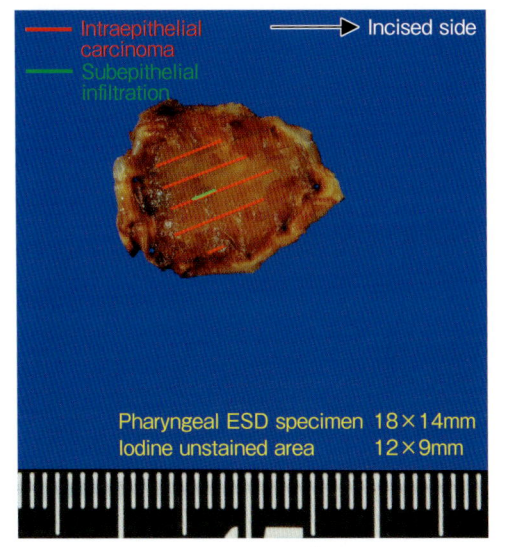

Macroscopic pathology (ESD-resected specimen)：A 0-Ⅱa+Ⅱb lesion of 12×9 mm is observed.

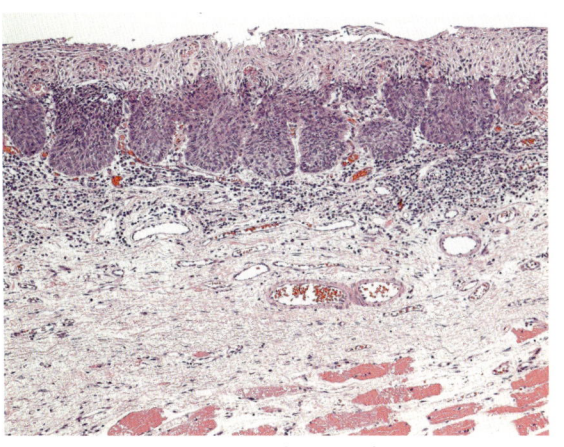

Pharyngeal ESD specimen 18×14mm
Iodine unstained area 12×9mm

— Intraepithelial carcinoma
— Subepithelial infiltration
▷ Incised side

Microscopic pathology（HE×100）：Subepithelial infiltration of 320 μm from the superficial layer （90 μm from the basal layer） is observed in the area coincident to the Ⅱa area.

Comment

With hypopharyngeal carcinoma, local treatment including endoscopic treatment is usually though to be indicated for the intraepithelial carcinoma（pTis）and subepithelial infiltration of 500 to 1,000 μm, although studies—including measurement methods—are limited at this time. As the invasion depth diagnosis of hypopharyngeal carcinoma is not yet established, diagnosis should be performed using the same method used for esophageal carcinoma. In the present case, the type B2 vessels and the avascular area, middle, are recognized as defined in the Japan Esophageal Society Classification of Magnified Endoscopy. As these findings would suggest an invasion depth of MM if the case was an esophageal carcinoma, subepithelial infiltration was suspected before treatment.

▶**Observation tips** When inserting the upper gastrointestinal endoscope, be sure to observe the laryngopharyngeal region to locate lesions by localized surface irregularities, erythema and color fading. With males in their 50s or older, you should also use of NBI or BLI. With these cases, the lesion can be located by searching for brownish areas.

(Shimizu, Y.)

Esophagus

See page 4 for explanation of abbreviations.

Esophagus

General Theory : How to Observe This Region with NBI or BLI

Tips on NBI Observation

■ Introduction

The esophagus is an organ covered with stratified squamous epithelium. In Japan, vast majority of malignant tumors in the esophagus are usually squamous cell carcinomas (SCCs).

Until recently, esophageal SCC was generally considered as a kind of gastrointestinal cancer most difficult to detect at an early stage. Nowadays, thanks to the widespread use of endoscopy and iodine staining, more than half of esophageal SCCs are detected at an early stage. Moreover, since most of the SCCs detected at an early stage are treated endoscopically, patients have experienced significant improvements in both quality of life (QOL) and prognosis.

Though iodine staining play a very important role in early detection of esophageal cancer, issues such as strong stimulation and allergic reaction discourage endoscopists from frequently using iodine staining in screening endoscopy.

The Narrow-Band Imaging (NBI) system overcomes these difficulties, providing a revolutionary solution to the early detection and diagnosis of esophageal SCCs.

There are two ways to perform esophageal observation using NBI the non-magnifying method and the magnifying method. As non-magnifying NBI procedure observation is more or less identical to conventional white-light imaging (WLI) procedure, we will highlight the points to keep in mind during examinations including NBI as well as WLI endoscopy. If a lesion is found in NBI non-magnifying observation, magnifying observation should be performed in order to diagnose the lesion qualitatively (differentiation, benign/malignant judgment) and quantitatively (extent, invasion depth). When discussing NBI magnifying observation, we will also refer to the differences between new and old systems/endoscopes.

In this section, superficial esophageal squamous cell (SESCC) carcinoma is defined as an SCC where high-grade intraepithelial neoplasia (HGIN) and carcinoma infiltration are limited to the submucosal layer.

■ I. Points to remember in NBI observation—and normal observation—of SESCC

1. Elimination of saliva and mucosa

If too much saliva or mucus, attaches to the esophageal wall during observation, you will not be able to inspect the esophagus with a clear view. In order to observe the entire esophagus without missing any details, it is important to first get rid of any saliva or mucus. One of the most effective ways to do this is to have the patient drink water or take pronase (Pronase MS® is covered by the Japanese Health Insurance System when it is used in dye-staining chromoendoscopy) before pharyngeal anesthesia.

2. Premedication

At our hospital, we apply sedatives liberally, as doing so can reduce the vomiting reflex of patients and ensure a clear view from the cervical esophagus. Sedation is also helpful if iodine is sprayed after WLI or NBI observation, as it can minimize potential discomfort to the patient that could be caused by the stimulus effect of the iodine solution.

＜Sedatives and doses＞
1) Routine examination
   ❶ Prepare a 10 ml solution combining 2 ml of midazolam (Dormicum® 10 mg)＋8 ml of saline. Intravenous administration of 2-3 ml (2-3 mg) of this solution.
   ❷ Prepare a 10 ml solution combining 1 ml of flunitrazepam (Rohypnol® 2 mg)＋9 ml of saline. Intravenous administration of 1-1.5 ml (0.2-0.3 mg) of this solution.
2) If iodine staining is scheduled：
   Intravenous administration of pethidine hydrochloride (Opistan®) 1A (35 mg) and 1.5-2.0 ml (0.3-0.4 mg) of the flunitrazepam solution combining 1 ml of flunitrazepam (Rohypnol® 2 mg) with 9 ml of saline.

3. Esophageal lavage

After inserting the scope, wash out the esophagus at a point roughly 25 cm from the upper incisors. Use 40-60 ml of Gascon® solution and apply it from the right wall, taking the direction of gravity into consideration.

Blood sticking to the walls of the esophagus can be a major obstacle to NBI observation. This means you need to be especially careful performing lavage when a easily-bleeding lesion is present or have to rinse away incoming blood after biopsy of a laryngopharyngeal lesion. After washing, suction out any lavage fluid that has accumulated in the esophagus, pull the scope back to a point about 20 cm from the upper incisors and start observation from the cervical esophagus.

4. Timing and procedure of NBI non-magnifying observation

At our hospital, we try to find a lesion in the esophagus especially while inserting the scope. After NBI observation of the laryngopharyngeal region, the scope is moved forward as is into the esophagus, which is also observed with NBI. If the pharyngeal reflex makes it difficult to perform observation while inserting the endoscope from the esophageal entrance to the cervical esophagus (about 18 cm from the upper incisors), then observe this region while withdrawing the endoscope.

The esophagogastric junction is observed with both NBI and WLI. Check for reflux esophagitis and Barrett's esophagus. If the latter is found, observe it with NBI magnifying observation.

As we generally use WLI for observation of the stomach and duodenum, we usually also use it in esophageal observation while withdrawing the endoscope. If we could not obtain reliable observation results of the region from the esophageal entrance to cervical esophagus during insertion, we will observe the region again with NBI.

Here are a few tips for observation of this region, as well as for observation of the esophagogastric junction.

Esophageal entrance to cervical esophagus：Observation during insertion is possible by inserting the endoscope slowly while insufflating air. If the reflex is strong, do not try to observe; instead, do it during scope withdrawal, by withdrawing the endoscope as slowly as possible while insufflating air. In the case that it becomes difficult to maintain sufficient space in the inner cavity, releasing patient's breath often help the observation if the patient is conscious.

Esophagogastric junction：Utilize the respiratory displacement of this region. In cases where observation is difficult due to the contraction of the lower esophageal sphincter, have the patient take a deep breath. This often makes it possible to ensure

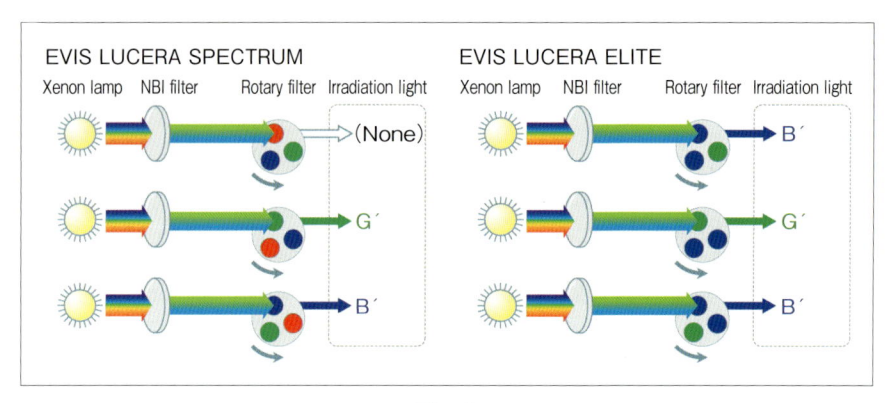

Fig. 1
With the new system (ELITE), NBI observation brightness can be significantly increased by a dedicated NBI filter assigned the blue light filter (B) to the red light filter (R), resulting in the "BGB" filter.

(Source : Olympus Medical Systems Corp.)

an enough visual field of view.

This technique takes advantage of the fact that the esophageal hiatus of the diaphragm relaxes during inspiration as well as increases negative pressure in the esophagus. When the esophagogastric junction prolapses toward the proximal side, quickly proceed to observation and photography.

5. **NBI non-magnifying observation**

Many superficial esophageal carcinomas present well-demarcated brownish areas under NBI non-magnifying observation. A multi-center randomized controlled trial has proven that NBI can detect SESCC with significantly high accuracy even without iodine staining[1].

However, due to the characteristics of the NBI filter in the light source, the brightness always decreases in NBI observation. Though not as dark as when observing the esophagus, the low level of brightness in NBI far-view observation in the stomach with a large inner cavity has often ever been brought up a practical issue.

To deal with this, the intensity of the light source in the new system (EVIS LUCERA ELITE, CV-290) has been almost doubled, and a new NBI filter has been installed (**Fig. 1**), making possible NBI observation with brightness equivalent to WLI (**Figs. 2a, b**). The new system also offers much improved image quality thanks to enhanced noise reduction function and the use of a higher-resolution 26-inch liquid crystal display (1,920×1,200 pixels, about 120% higher than the previous 21-inch monitor). This enables observation of the intraepithelial papillary capillary loops (IPCLs) even without magnification (inside the yellow ellipse in Fig. 2b).

To clearly image the brownish area that indicates SESCC in NBI non-magnifying observation, we recommend slightly reducing the amount of insufflation. This increases the vascular density of the lesion, resulting in an increase in the hemoglobin quantity per area. This, in turn, means that there will be a bigger difference in the amount of NBI light absorbed by the lesion compared to the surrounding mucosa, producing an image with higher contrast and clarity.

6. **NBI magnifying observation**

Like iodine staining, diagnosis of the presence of a SESCC (including high-grade intraepithelial neoplasia : HGIN) based on the brownish area observed with the NBI is not infallible. Low grade intraepithelial neoplasia (LGIN) as well as non-neoplastic lesions, such as inflammatory lesions and heterotopic gastric mucosa, also present a

a : WLI observation (new system)　　b : NBI non-magnifying observation (new system)

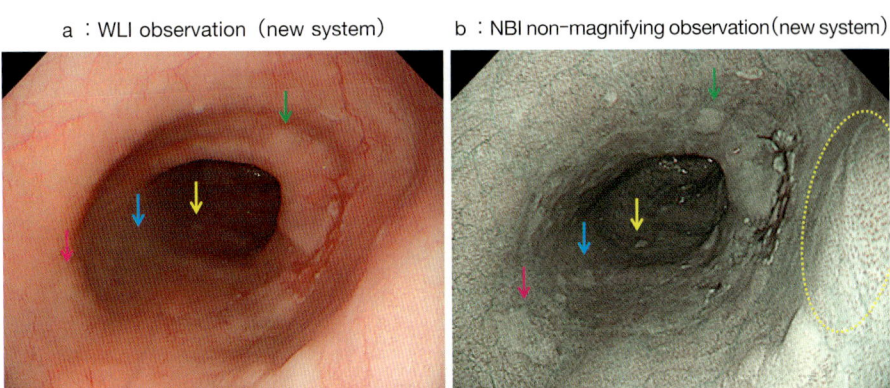

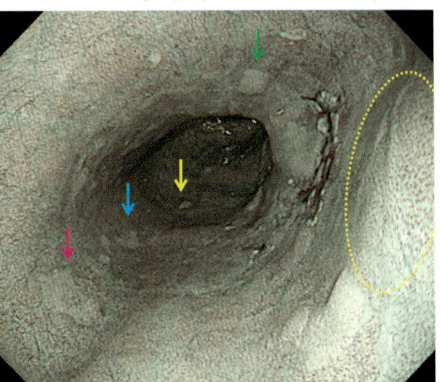

Fig. 2
NBI light can enhance structural changes in the superficial layer by the effectiveness of its scattering/absorption characteristics. NBI images produced by the new system, which features doubled light intensity, can image the glycogenic acanthosis from the near view to the far view more distinctly than WLI (arrows).

Endoscope : GIF-H290 (Olympus)
Light source : EVIS LUCERA ELITE (Olympus)
NBI setup : Structure enhancement A7, color mode 1

NBI magnifying observation
(Near Focus, new system)

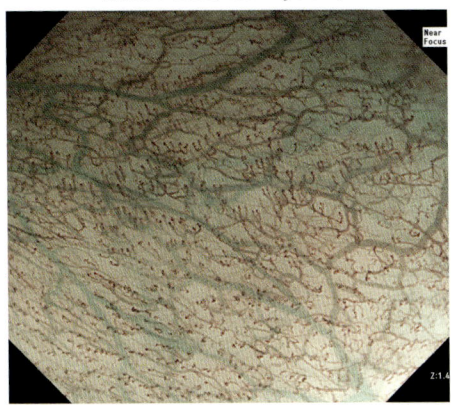

Endoscope : GIF-H290 (Olympus)
Light source : EVIS LUCERA ELITE (Olympus)
NBI setup : Structure enhancement A7, color mode 1

Fig. 3　Normal IPCL Image

brownish area. Magnifying observation is generally believed to be the most effective way to differentiate these lesions.

Heterotopic gastric mucosa has a surface pattern similar to the gastric mucosa. As this can be seen with low to medium magnification, differentiation from esophageal carcinoma, which does not have this pattern, is relatively easy. To differentiate SESCC from an inflammatory lesion or low-grade intraepithelial neoplasia (LGIN), it is necessary to evaluate the morphological changes of the IPCLs.

IPCLs consist of loop-structured micro-vessels found at the terminal position 3 to 4 branches after the arborizing vessels which are mainly located immediately above the muscularis mucosa and are histologically localized in the epithelial papilla (**Fig. 3**). Many squamous cell carcinomas have all of the four morphological change of IPCL (known as the tetralogy), which consist of three morphological changes found by

a：WLI observation (new system)

b：NBI non-magnifying observation (current system)

c：NBI non-magnifying observation (new system)

Endoscope：GIF-HQ290 (Olympus)
Light source：EVIS LUCERA ELITE (Olympus)

Endoscope：GIF-H260Z (Olympus)
Light source：EVIS LUCERA SPECTRUM (Olympus)
NBI setup：Structure enhancement A8, color mode 1

Endoscope：GIF-HQ290 (Olympus)
Light source：EVIS LUCERA ELITE (Olympus)
NBI setup：Structure enhancement A7, color mode 1

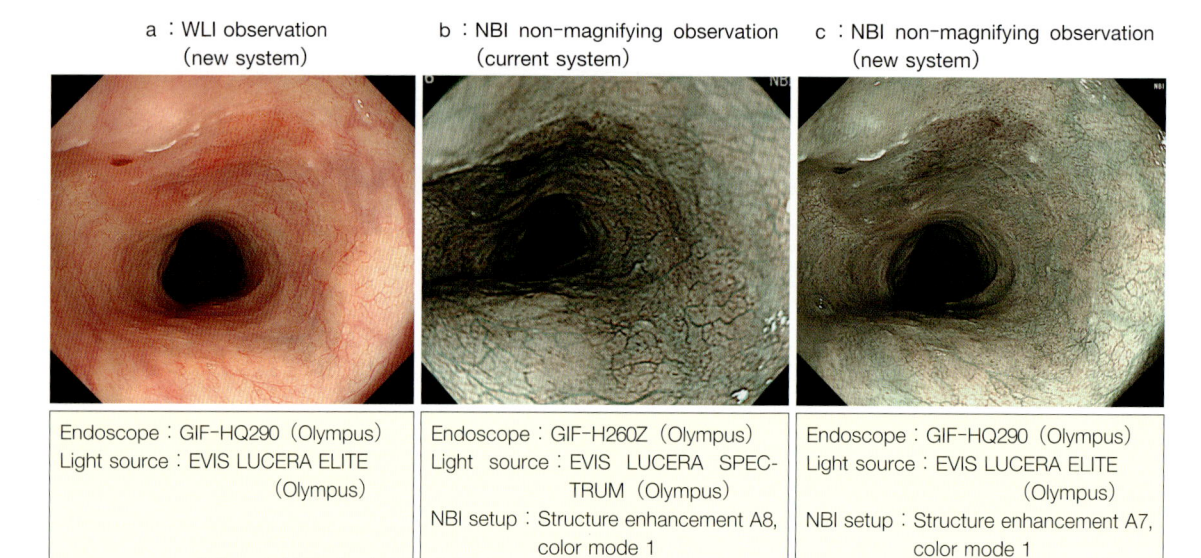

Fig. 4

a：A flat erythematous lesion is recognized in the 12 o'clock direction of the middle esophagus and a slightly erythematous region is also observed in the 10-11 o'clock direction. This lesion's demarcation is not very clear.

b, c：With both the current and new systems, this lesion presents a brownish area under NBI non-magnifying observation. The image produced by the new system is obviously brighter throughout the entire area than the image produced by the current system. The improved brightness enables observation of a much wider area of the esophageal mucosa, providing a clear view all the way to the distal side far away from the lesion. With the new system, the brownish area in the 10-11 o'clock direction is imaged relatively clearly, and the demarcation on the distal side of the lesion is visible, whereas they are obscure due to the poor light intensity of the current system.

NBI magnifying observation (Near Focus, new system)

Endoscope：GIF-HQ290 (Olympus)
Light source：EVIS LUCERA ELITE (Olympus)
NBI setup：Structure enhancement A7, color mode 1

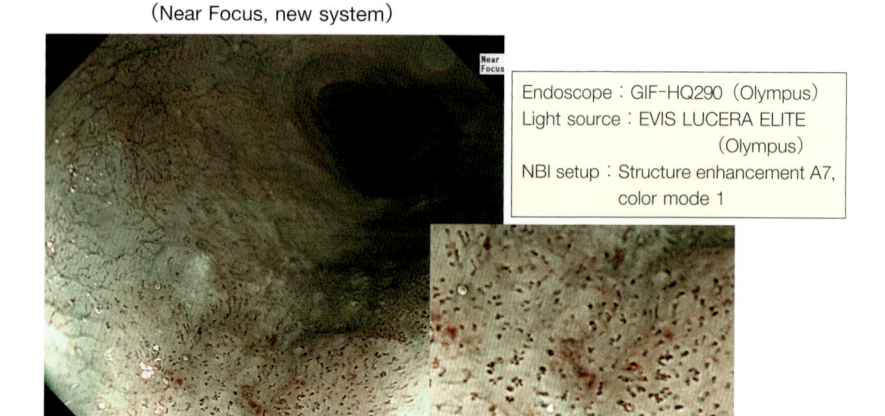

Fig. 5

In NBI magnifying observation in the Near Focus mode, the background mucosa between vessels in the lesion is shown in a pale brownish color (intervascular background coloration), and all of the tetralogy features—dilation, tortuosity, changes in caliber and various shapes—are recognized in the IPCLs.

a：NBI magnifying observation
(Near Focus, new system)

b：NBI magnifying observation (Near Focus
+electronic zoom 1.4×, new system)

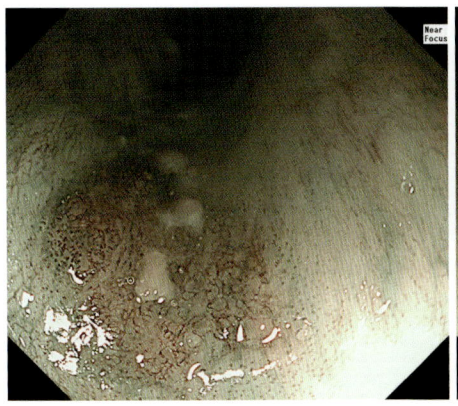

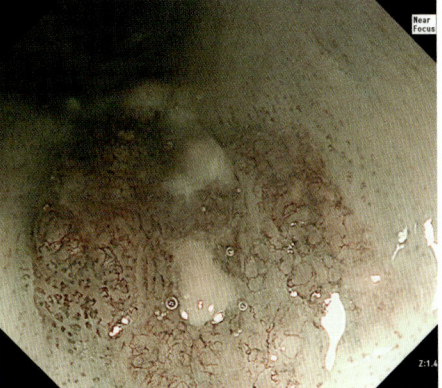

Fig. 6
a : Abnormal vessels with remarkable elongation and poor loop formation can be seen from the center to the right (vicinity of the erosion). These are considered corresponding to the B2 vessels.
b : 1.4×electronic zoom enables more detailed observation of the morphological changes in the abnormal vessels and also shows a region in which the vascular density is relatively low (vicinity of the erosion).

Endoscope：GIF-HQ290 (Olympus)
Light source：EVIS LUCERA ELITE
(Olympus)
NBI setup：Structure enhancement A7,
color mode 1

NBI magnifying observation
(Near Focus, new system)

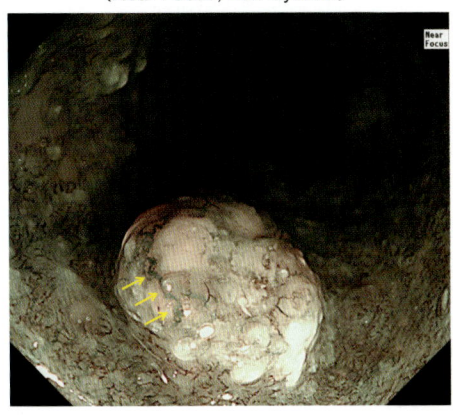

Endoscope：GIF-HQ290 (Olympus)
Light source：EVIS LUCERA ELITE
(Olympus)
NBI setup：Structure enhancement A7,
color mode 1

Fig. 7
Greenish, highly-dilated abnormal vessels (yellow arrows) can be seen in the type 0-I protruded lesion. They seem to be equivalent to the B3 vessels.

observation of individual IPCLs, including dilation, tortuosity and changes in caliber, plus various shapes found by comparison of multiple IPCLs. These four elements are helpful in differentiating HGIN and invasive SCC from LGIN or inflammatory lesions (**Figs. 4, 5**)[2].

Additional morphological changes in the IPCLs are correlated with the invasion depth of the carcinoma. In our clinical study, no significant difference in the accuracy of preoperative diagnosis was shown between EUS and NBI magnifying endoscopy[3]

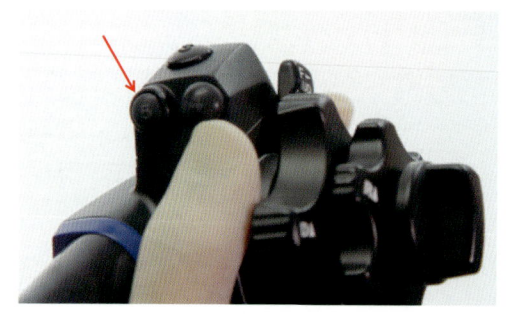

Fig. 8 Close-up Magnification of GIF-HQ290
Near Focus button (red arrow)

and both of them showed a significantly higher accuracy than WLI endoscopy. The Japan Esophageal Society (JSC) recently proposed a new magnification endoscopy classification for SESCC based on the two classifications proposed by Inoue et al[4] and Arima et al[5], which have long been used in clinical practice. Created specifically to support SESCC diagnosis including invasion depth[6] (see Table on page 57), the new classification is applicable to localized lesions suspected to be SCCs. The new dual focus endoscope (GIF-HQ290), released together with the new system, uses a low magnification but its high image quality can visualize the abnormal IPCLs in a tumor lesion as well as IPCLs in the normal region (**Fig. 3**) to abnormal IPCLs (JES Classification B1 : **Fig. 5**, B2 : **Figs. 6a, b**, B3 : **Fig. 7**).

The features of the dual focus endoscope are summarized in the following three points.

❶ **Simplified magnification technique** : While the conventional magnifying endoscope used a lever for magnification, the new scope can switch between two focus settings which are ordinal observation (Normal mode) and close-up observation (Near mode) using a single button on the scope operation part (**Fig. 8**). A single push of the button switches to a medium magnification image (max. 45× with high-definition TV monitor in scan mode 3) in the near focus mode. Combining that with electronic zooming (1.4×, 1.6×, 2.0×) can further increase magnification, though there will be some degradation in image quality.

Note : Pushing the button twice engages the electronic zoom setting.

❷ **Easy focusing** : The depth of focus is deeper than that of a conventional magnifying endoscope (3-7 mm) so it is easy to obtain an in-focus merely by the approach to a region of the interest, which means that there is theoretically no need to attach a hood. Less chance of contacting the lesion can reduce the risk of the bleeding that can severely hamper NBI observation.

❸ **Reduced diameter** : Compared to the H260Z scope, which has a distal-end diameter of 10.8 mm (12.8 mm when the hood is attached), the HQ290 is much slimmer, with a distal-end diameter of just 10.2 mm. This means that the HQ290 imposes much less of a strain on the patient during insertion, so it can be suitable for routine endoscopy, as well. In addition, as it is also equipped with an auxiliary water function (water jet), it can also be used in endoscopic treatment procedures such as ESD. The reduction in diameter can also be expected to improve operability during treatment as well as during observation.

The reduced scope diameter and simplified magnification method also mean that the GIF-HQ290 can be expected to be highly effective in simplified magnifying procedure during screening endoscopy. It has been pointed out that while the magnification ratios are sufficient for SESCC, they are not sufficient for magnifying endoscopic diagnosis of early gastric adenocarcinoma. Consequently, we are positioning this endoscope as a new category of endoscope, placed at halfway between conventional routine endoscopy and magnifying endoscopy for detailed observations in upper GI tract. We also believe that it will be useful in a wide range of clinical practices down to small clinics.

Although the clinical utility of the magnifying endoscope for upper GI carcinoma has been demonstrated in a large number of clinical studies, it is not yet in widespread use, even in large and/or specialized hospitals. As this endoscope is also applicable in routine endoscopy, we hope that it will lead to a dissemination of magnifying endoscopic diagnosis and an increase in the early detection rate of esophageal SCC. We also expect it to contribute to improving the QOL and prognosis of esophageal SCC patients.

Conclusion

In this section, we have outlined NBI endoscopic observation, focusing on SESCC and in the esophagus, highlighting various issues. We provided tips on everything from preparation and dealing with obstacles to insertion or observation to endoscopic diagnosis with non-magnifying or magnifying procedure. We also looked at some of the advantages of the new endoscopy system and novel endoscope.

References

1) Muto, M., Minashi, K., Yano, T. et al. : Early detection of superficial squamous cell carcinoma in the head and neck region and esophagus by narrow band imaging : a multicenter randomized controlled trial. J Clin Oncol 2010 ; 28 : 1566-1572
2) Inoue, H., Honda, T., Yoshida, T. et al. : Ultra-high magnification endoscopic observation of carcinoma in situ of the esophagus. Dig Endosc 1997 ; 9 : 16-18
3) Goda, K., Tajiri, H., Ikegami, M. et al. : Magnifying endoscopy with narrow band imaging for predicting the invasion depth of superficial esophageal squamous cell carcinoma. Dis Esophagus 2009 ; 22 : 453-460
4) Inoue, H. : Magnification endoscopy in the esophagus and stomach. Dig. Endosc 2001 ; 13 : S40-S41
5) Arima, M,, Tada, M., Arima, H. : Evaluation of microvascular patterns of superficial esophageal cancers by magnifying endoscopy. Esophagus 2005 ; 2 : 191-197
6) Oyama, T., Monma, K. and Makuuchi, H. : Magnifying endoscopic diagnosis of esophageal squamous cell carcinoma—introducing the JES classification (in Japanese, title translated). Shokaki Naishikyo (Endoscopia Digestiva) 2012 ; 24 : 466-468.

(Goda, K., Dobashi, A., Tajiri, H.)

Esophagus

General Theory : How to Observe This Region with NBI or BLI

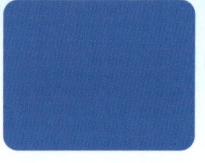

Tips on BLI Observation

I. Features of the LASEREO system

With the development of a new endoscopy system using laser light as the light source, the LASERO system, Blue Laser Imaging (BLI) has been added to the various digital image enhancement techniques already available. One of the most important features of this system is the clarity of white-light images, which has made it easy to observe delicate color tone changes. The BLI mode images are also bright, making it possible to obtain sharp, bright close-up images even in magnifying observation, as well as to capture still photos with little, if any, blurring.

The BLI setup we use in esophageal observation consists of structure enhancement set to B8 and color enhancement set to C1. We do not use the BLI-bright mode in the esophagus.

II. Precise observation of lesions

Since esophageal lesions include lesions with faded colors or poor color tone change, as well as ones with clear, red vascular proliferation, they should first be observed with white light to check the extent of the lesion, the morphology of the margins, the degree of thickening and depression, and the surface structure. After white light observation, switch the light source to BLI and observe the microvessels with magnifying observation. The following are some basic points you should try to keep in mind when observing lesions :

❶ With superficial esophageal carcinoma, there is a very close relation between the type and invasion depth and between the invasion depth and lymph node metastatic rate.
❷ Types 0-Ⅰ and 0-Ⅲ lesions have a high probability of being SM cancers.
❸ The invasion depth of a type 0-Ⅱ lesion is assessed based on the depth of depression, shape of demarcation and the presence of internal irregularities.
❹ EP/LPM carcinomas form shallow depressions with an inner surface that is either flat or very finely granulated.
❺ MM/SM1 carcinomas often form depressions accompanied by granular elevations and/or certain degree of thickness.
❻ SM2 carcinomas are often accompanied by nodes, pleated thickening and/or deeper depression.
❼ Type 0-Ⅱa lesions have a standard height of about 1 mm and are whitish with a clear rise. Lesions with aggregated papillary protrusions are often well-differentiated carcinomas.
❽ Type 0-Ⅱc lesions with marginal elevations, type 0-Ⅱa lesions with an unclear rise, and type 0-Ⅰs lesions that resemble submucosal tumors have a high probability of being MM or deeper carcinomas.

III. Detailed endoscopic observation using a magnifying endoscope

For smooth detailed observation, it is important to set up your environment so that you can focus on the examination procedure.
❶ Attach the hood to the distal end.
Since the esophagus is strongly affected by both respiratory movement and heartbeat, and as it lies in a tangential direction to the lumen, a distal hood is indispensable for esophageal observation. The MB46 Black Hood manufactured by Olympus or the Slit & Hole Type (M) Elastic Touch manufactured by Top Corporation can be used for this purpose. The hood is attached by inserting it deeply until it is not visible in the field of view

Table Magnifying Endoscopy Classification of Superficial Esophageal Carcinomas by Japan Esophageal Society (Excerpt)

Type A : Lesions with no or slight vascular morphological change
Changes in the intraepithelial papillary capillary loops (IPCLs) are not detected or are very minor.
Type B : Lesions with advanced degree of vascular morphological change
B1 : Loop-like abnormal vessels with all of the following present : dilation, tortuosity, irregular diameters and/or irregular shapes B2 : Abnormal vessels with poor loop formation. B3 : Highly dilated irregular vessels (Note 6). Avascular area (AVA) : An area with no vessels or that is sparsely populated by vessels encircled by type B vessels is called an AVA. An AVA is classified as AVA-small when the size is less than 0.5 mm, AVA-middle when it is between 0.5 mm and 3 mm, and AVA-large when it is 3 mm or more. However, note that an AVA composed exclusively of B1 vessels is equivalent to the invasion depth of T1a-EP/LPM regardless of the size.
Additional remark 1 : A lesion with irregular, finely reticular vessels may be observed. Such a lesion is classified as an "R" lesion because it is often a poorly differentiated esophageal carcinoma, miscellaneous carcinoma and lesions showing INFc infiltrative patterns. Note 6 : Irregular vessels at least three times larger than B2 vessels, and with diameters of at least 60 μm.

[Quoted from Reference 3)]

of a normal observation image. If the hood projects by 1–2 mm from the distal end of the endoscope, that is usually sufficient.

❷After washing the lumen, suction out all the fluid.
Start observation by observing the oral cavity and pharynx, and then advance the endoscope while carefully observing the esophageal entrance and cervical esophagus, as there is often more than just one lesion. To avoid missing lesions in the cervical esophagus and/or upper esophagus, do not perform suction or advance the endoscope forcibly in these regions. Instead, hold the endoscope steady, inject Gascon® solution to wash the region and then suction the fluid in the lumen carefully. Be sure to suction this region well as the fluid tends to pool easily around the lesion on the left side of the esophagus if the endoscope is pushed against it for magnifying observation. In addition, as there is a risk of reflux of fluid inside the stomach, be sure to suction fluid from inside the stomach.

❸Displace the distal end by separating it from the lesion, without sliding.
When the endoscope reaches the region of interest, twist the endoscope to bring it toward the anterior wall to enable fine control. When moving on to the next field of view, move the endoscope by separating it from the lesion, without sliding the scope while the distal end is applied to the lesion. Otherwise, bleeding could interfere with the diagnosis.

❹When the lesion extends over a broad area, switch the magnification from medium to high and vice versa to find the optimum observation position, and observe the lesion by controlling the orientation.

❺Fine-adjust the focus by moving your right hand a little. Adjust the distance from the lens while repeating short insufflations.

Ⅳ. JES classification of microvessels based on magnifying endoscopy and interpretation of microvessels

The Japan Esophageal Society (JES) proposed a new classification for the magnifying endoscopy of superficial esophageal carcinoma based on the Inoue classification[1] and the Arima classification[2] (**Table**[3]). **Figs. 1** and **2** show the BLI magnifying observation images that correspond with the classification.

❶A type B1 vessel refers to an irregular vessel with a slight loop. It roughly corresponds with the vessels associated with EP/LPM carcinomas.
Destruction of the vascular morphology, irregular vascular diameters and disorganization are

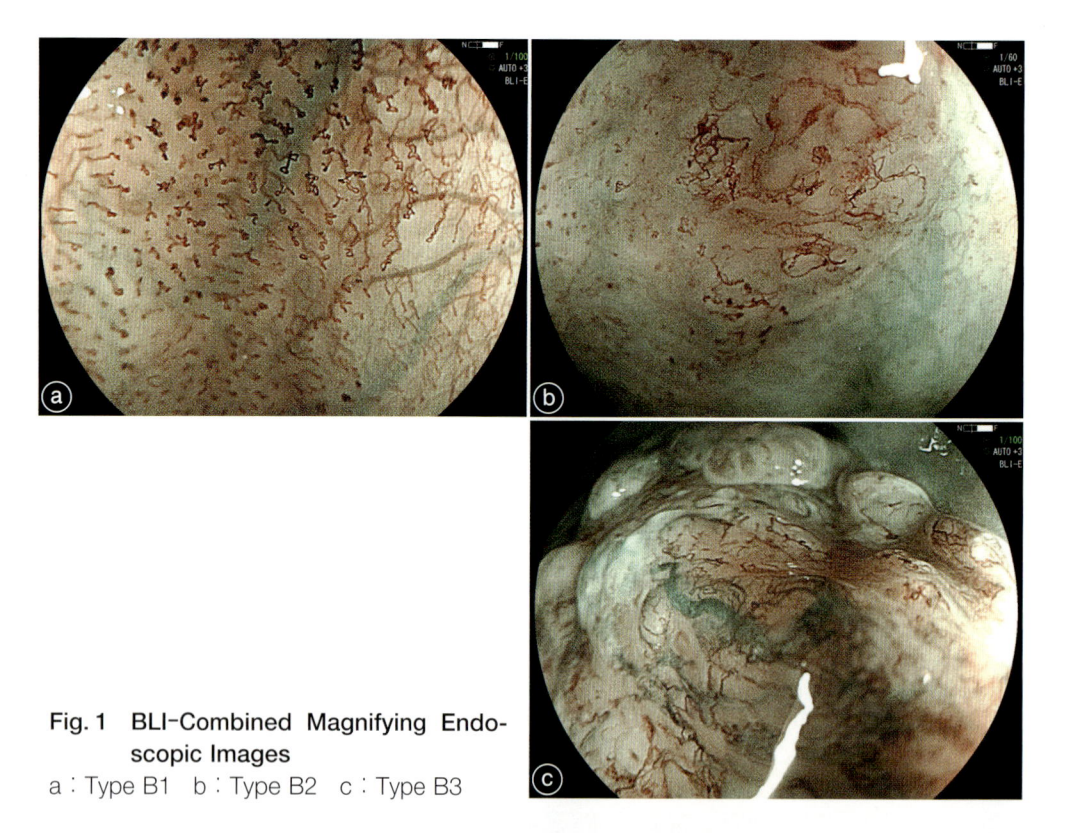

Fig. 1 BLI-Combined Magnifying Endoscopic Images
a : Type B1   b : Type B2   c : Type B3

Fig. 2 BLI-Combined Magnifying Endoscopic Images
a : AVA-small   b : AVA-middle (arrows)

observed with the vessel. Vessels with a destroyed filamentous vessels, a crushed dot shape and spiral vessels in the papillary protrusion are typical B1 vessels.

❷A type B2 vessel refers to a vessel that deviates from the loop structure. It is observed in invasion depths at the LPM or deeper levels. Multi-layered (ML) vessels with a destroyed loop structure and irregularly branched (IB) vessels are typical B2 vessels.

❸A type B3 vessel refers to a thick irregular vessel with a diameter of over 60 μm. It is often recognized with SM2 or deeper carcinomas.

❹The avascular area (AVA) means the size of the tumor mass composed of the invaded section. Generally, AVA-small corresponds to the EP/LPM carcinomas, AVA-middle to the MM/SM1 carcinomas and AVA-large to the SM2/SM3 carcinomas[3].

❺Fine frizzy reticular (R) vessels with noticeably irregular diameters are observed with poorly differentiated carcinomas that do not form clear tumorous masses, esophageal

a, b : conventional endoscopic images. The posterior wall side where a faded, yellowish flat thickened plane has formed is referred to as part A and the left side wall where coarse granular protrusions have aggregated is referred to as part B.

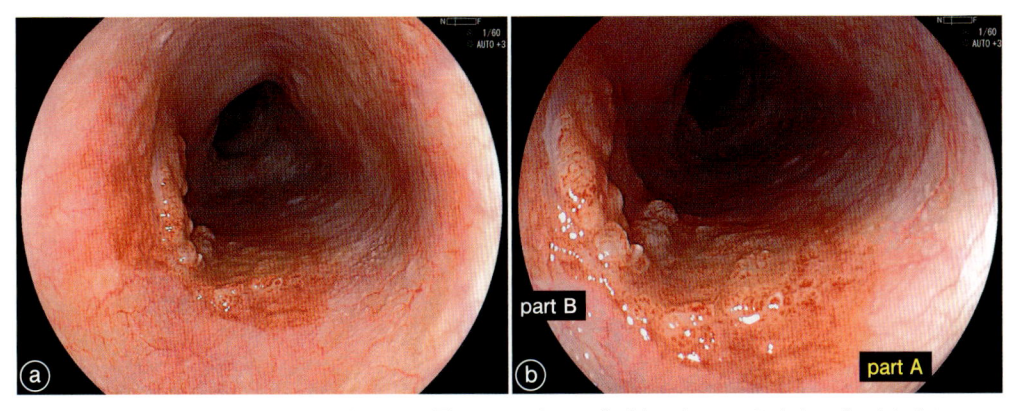

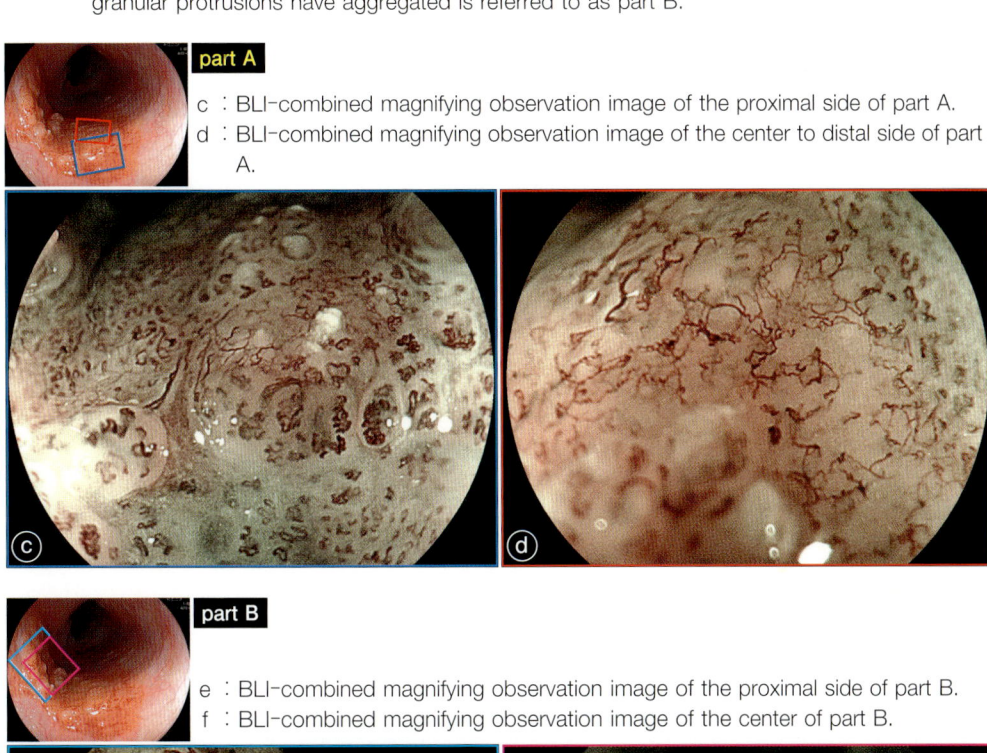

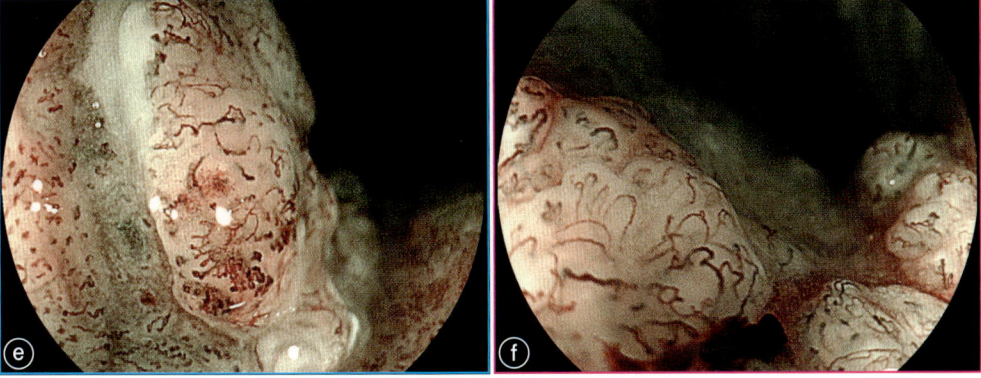

part A
c : BLI-combined magnifying observation image of the proximal side of part A.
d : BLI-combined magnifying observation image of the center to distal side of part A.

part B
e : BLI-combined magnifying observation image of the proximal side of part B.
f : BLI-combined magnifying observation image of the center of part B.

Fig. 3　Type 0-Ⅱa+Ⅰs+Ⅱc Esophageal Carcinoma（pT1b-SM1）

g : Iodine stained image.
h : Iodine stained image of a freshly resected specimen obtained by ESD.

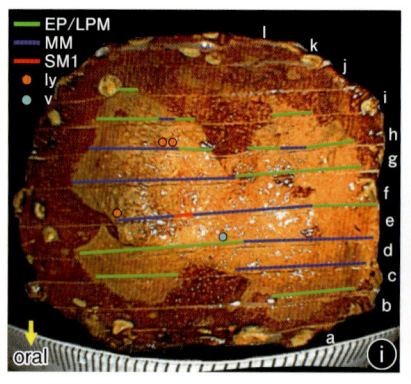

i : Construction diagram showing mod＞por SCC, pT1b-SM1, ly1, v1, INFb.

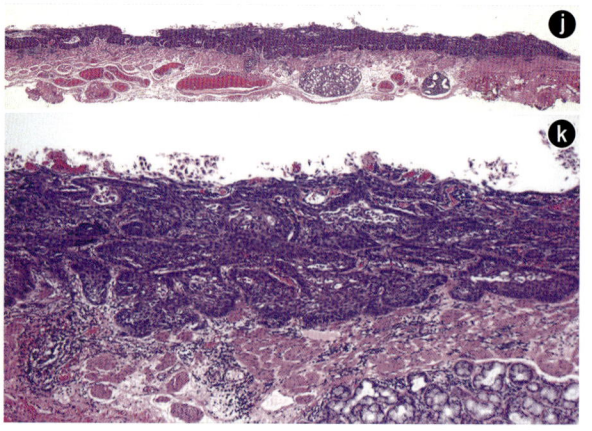

j , k : Histopathological images of flat thickening of part A.

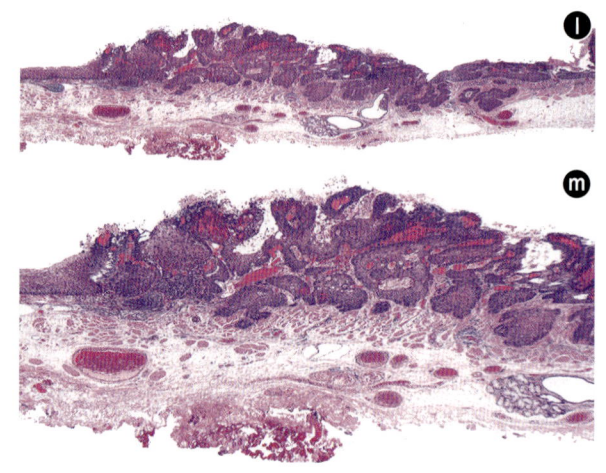

l , m : Histopathological images of coarse granular protrusions of part B

Fig. 3　Type 0 - Ⅱa＋Ⅰs＋Ⅱc Esophageal Carcinoma (pT1b-SM1)

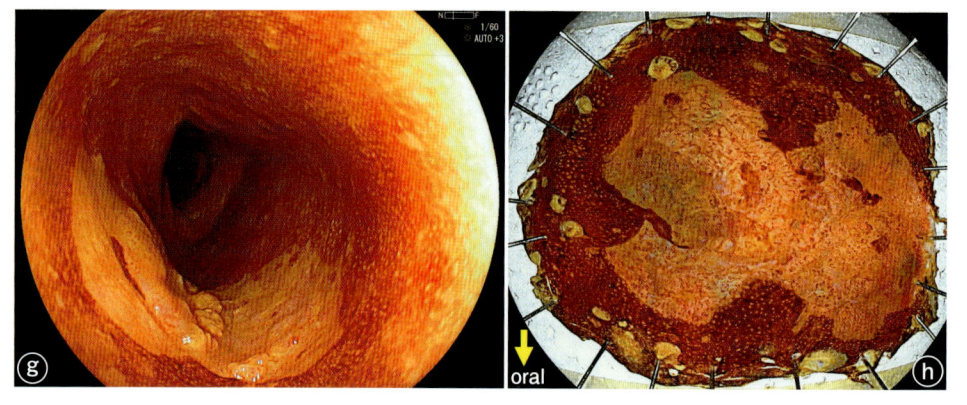

carcinomas, miscellaneous carcinoma and lesions showing INFc infiltrative patterns. They have relatively low vascular density and are often observed in faded-color areas. They may also be seen on part of the surface of Ⅱc lesions.

V. Case presentations (Fig. 3)

This is a semi-circumferential lesion extending from the posterior wall of the upper thoracic esophagus towards the left side wall (**Fig. 3a**). As the posterior wall side of the slightly erythematous shallow Ⅱc depression has a thickened flat surface with a slightly faded yellowish color, while the left side wall has an aggregation of coarse granular protrusions with a relatively clear rise, this lesion is diagnosed as a type 0-Ⅱa+Ⅰs+Ⅱc esophageal carcinoma. The posterior wall side is referred to as "part A" and the left side wall is referred to as "part B" (**Fig. 3b**). With BLI-combined magnifying observation, B1 vessels with irregular shapes leaving the trace of loop structure, dilation and tortuosity are observed in the shallow Ⅱc region on the proximal side of part A and the rising section of the flat thickened surface, while B2 vessels with destroyed loops are observed in the thickened section in the deeper position (**Fig. 3c**). It is also observed that B2 vessels with a destroyed loop structure and noticeable diameter irregularities form an irregular network on the flat thickened surface (**Fig. 3d**). The coarse granular margin of part B in the left wall direction, on the other hand, features a mix of sections showing traces of loops and B2 vessels stretched by the disappearance of the loops (**Fig. 3e**). In the granular protrusions in the deeper position, the aggregation of B2 vessels have been distorted by stretching of the loop (**Fig. 3f**). For the shallow Ⅱc regions around the lesion, all of the cT1a-EP/LPM, flat thickening and granular protrusion are diagnosed as cT1a-MM/T1b-SM1. We diagnosed this lesion as cN0M0 with EUS, CT and US, and treated it with endoscopic submucosal dissection (ESD) to it. The histopathological study of the lesion showed mod＞por SCC, pT1b-SM1, ly1, v1, INFb (**Fig. 3i**). The lesion was found to be an SM1 carcinoma, with part A presenting a flat thickened surface that included the cancer nest, which penetrated the muscle layer and was stretched out like a sheet (**Figs. 3j, k**), while part B presented tumor masses of various sizes that infiltrated both upward and downward (**Figs. 3l, m**). The carcinoma was additionally treated with surgery. Following surgery, there were no signs that any remnant of lesion was still present. As a result, the diagnosis updated to pN0.

Conclusion

The superficial esophageal carcinoma is composed of various elevations and depressions, and often extends across a wide area. The entire lesion should first be observed to evaluate if there is any region composed of B2 vessels. If a region encircled by B2 vessels is found, reduce the magnification ratio and check the position of the lesion where this region was found. We believe that, to decide the treatment policy based on precise invasion depth diagnosis and invasion mode evaluation, it is important to evaluate the microvascular images observed in each position and to develop an eye that will not miss infiltrations.

References

1) Inoue, H., Ishigaki, T, Misawa, M. et al.: Invasion depth diagnosis of superficial esophageal carcinoma—NBI-combined magnifying endoscopy (in Japanese, title translated). I To Cho (Stomach and Intestine) 2011 : 46 : 664-675
2) Arima, M. and Arima, H.: Precise diagnosis of esophageal squamous cell carcinoma using image-enhanced magnifying endoscopy (in Japanese, title translated). Shokaki Naishikyo (Endoscopia Digestiva) 2011 : 23 : 695-702
3) Arima, M., Arima, H., Yamada, T. et al.: Diagnosis of initial invasion images of esophageal mucosal carcinoma—from the standpoint of normal endoscopy (in Japanese, title translated). I to Cho (Stomach and Intestine) 2012 : 47 : 1349-1358

(Arima, M., Tsunomiya, M., Yoshii, T.)

Case 9 **Glycogenic acanthosis (GA)**

Male in 60s *Purpose* Screening *Location* Middle esophagus

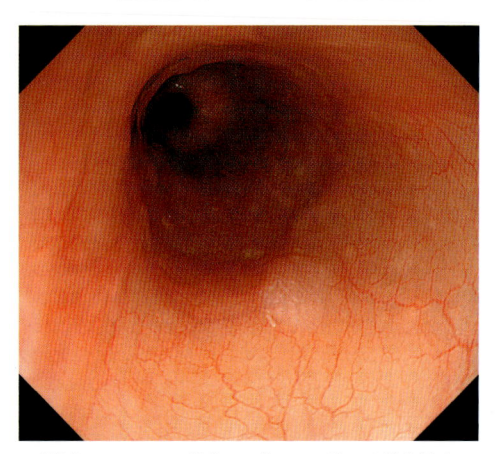

WLI non-magnifying observation: Whitish flat elevated lesion in middle esophagus.

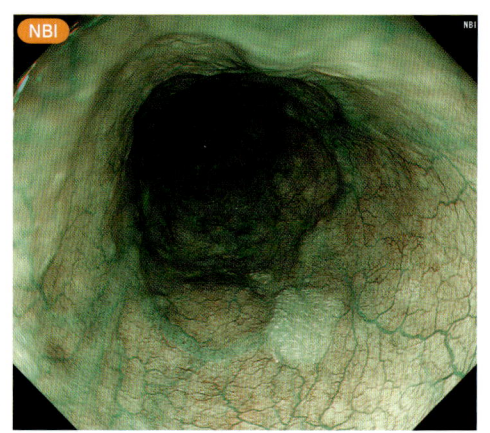

NBI non-magnifying observation: Whitish flat elevated lesion in middle esophagus.

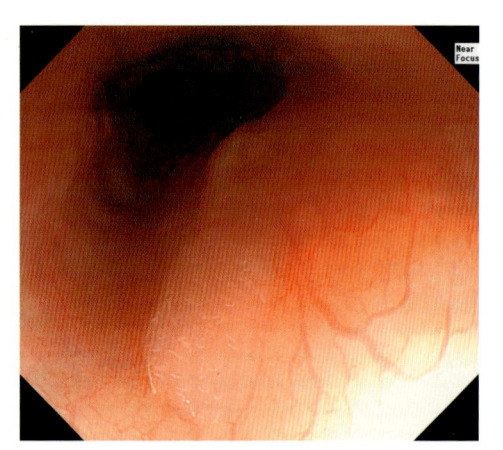

WLI magnifying observation (Near Focus): No vessels. Only whitish microstructures are observed in the lesion.

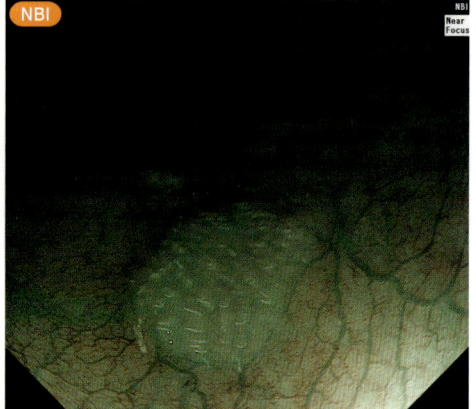

NBI magnifying observation (Near Focus): No vessel observed in the lesion even with NBI.

Scope : GIF-HQ290 (Olympus)　　Light source : EVIS LUCERA ELITE (Olympus)
NBI setup : Structure enhancement B8, color mode 2

Comment

A whitish elevated flat lesion with a diameter of around 5 mm is observed on the posterior wall of the middle esophagus. It also looks whitish when imaged with NBI non-magnifying observation. No vessels can be seen in either WLI or NBI magnifying observation, but white microstructures with regular organization are recognized. As white microstructures are observed on the surface of this whitish elevated lesion and it is not accompanied with atypical vessels, it can be diagnosed as a glycogenic acanthosis (GA).

▶**Observation tips** With both WLI and NBI, the GA is observed as a white turbid flat elevated lesion with no recognizable vessels. Staining it densely with iodine and observing it under magnification shows a regular arrangement of fine white dot-like patterns. As the region is well demarcated, it is difficult to differentiated from epithelial tumors, particularly superficial esophageal carcinoma with an upward growth tendency. Differentiation between the carcinoma and GA is possible because the former is accompanied with atypical vessels and is not stained by iodine spraying, while no vessels of any kind—including atypical ones—can be detected in the latter and it is stained densely by iodine spraying. Another point for differentiation is that many GA cases are multiple occurrence cases.

The histopathological image shows hyperplasia of squamous epithelium containing glycogen and a thickening change in the mucosal epithelium where prickle cells with bright, rich cytoplasm are growing[1].

Reference　1) Iriguchi, Y. et al. : I To Cho (Stomach and Intestine) 2012 ; 47 (Extra issue, "Glossary of Gastric and Intestinal Terms with Illustrations 2012" [in Japanese, title translated]) : 676

(Morita, S., Muto, M.)

Case 10 Esophageal papilloma

Male aged 67 |Purpose| Follow-up after ESD of Barrett's esophageal carcinoma
|Location| Lower thoracic esophagus

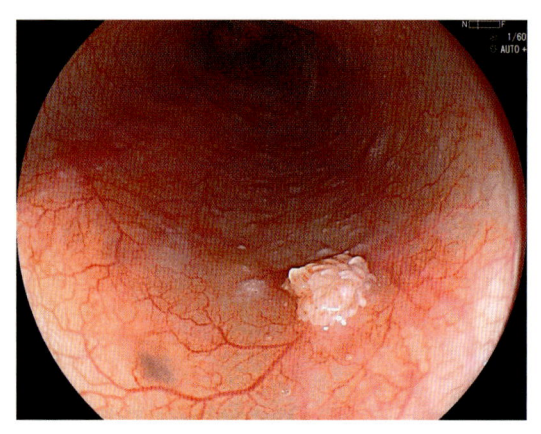

White-light observation : A whitish, mulberry-like, semi-pedunculated elevated lesion with a size of 3 mm is recognized on the posterior wall at 35 cm from the upper incisors.

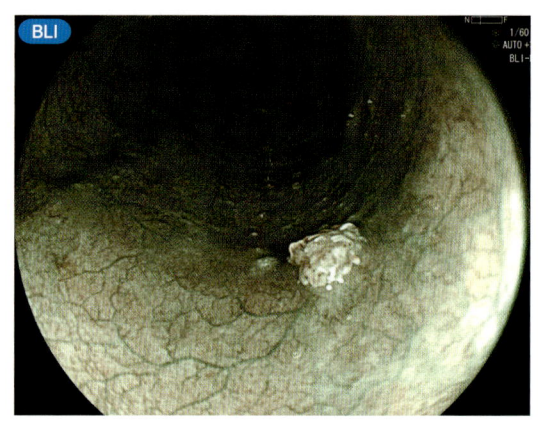

BLI-combined observation : The lesion is imaged as a whitish area.

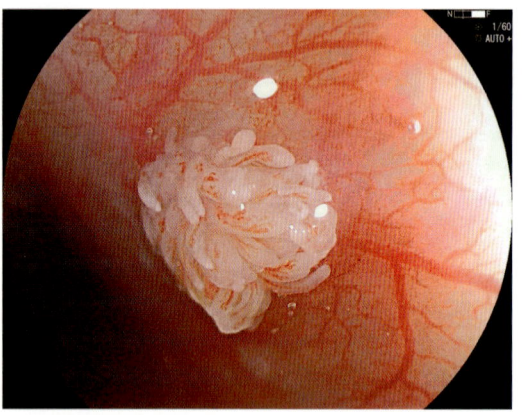

White-light low-magnification observation : An aggregation of thin papillary protrusions that look transparent, whitish and soft is observed.

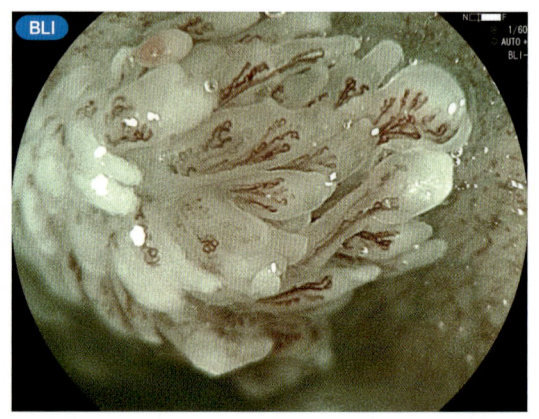

BLI-combined magnifying observation : Dilated, branched microvessels are observed in the papillary protrusions.

Scope：EG-L590ZW（Fujifilm） Light source：LASEREO（Fujifilm）
BLI setup：Structure enhancement B8, color enhancement C1

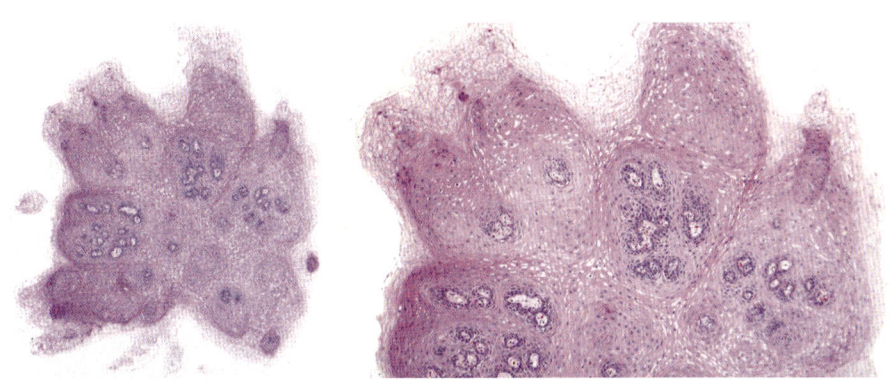

Histopathological image of biopsy section: Granules of widely variable sizes, accompanied with papillary growth of hyperplastic stratified squamous epithelium, have aggregated on the cut surface. No cellular atypia or nuclear division is observed.

Comment

Since esophageal papilloma is often accompanied by esophageal hiatal hernia and reflux disease, it is considered to be caused by the chronic stimulation of a disease. The relationship with the human papilloma virus (HPV) infection has been discussed, but the frequency of HPV infection is regarded to be low. It presents a shape like a finely lobed sea anemone or semicircular or mulberry-like morphology. The main target of differentiation of such a lesion in which papillary protrusions have aggregated is a very well-differentiated type 0 - II a esophageal carcinoma, which often presents a similar vascular morphology to a papilloma, making it hard to differentiate.

▶**Observation tips** The lesion is usually whitish with a hint of transparency. In the lower esophagus, however, it looks reddish because of dilation and tortuosity of microvessels in the granules. In magnifying observation, small vessels are observed in the center of each of the lobed protrusions while vessels branched like leaf veins are observed in flat elevations.

(Arima, M.)

Case 11 NERD

Female in 60s *Purpose* Annual periodical checkup *Location* Esophagogastric junction
Non-erosive reflux disease (Grade M according to the Los Angeles Classification revised version)

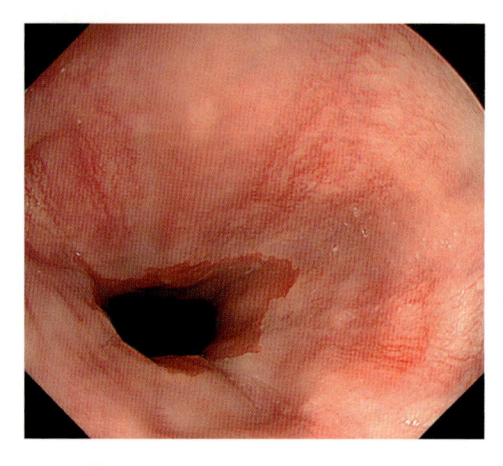

WLI observation : In the esophagogastric junction (EG-J), white turbid areas in radial locations (12, 2, 5 and 8 o'clock directions) are observed, while visibility of the lower esophageal palisade vessels in the corresponding regions is reduced.

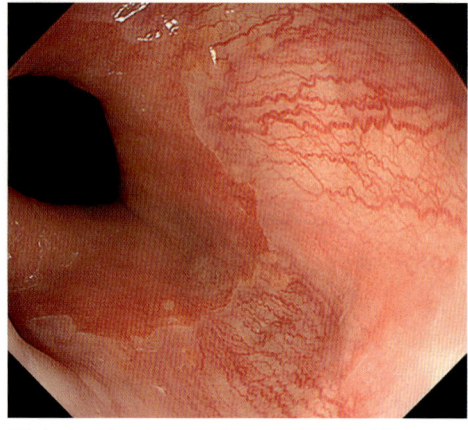

Dilated palisade vessels are observed between the white turbid areas in the 2 o'clock direction of the EG-J.

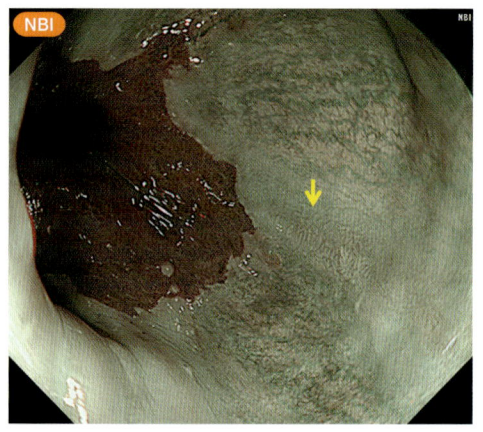

NBI non-magnifying observation : In addition to the white turbid area, dilated IPCLs are observed in the 3-4 o'clock direction (arrow).

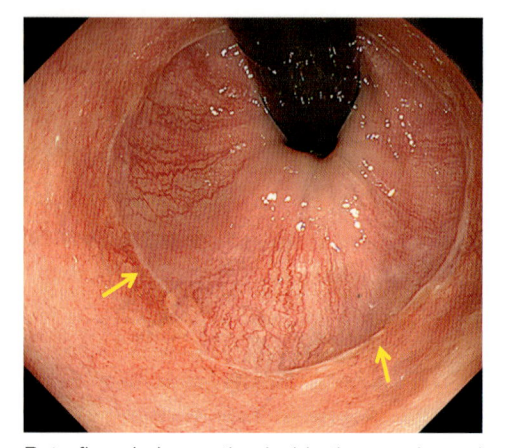

Retroflexed observation inside the esophageal hiatal hernia : Dilated palisade vessels are observed between white turbid mucosa in radial locations (arrows)

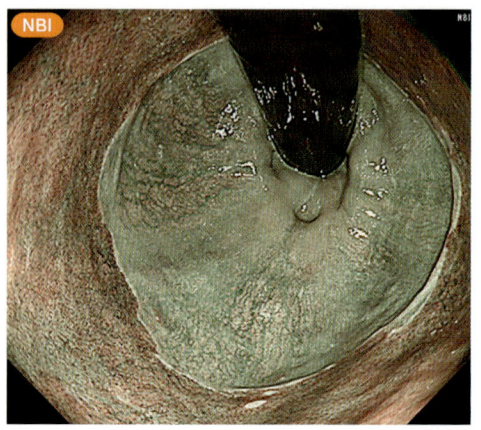

NBI non-magnifying observation, retroflexed observation in the esophageal hiatal hernia : The white turbid areas are enhanced.

Scope：GIF-HQ290（Olympus）　　Light source：EVIS LUCERA ELITE（Olympus）
NBI setup：Structure enhancement of A7, color mode 1

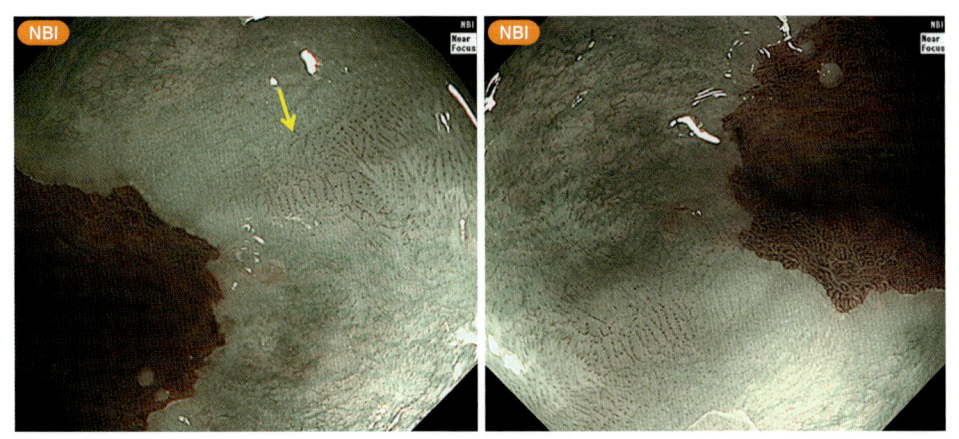

NBI magnifying observation（Near Focus, white turbid area in the 7 o'clock direction corresponding to the 3-4 o'clock direction in the right figure in the center row on the page on the left）：In the lesion corresponding to the white turbid area, superficial vessels dilated in micro-dot shape are visible in contrast to the non-turbid areas in between（arrow）. The superficial vessels in the micro-dot shape are arranged regularly and present a stripe pattern.

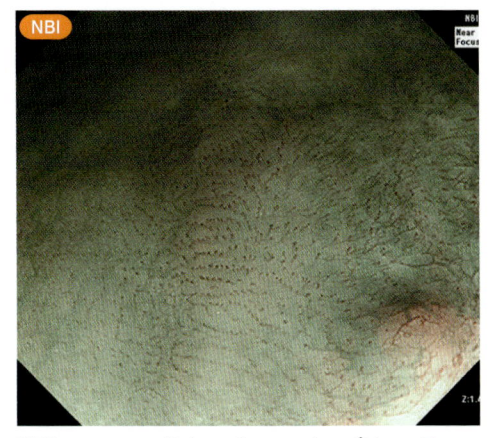

NBI non-magnifying observation（Near Focus ＋1.4×electronic zoom）：No obvious irregularity is observed with the dilated microvessels. They grow in regular arrangement.

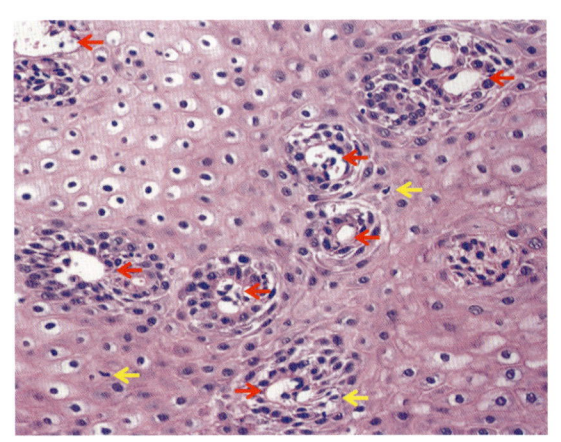

Biopsy specimen（HE）：Together with the dilation and proliferation of intraepithelial papillary vessels（red arrows）, a very small number of intraepithelial lymphoid infiltrations（yellow arrows）are observed.

Comment

As the name implies, non-erosive reflux disease（NERD）is not accompanied by erosion. It is not possible to use color tone changes such as white turbidity as a predictive factor because of the problem of low coincidence between results of different observers. However, recent clinical studies using the NBI magnifying endoscopy have revealed that the dilation or proliferation of IPCLs can be an endoscopic predictive factor for NERD. By making it possible to start NBI magnifying observation at the touch of a button, the new system's magnifying endoscope has the potential to help facilitate quick, objective NERD diagnosis.

(Dobashi, A., Goda, K., Tajiri, H.)

Case 12 NERD

(Endoscopic classification : Los Angeles Classification revised version)

Case 1 NERD, Grade M

BLI setup : Structure enhancement B8, color enhancement C1

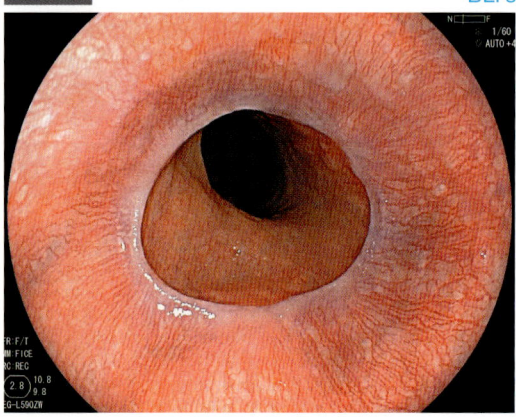

White-light observation : A slightly white turbid mucosa is observed on the esophageal mucosa immediately above the esophagogastric junction.

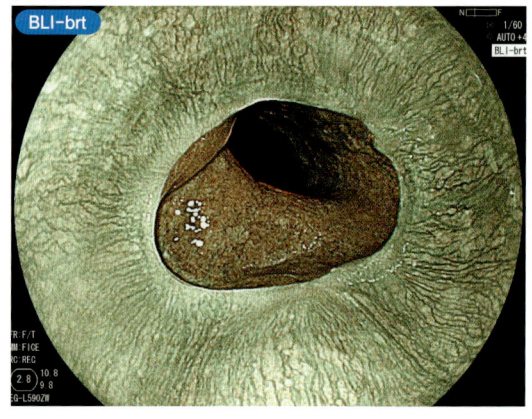

BLI-bright mode observation : The palisade vessels in the lower esophagus can be observed more clearly than under white-light observation.

Case 2 NERD, Grade M

BLI setup : Structure enhancement A4, color enhancement C1

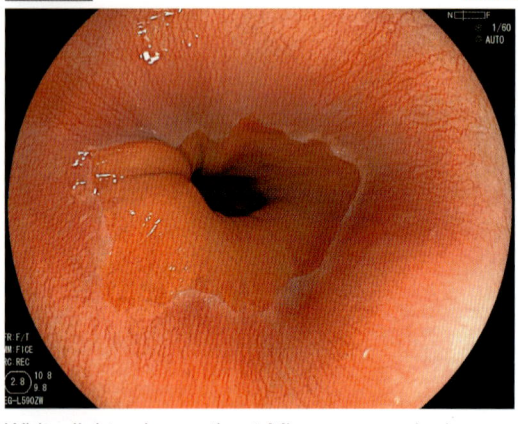

White-light observation : Minor mucosal damage composed of white turbidity is observed on the esophagogastric junction.

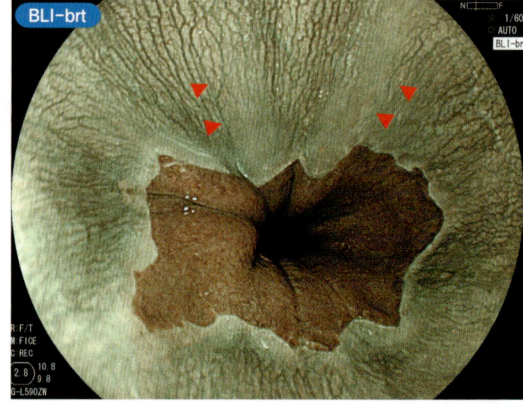

BLI-bright mode observation : Mucosa thickened by inflammation is traversing toward the proximal side (red arrowheads).

Case 3 NERD, Grade M

BLI setup : Structure enhancement B6, color enhancement C1

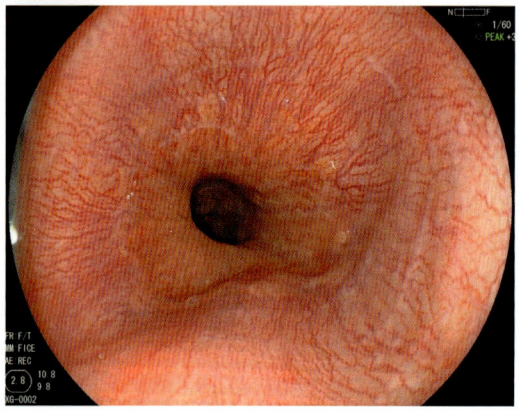

White-light observation : The esophagogastric junction is made unclear due to the inflammation.

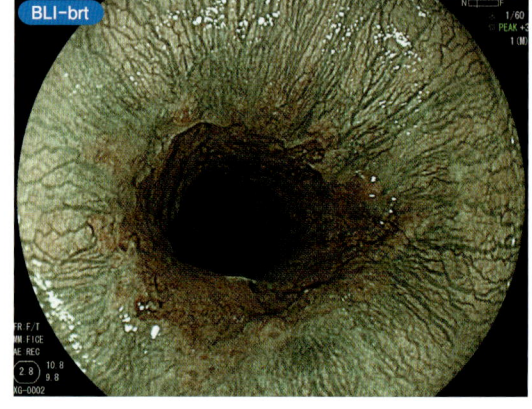

BLI-bright mode observation : The thickened esophageal mucosa at the bottom end of the esophagus can be clearly observed.

Scope：EG-L590ZW（Fujifilm）　Light source：LASEREO（Fujifilm）
BLI setup：Specified for each case

Case 4　NERD, Grade M

BLI setup：Structure enhancement A4, color enhancement C1

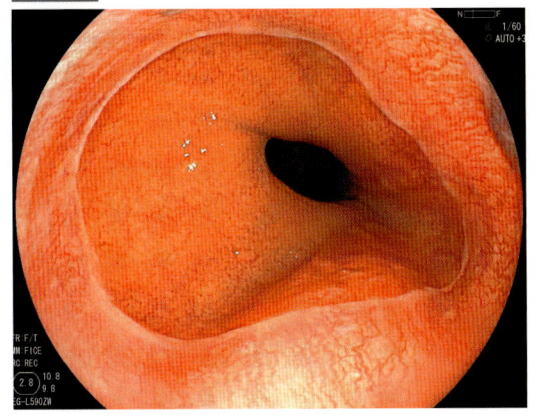

White-light observation：Minor mucosal damage composed of white turbidity is observed on the esophagogastric junction.

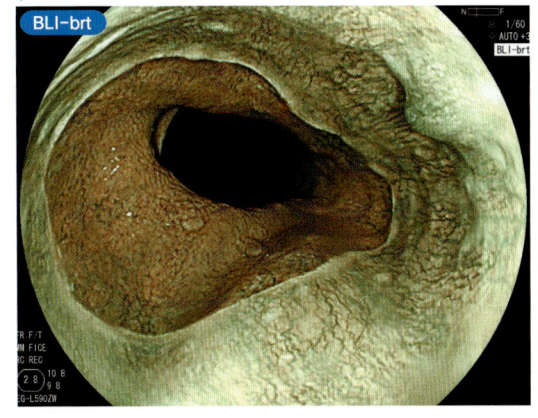

BLI-bright mode observation：The mucosa in the 6 o'clock direction is thickened, obscuring the view of the palisade vessels.

Comment

In white-light observation, the high overall brightness facilitates lower esophageal observation under deep inspiration, allowing minute changes in the mucosa to be observed. Switching to BLI observation improves the visibility of the palisade vessels in the lower esophagus. As NERD often appears as a normal condition when observed in endoscopy, it is important to formulate a diagnosis from a comprehensive viewpoint, taking into account subjective symptoms, as well.

▶**Observation tips**　Have the patient take a deep breath to expand the esophagogastric junction and lower esophagus so that you can observe them more easily. Since the endoscopic findings accompanying the NERD are defined as Grade N without mucosal changes, erythema on the esophagogastric junction or Grade M with white mucosal thickening, it is important to note even slight changes in color tone.

(Yamamoto, F., Miyahara, R., Goto, H.)

Case 13 GERD

Male in 50s **Purpose** Detailed examination of heartburn and epigastric pain
Location Esophagogastric junction-lower esophagus Gastroesophageal reflux disease (Grade B according to the Los Angeles Classification)

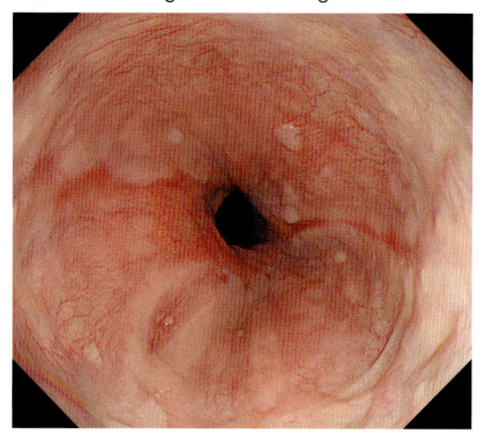

WLI observation: Linear erythematous depressions of about 3 cm (GERD, Grade B) in length and thickened white radiating turbid areas can be seen in the 3 and 9 o'clock directions of the esophagogastric junction. Tongue-shaped columnar epithelium extending from the gastric mucosa are also observed in the 6-9 o'clock direction.

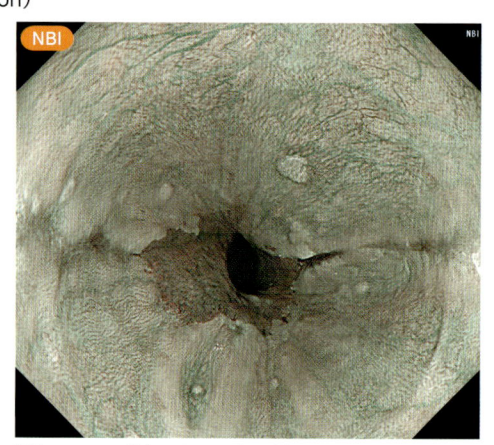

NBI non-magnifying observation: The tongue-shaped columnar epithelium is visualized as a brownish area more distinctly than WLI.

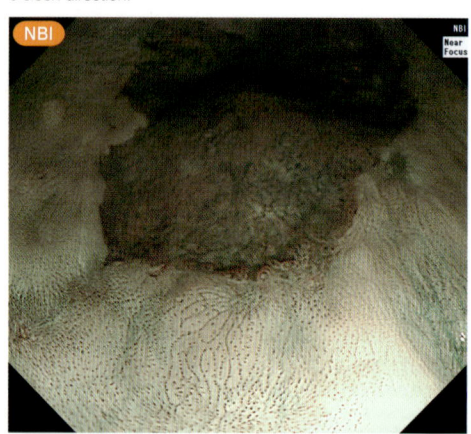

NBI magnifying observation (Near Focus): Increase in a number of dilated IPCLs are seen as dots in the white turbid esophageal epithelium in the vicinity of the squamocolumnar junction. Despite increase in a number of the dilated IPCLs, their regularity of their arrangement is maintained.

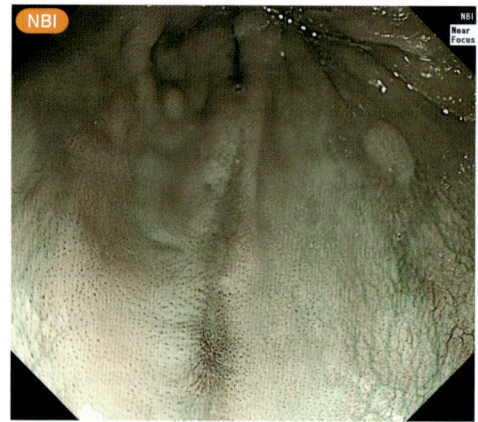

NBI magnifying observation (Near Focus): The number of IPCLs and their degree of dilation increases gradually in the transition from the right end to the normal area→white turbid area →linear erythematous area (6 o'clock direction).

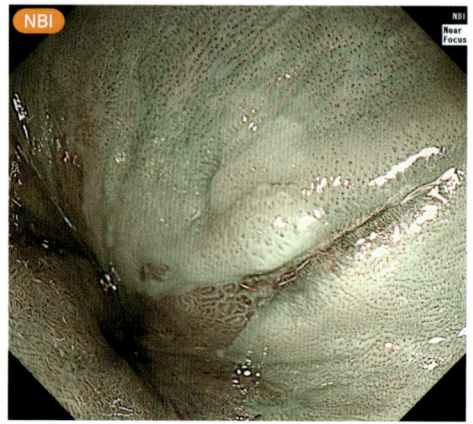

NBI magnifying observation (Near Focus): Noticeable increase in a number of dot-shaped dilated IPCLs is observed around the erosion in the 3 o'clock direction. The IPCL arrangement is regular.

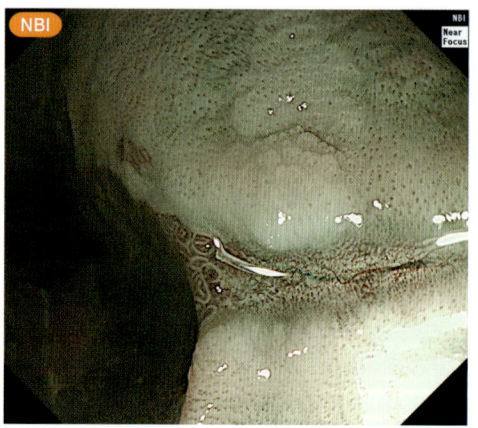

NBI magnifying observation (Near Focus+1.4×electronic zoom): The bottom part of the erosion presents increasing in a number of microvessels but does not show irregularities in diameter or shape.

Endoscope：GIF-HQ290（Olympus） Light source：EVIS LUCERA ELITE（Olympus）
NBI setup：Structure enhancement A7, color mode 1

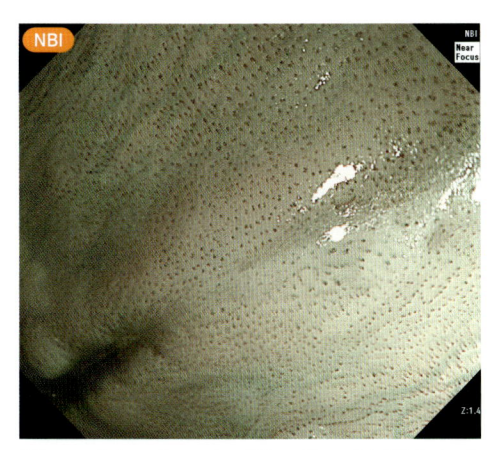

NBI magnifying observation（Near Focus＋1.4×electronic zoom）：Significant increase in a number of regularly arranged dot-shaped dilated IPCLs is observed in the longitudinal white turbid area on the proximal side of the erosion.

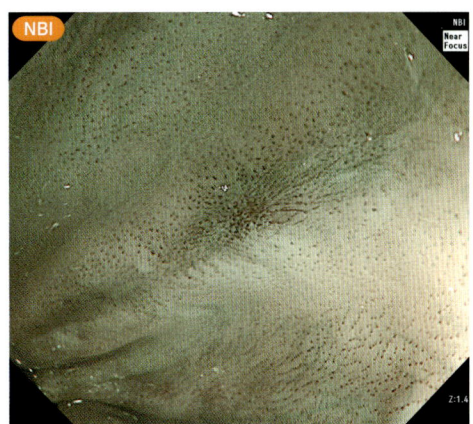

NBI magnifying observation（Near Focus＋1.4×electronic zoom）：Dot-shaped or linear elongation of the IPCLs is recognized at the most proximal portion of the erosion. There are no irregularities in diameter or shape.

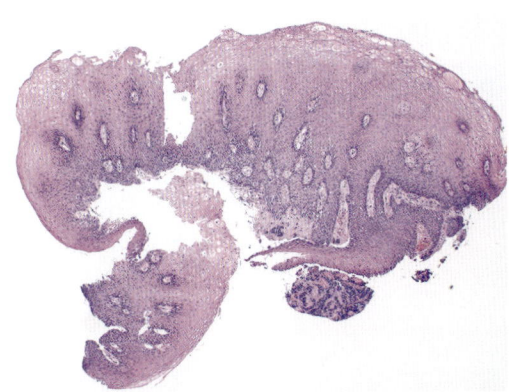

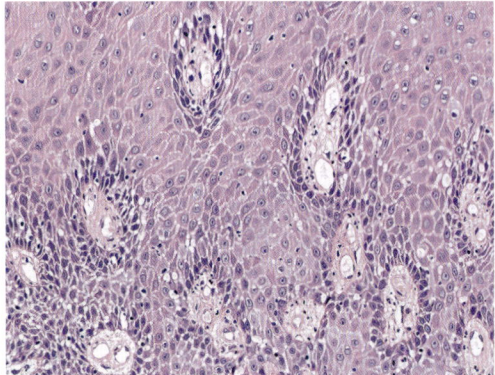

Histologic findings of the biopsy specimen obtained from the erosion：A large number of dilated intrapapillary capillaries are observed in the stratified squamous epithelium layer, and inflammatory cellular infiltration is seen in the vascular stroma and between squamous epithelial cells.

Comment

The Los Angeles Classification, which is based on the degree of mucosal break, is commonly used in endoscopic diagnosis of reflux disease. As this case has an erosion accompanied with linear erythema（mucosal break）with a length over 5 mm, we diagnosed it as a Grade B reflux esophagitis. Although diagnosis is usually possible with conventional WLI endoscopy, it may be necessary to diagnose the benign/malignant differentiation when the erythematous or white turbid or when an erosion or ulcer has an irregular shape. The findings in the NBI magnifying observation of reflux disease include：①It is accompanied by increasing in dilated IPCLs like the NERD, but the arrangement is regular and few irregularities（in diameter or and shape）are observed；②There is no clear demarcation in the transition between the center of the inflammation（with white turbid area, erosion, etc.）and the surrounding normal mucosa；the extent of dilation and increase in a number of the IPCLs reduces gradually as far as the normal IPCLs is observed.

(Goda, K., Dobashi, A., Tajiri, H.)

Case 14 GERD

(Endoscopic classification：Los Angeles Classification revised version)

Case 1 GERD (Grade A)　Female in 50s　**Purpose** Screening

BLI setup：Structure enhancement A8, color enhancement C1

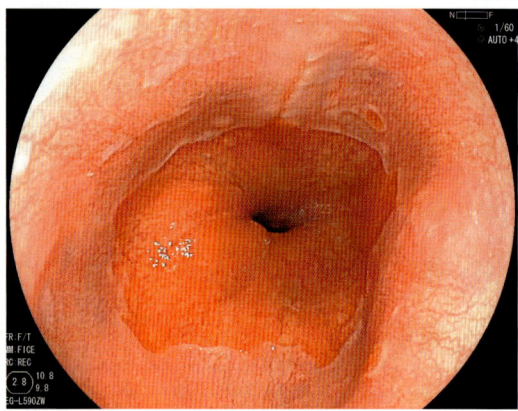

White-light observation of esophagogastric junction：Erythematous erosion can be seen extending in a line in the 12 o'clock direction of the image.

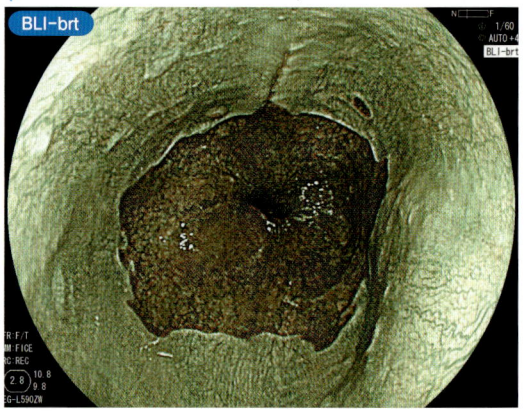

BLI-bright mode non-magnifying observation：The erythematous erosion appears brownish.

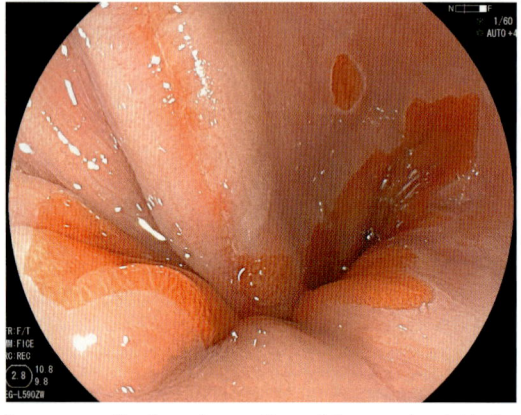

Low-magnification observation of the erosion：Erythematous erosion and white mucosal damage in the surrounding area are observed.

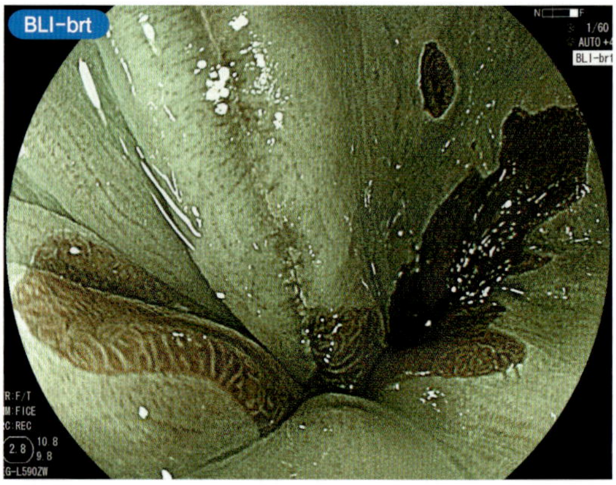

BLI-bright mode low-magnification observation of the area around the erosion.

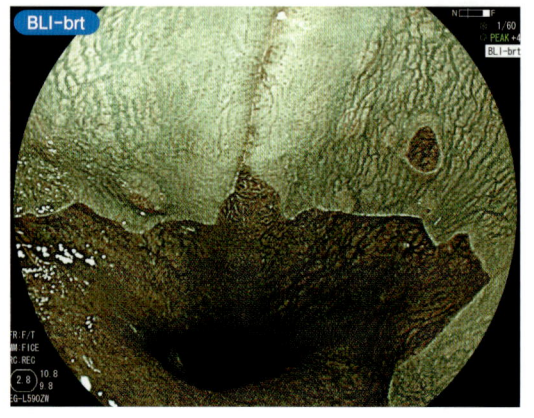

BLI-bright mode low-magnification observation of the erosion：The mucosa around the erosion has thickened and the palisade vessels are not visible.

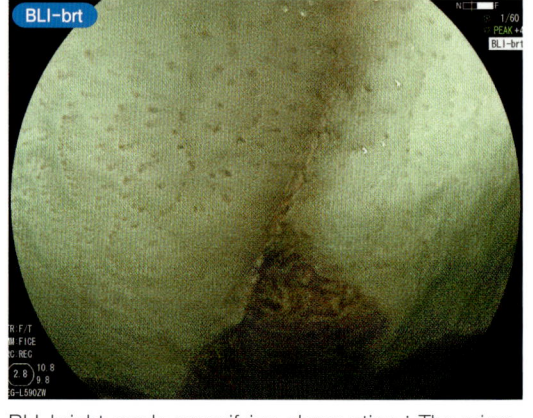

BLI-bright mode magnifying observation：The microvessels around the erosion show low density and no neoplastic changes are observed.

Endoscope：EG-L590ZW（Fujifilm）　Light source：LASEREO（Fujifilm）.
BLI setup：Specified for each case.

Case 2　GERD（Grade A）　　　　　BLI setup：Structure enhancement B8, color enhancement C1

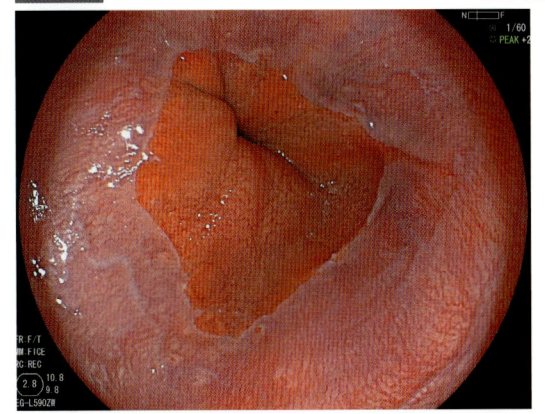

White-light observation：Erythematous mucosal damages are recognized in the 3 and 12 o'clock directions of the image.

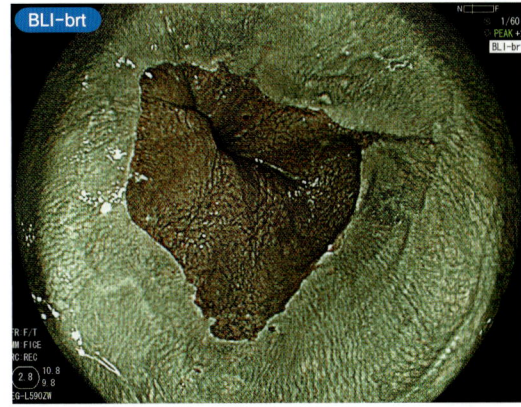

BLI-bright mode observation：The mucosal damage in the 12 o'clock direction of the image can be recognized more clearly. It appears brownish in color and is coincident with the region observed with the white light.

Comment

GERD (gastroesophageal reflux disease) is diagnosed by the erythema or white mucosal damage observed in white-light observation. It is recognized as a lesion extending in the longitudinal direction toward the proximal side. Depending on the degree of inflammation, its appearance can vary from a simple color tone change to a lesion with loss of epithelium and attaching of slough. The mucosal disorder is easy to confirm because both white-light and BLI observation provide a bright field of view, while BLI also enhances the contrast.

▶**Observation tips** As with cases of Barrett's esophagus, have the patient breathe in deeply to expand the lower esophagus and observe the esophagogastric junction. In general, the typical endoscopic finding indicating GERD is erosion with a linear, grooved or branch-like shape extending in the longitudinal direction from the junction or from the lower esophagus. The degree of erosion decreases as it extends towards the proximal side, and it is rare that the lesion reaches the upper esophagus.

(Yamamoto, F., Miyahara, R., Goto, H.)

Case 15 Type 0-I superficial esophageal carcinoma

Male in 60s Purpose Follow-up of reflux disease Location Upper/middle esophagus
Macroscopic type 0-I + IIb

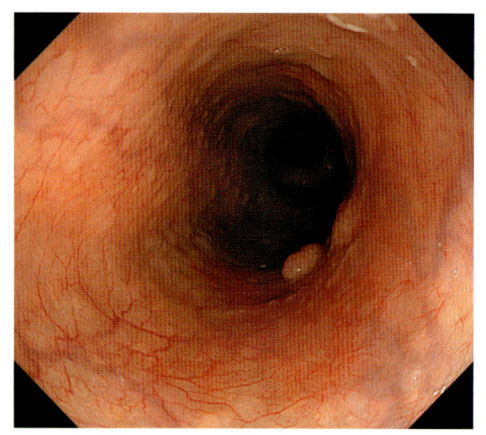

WLI non-magnifying observation : Whitish elevated lesion accompanied by an erythematous flat lesion in the middle esophagus.

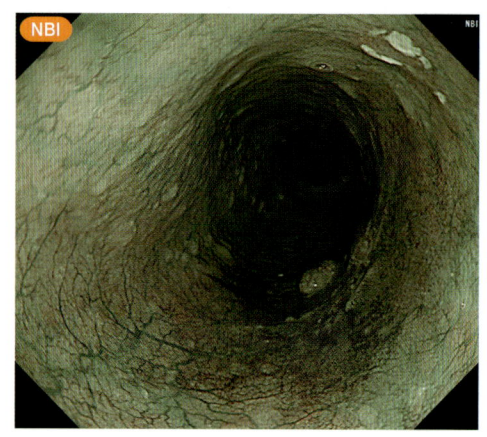

NBI non-magnifying observation. Protruded region accompanied by a flat brownish area in the middle esophagus.

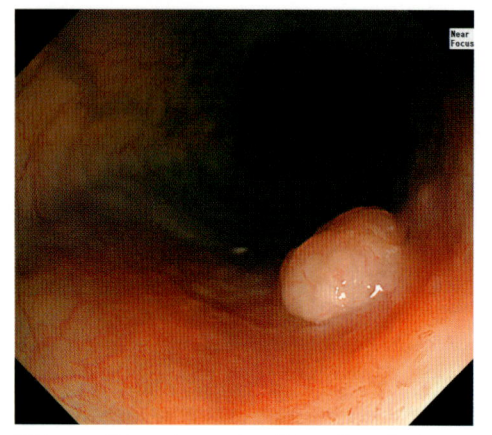

WLI magnifying observation (Near Focus) : In the area surrounding the elevation, normal vessels have disappeared and atypical vessels are observed.

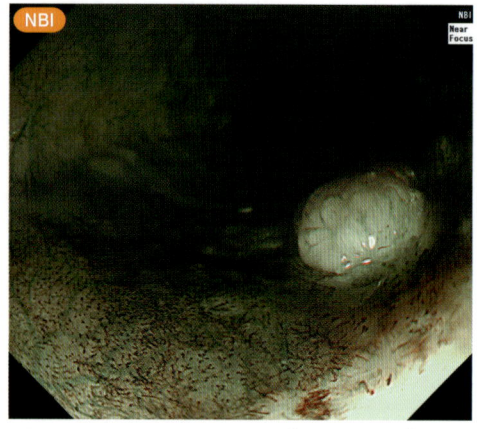

NBI magnifying observation (Near Focus) : NBI enables clear observation of the loss of normal vessels and the atypical vessels.

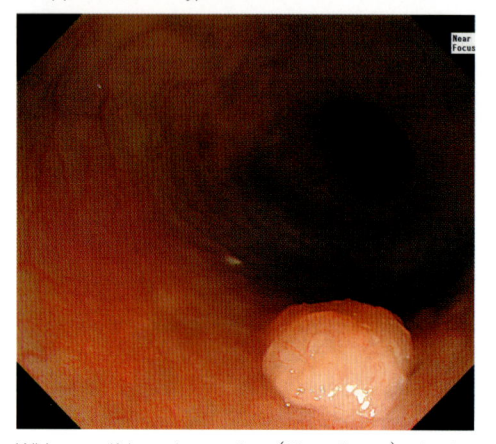

WLI magnifying observation (Near Focus) : In the elevated region, atypical vessels that are dilated and stretched are observed though the density is low.

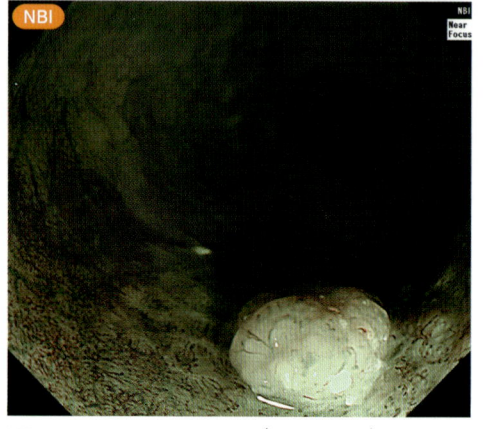

NBI magnifying observation (Near Focus) : The NBI makes possible observation of atypical vessels more clearly.

Endoscope：GIF-HQ290（Olympus）　Light source：EVIS LUCERA ELITE（Olympus）
NBI setup：Structure enhancement B8, color mode 2

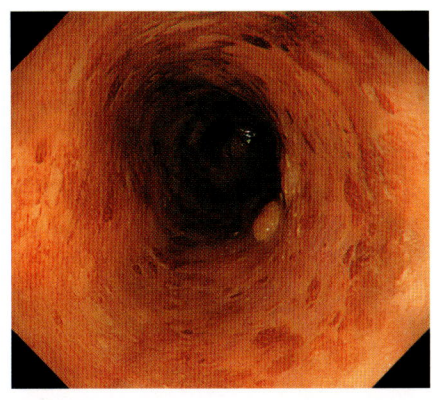

Non-magnifying iodine-stained observation：Iodine does not stain the lesion.

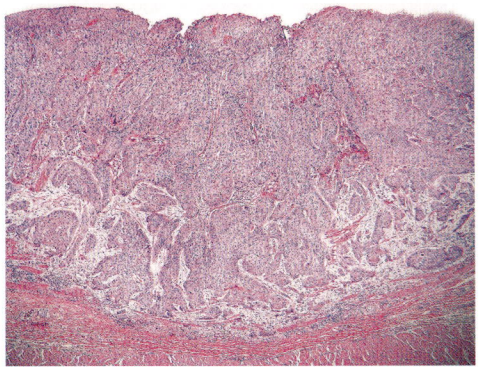

The carcinoma invades the deep part of the submucosal layer in the 0-Ⅰ elevated region, and is diagnosed as SM3.

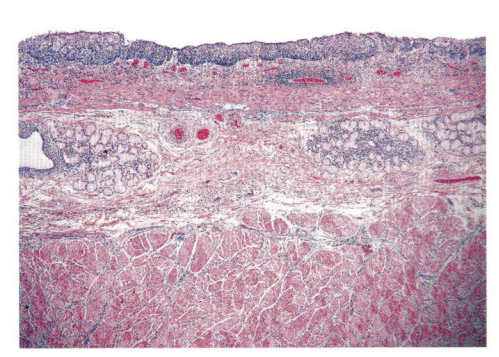

The 0-Ⅱb flat region in the surrounding area is LPM.

Comment

This is a case of 0-Ⅰ esophageal carcinoma accompanied by a 0-Ⅱb lesion in the surrounding area. With this case, an elevated white lesion was recognized in the middle part of the esophagus. In magnifying observation of the elevated lesion, normal vessels were not visible, but dilated or stretched atypical vessels were present. Because of the presence of atypical vessels and the fact that it could not be stained with iodine, the lesion was diagnosed as a tumor. Invasion depth diagnoses based on the morphology of vessels on the tumor surface as established by Arima, Inoue et al.[1,2] are difficult to apply to elevated lesions. In this case, the tumor is a 0-Ⅰ lesion, and can be seen to have a high elevation when observed macroscopically. Its invasion depth is estimated at SM2 or deeper. Pathologic diagnosis classified it as an SM3 lesion.

Since lesions with noticeable protrusions are often accompanied by flat lesions, we also observed the lesion in the far view mode to make sure we didn't miss anything. In this case, too, we found an erythematous flat lesion with no normal vessels visible in the area around the elevation. It was recognized as a brownish area in NBI non-magnifying observation. Low-magnifying observation showed proliferation of dilated and tortuous atypical vessels, which can be found more easily in combination with NBI. When iodine staining was applied, this region remained unstained. Based on these findings, the lesion was diagnosed as a tumor. Individual vessels could be seen to form loops on the extremities and the invasion depth seemed to be EP/LPM. Pathological diagnosis classified it as LPM.

▶**Observation tips**　A lesion can be diagnosed as a tumor if a brownish area with atypical vessels is observed in NBI observation. While detection of a tumor is quite easy with an elevated lesion, the flat lesions that develop around it tend to be missed. To avoid missing any flat lesions that may be present, observe the lesion using a relatively far view to see if the brownish area extends around the lesion.

Reference　1) Inoue H.：Dig. Endosc. 2001；13：S40-S41
　　　　　　　2) Arima, M. et al.：Shokaki Naishikyo（Endoscopia Digestiva）2005；17：2076-2083

（Morita, S., Muto, M.）

Case 16 Type 0-Ⅰs superficial esophageal carcinoma

Male aged 75 *Purpose* Detailed examination of esophageal carcinoma *Location* Midthoracic esophagus
Macroscopic type 0-Ⅰs

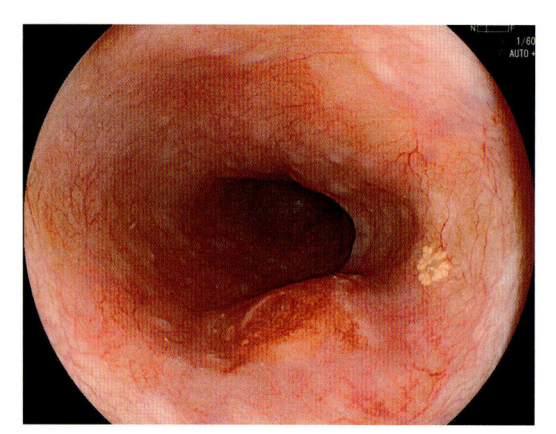

White light observation : An elevated lesion with a size of 20 mm and a not very well demarcated rise is observed on the posterior wall at a point 30 cm from the upper incisors. An exposed tumor is recognized on the top surface of the elevation, but the rising section is covered with squamous epithelium. Ectopic sebaceous glands are observed on the right side of the tumor.

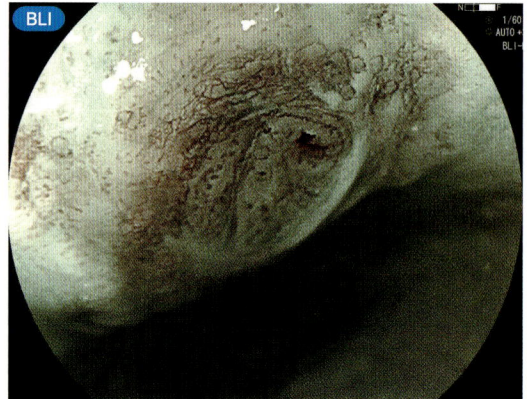

BLI low-magnification observation : The top section forms a shallow depression, and multiplied brownish type B2 vessels are observed in the margins.

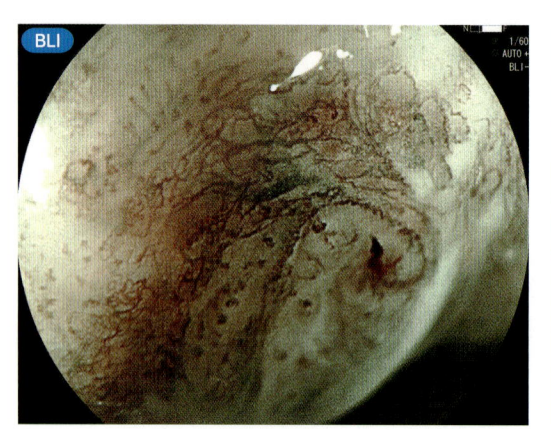

BLI high-magnification observation : Dark-greenish irregular vessels (type B3) thicker than the B2 vessels are observed.

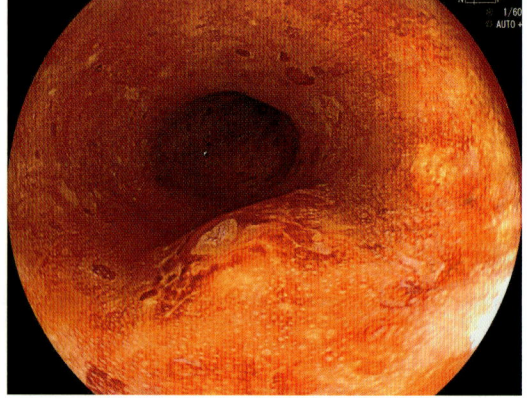

Iodine-stained image : Most of the lesion is stained, but the top section is unstained.

Endoscope：EG-L590ZW（Fujifilm）　Light source：LASEREO（Fujifilm）
BLI setup：Structure enhancement B8, color enhancement C1

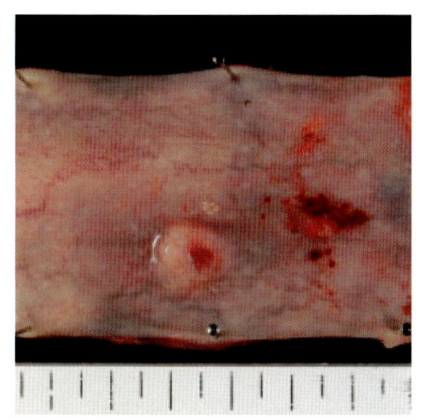

Macroscopic view of freshly resected specimen

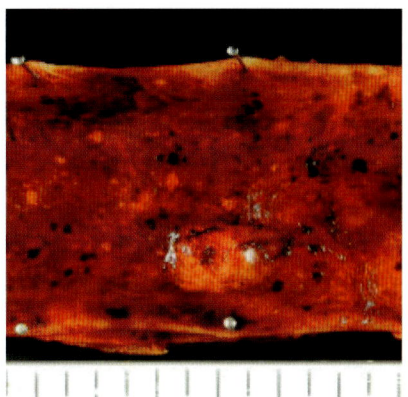

Iodine-stained view of freshly resected specimen

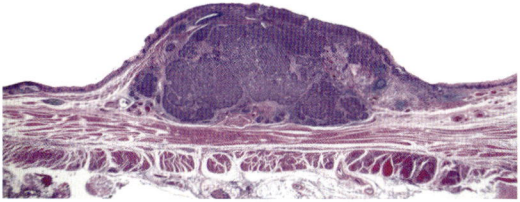

Histopathological image：Moderately differentiated, pT1b-SM3, ly2, v1, INFb, pN0, 20×12 mm

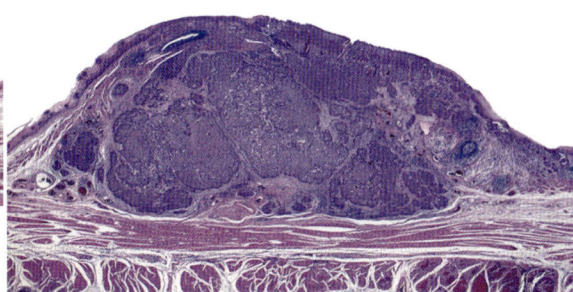

Comment

This case is a type 0-Ⅰs esophageal cancer with a gentle rise. Most of the lesion was covered with epithelium except for the top section where the epithelium had thinned and a shallow depression had formed. The tumor had invaded the margins of the depression in the area bordering the exposed part of the tumor, so small brownish B2 vessels could be observed in the region. High-magnification observation found thick, dark greenish irregular B3 vessels interspersed with the brownish B2 vessels. Based on normal observation, this lesion was suspected to be SM2/SM3 with disease type diagnosis；however, under magnification, B3 vessels were found to be present, suggesting deep SM invasion.

Even though the lesion surface was covered with squamous epithelium, tumorous vessels could be observed in the area where the epithelium had thinned due to tumor invasion. The dark greenish vessels indicated that penetration was quite deep.

▶Observation tips　To magnify a lesion, twist the endoscope and bring it toward the anterior wall. This facilitates angulation, making the operation easier. To avoid bleeding when moving on to the next field, carefully separate the endoscope from the lesion before moving it. Do not slide the endoscope while the distal end is applied to the lesion.

(Arima, M.)

Case 17 Type 0-Ⅱa superficial esophageal carcinoma

Male in 70s   *Purpose* Follow-up of endoscopic treatment of esophageal carcinoma
Location Abdominal esophagus   *Macroscopic type* 0-Ⅱa

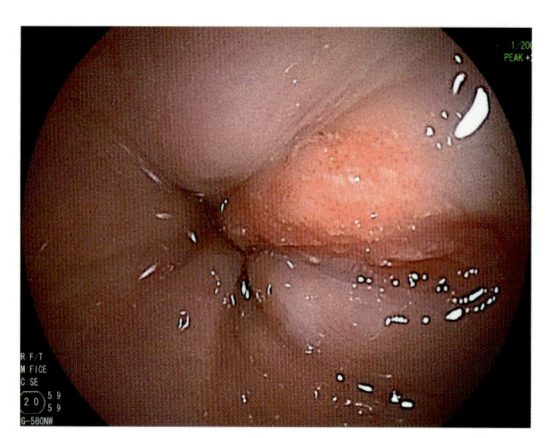

Transnasal endoscope (white-light observation): An erythematous, low elevated lesion is observed on the right side wall of the abdominal esophagus.

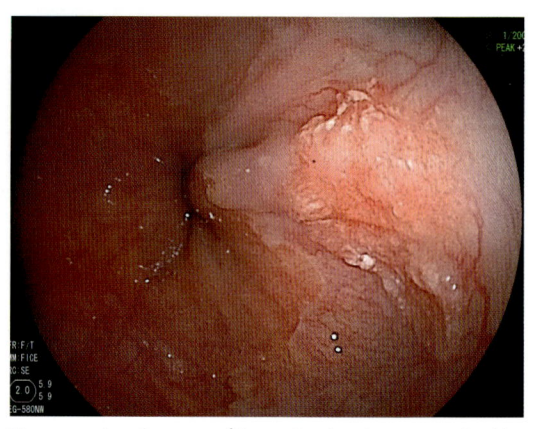

Transnasal endoscope (the region has been stretched by deep inspiration): The level is that of the palisade vessels. Fine slough can be seen attached to the superficial layer.

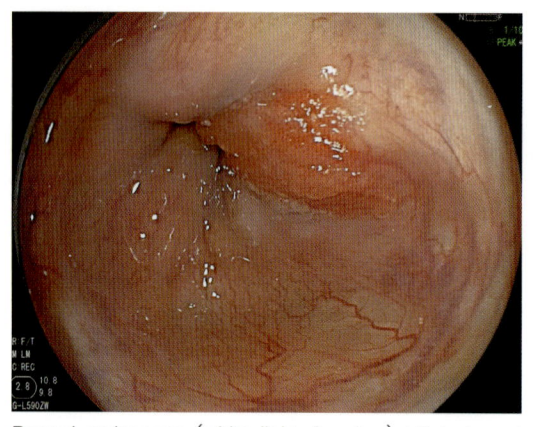

Peroral endoscopy (white-light, far view): Dot-shaped B1 vessels are vaguely recognizable on the superficial layer.

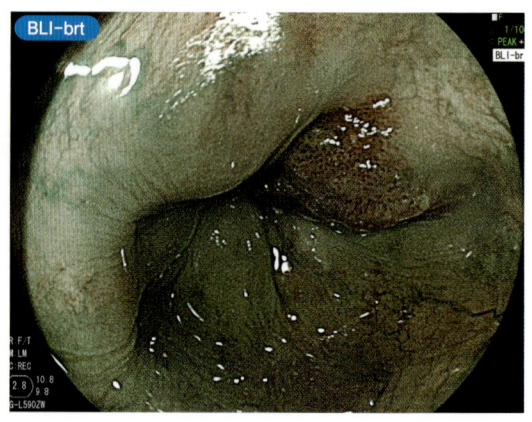

Peroral endoscopy (BLI-bright, far view): A well-demarcated brownish area and dot-shaped vessels are observed.

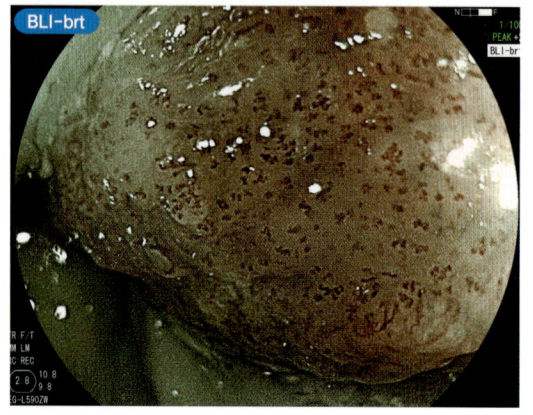

Magnifying endoscope (medium magnification, BLI-bright mode): B1 vessels and a brownish intervascular background coloration are clearly recognizable.

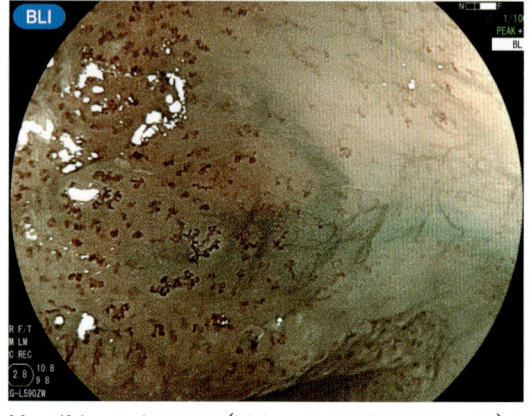

Magnifying endoscope (high magnification, BLI mode): On the proximal-side demarcation, dense proliferation of dilated, tortuous B1 vessels with irregular diameters and shapes is observed in the cancerous lesion (on the left side).

Endoscope: EG-580NW transnasal endoscope (Fujifilm), EG-L590ZW peroral endoscope (Fujifilm)
Light source: LASEREO (Fujifilm) BLI setup: BLI mode: Structure enhancement A6, color enhancement C1, BLI-bright mode; Structure enhancement A6, color enhancement C1

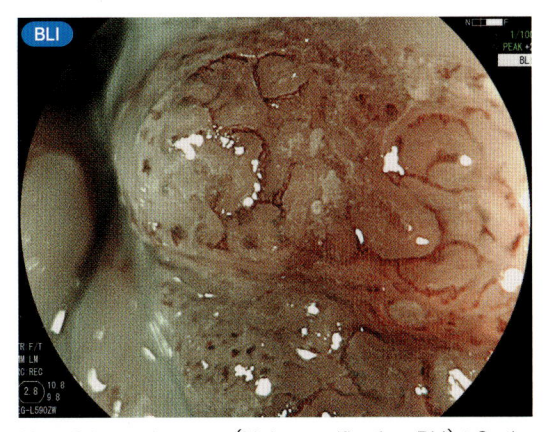

Magnifying endoscope (high magnification, BLI): On the elevated region on the distal side, the mixed presence of AVA-s and dot-shaped vessels is observed.
The lesion is diagnosed as a squamous cell carcinoma with a T1a-LPM invasion depth.

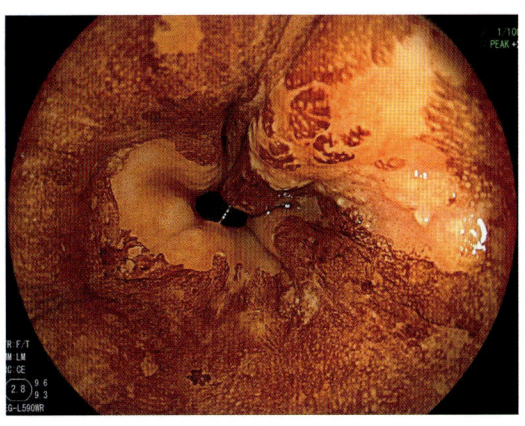

Iodine stained observation: A 1/6-circumferential area is not stained by iodine. A squamocolumnar junction (SCJ) is observed on the immediately distal side of the lesion; however, the lesion does not overlap the SCJ.

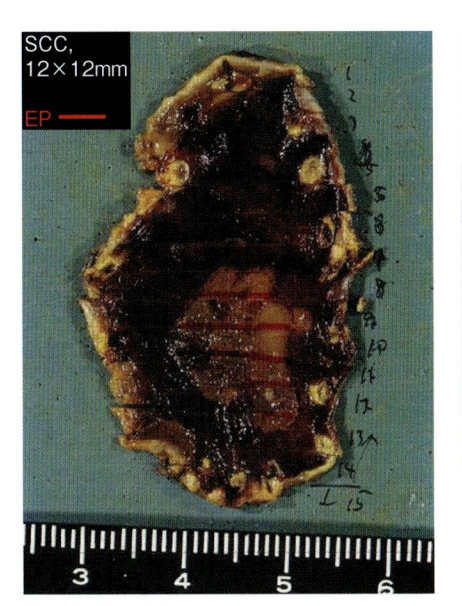

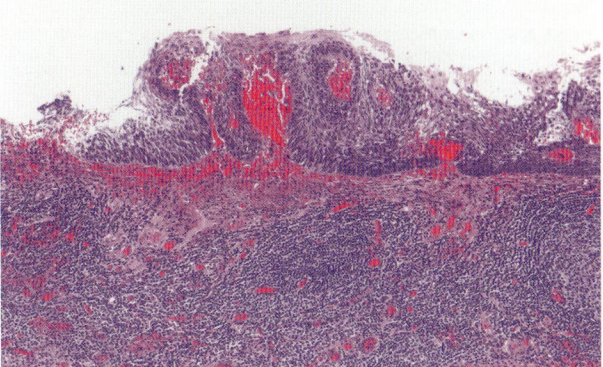

Microscopic pathology: Squamous cell carcinoma with a T1a-EP invasion depth.

Resected specimen mapping: Non-stained area with a size of 12×12 mm.

Comment

This is an erythematous, low-elevated lesion localized on the immediately proximal side of an SCJ. Although the location might have required differentiation from Barrett's esophageal carcinoma, BLI magnifying observation made it possible to diagnose it as a squamous cell carcinoma at a glance.

▶**Observation tips** Having the patient take a deep breath stretches the wall in the vicinity of the esophagogastric junction, making it easy to view the overall image of a lesion in this region. In white-light observation, a squamous cell carcinoma is frequently indicated by surface roughness and attaching of fine slough, while Barrett's adenocarcinoma is often shown as glossy, localized erythema. The microvascular pattern on the superficial layer can be observed in the white-light near view observation, while BLI magnifying observation facilitates the recognition of atypical vessels. This advantage can also be applied to invasion depth diagnosis.

(Kawada, K., Kawano, T.)

Case 18 **Type 0 - Ⅱb superficial esophageal carcinoma**

Male aged 76　*Purpose* Follow-up after endoscopic treatment of esophageal carcinoma
Location Upper thoracic esophagus　*Macroscopic type* 0-Ⅱb

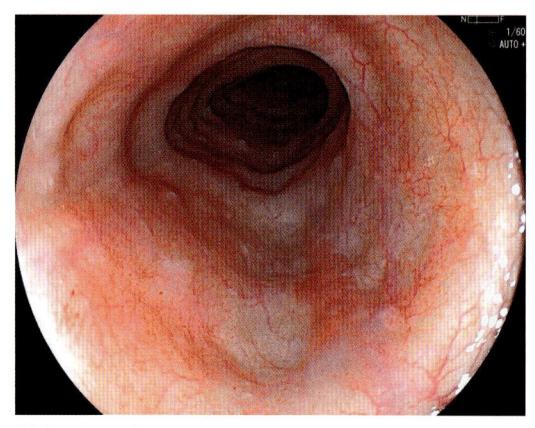

White-light observation : A fine erythematous area with a size of 10 mm is found on the right of the posterior wall extending in the vertical direction at 25 cm from the upper incisors. The vessels visible in the surrounding area are interrupted at the margins of the lesion. No difference in height from the normal mucosa is detected.

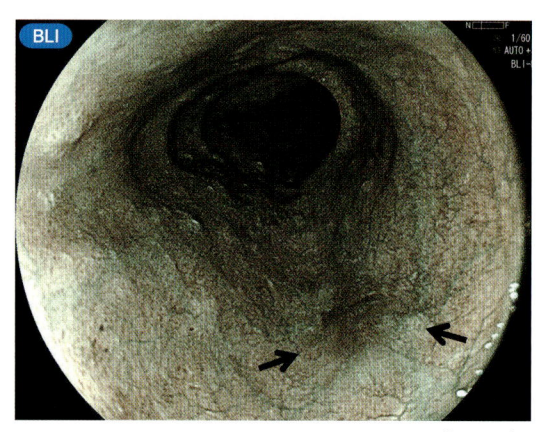

BLI observation : A brownish area is observed (arrows).

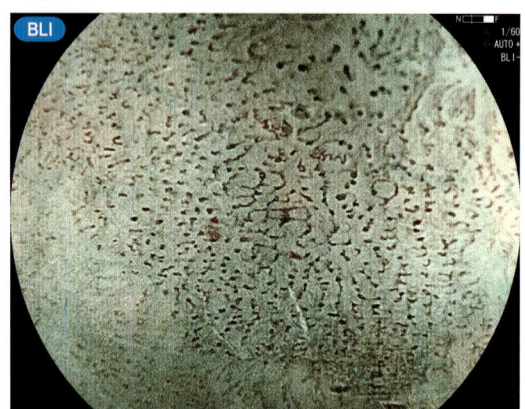

BLI magnifying observation : Irregularly shaped B1 vessels are observed in the same area as the erythematous area. Irregular arrangement and increased density with traces of loop structures are observed.

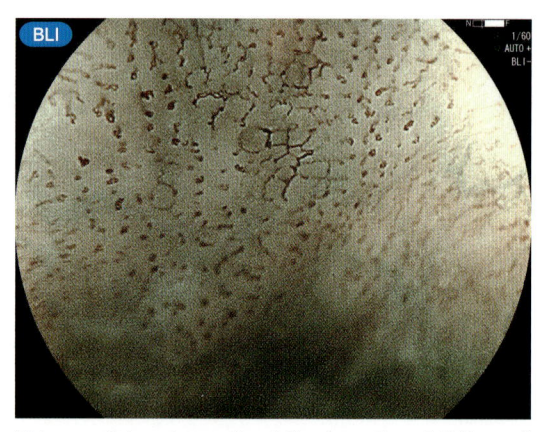

BLI magnifying observation : The formation of AVA-small are aggregated in a small ring shape of about 100 μm is observed.

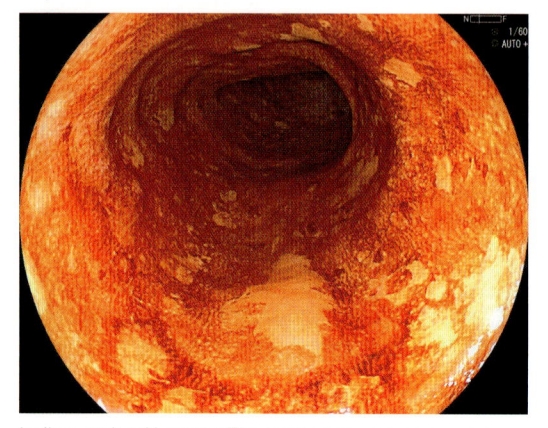

Iodine-stained image : The erythematous area presents an unstained area.

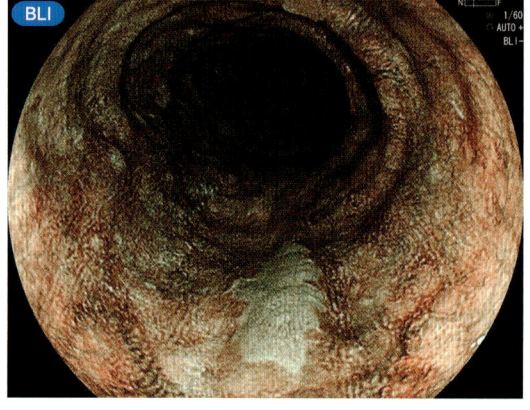

BLI combined iodine-stained image : The lesion looks pale greenish.

Endoscope：EG-L590ZW（Fujifilm）　Light source：LASEREO（Fujifilm）
BLI setup：Structure enhancement B8, color enhancement 1

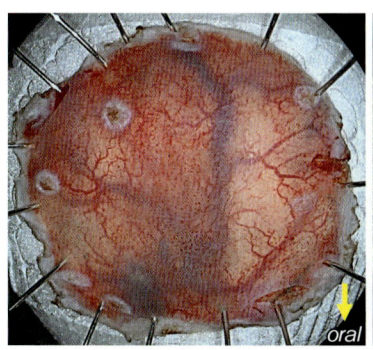

White-light observation of fresh specimen resected with ESD

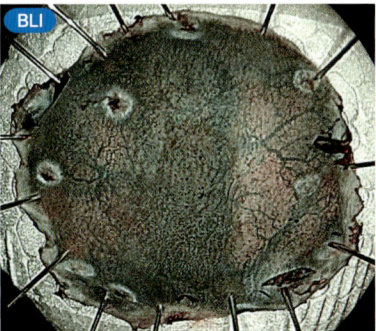

BLI observation of freshly resected specimen

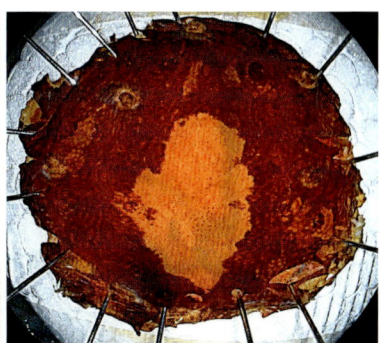

Iodine-stained image of freshly resected specimen：The lesion size is 12×9 mm.

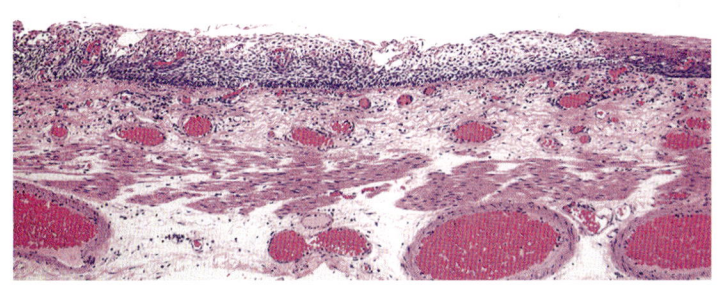

Histopathological image：The lesion is a pT1a-EP transmural intraepithelial carcinoma. There is no height difference on the boundary between the normal mucosa and the carcinoma, and the type is 0-Ⅱb.

Comment

Even when the lesion is a 0-Ⅱb esophageal carcinoma, it is often recognized as a vaguely erythematous area, if it is an intraepithelial carcinoma with near-transmural development. When a lesion is recognized as a reddened area, abnormal vessels are usually observed in magnifying observation. In this case, BLI magnifying observation showed a region containing an aggregation of very small AVAs encircled by type B1 vessels that showed traces of loops, as well as abnormal vessels which cannot be easily distinguished between types B1 and B2. As the small AVAs encircled by the unidentified abnormal vessels often present papilla-like structures, the lesion can be diagnosed as an EP carcinoma.

▶**Observation tips** With the AVAs in this case, B1 vessels are extended and connected with the surrounding area, forming multiple small AVAs. The relative regularity of the vessel diameters suggests that it is a lesion with poor invasion tendency.

(Arima, M.)

Case 19 **Type 0-IIc superficial esophageal cancer**
—Comparison of NBI/BLI observations

Male in 70s Purpose Follow-up after gastrectomy for gastric cancer
Location Left wall of mid-thoracic esophagus Macroscopic type 0-IIc

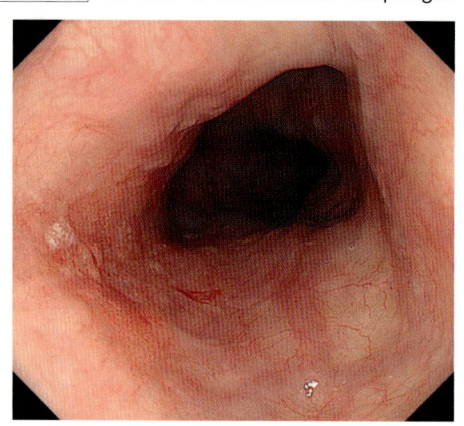

WLI observation (ELITE): A reddish depressed lesion is observed on the left-side wall of the mid-thoracic esophagus. The lesion is accompanied by granular elevations on the proximal side.

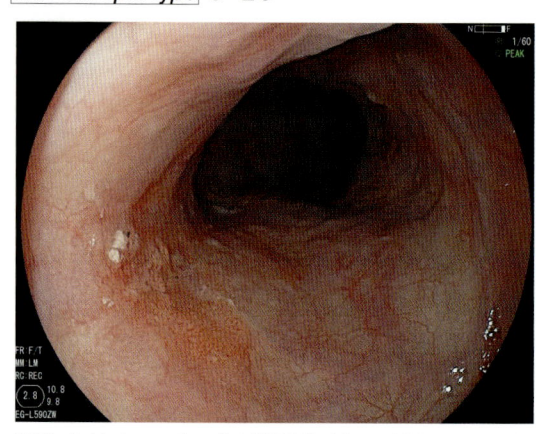

White-light observation (LASEREO): The reddish color and the loss of vascular pattern can be recognized more clearly than with the ELITE.

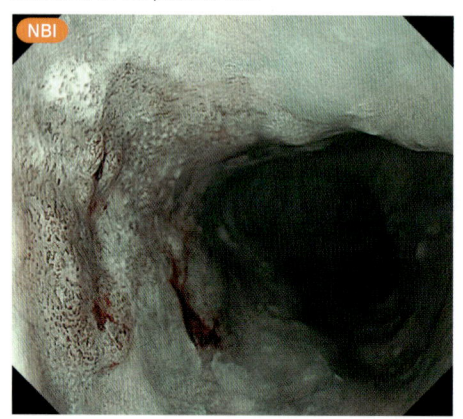

NBI observation (low magnification): The lesion is observed as a brownish area. Dilated dot-shaped vessels are observed on the proximal side of the lesion. The contours are imaged more sharply than in BLI.

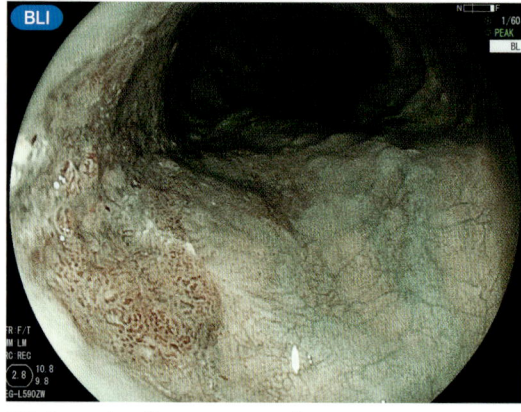

BLI observation (low magnification): A brownish area similar to that observed in NBI can be seen. However, the dot-shaped dilated vessels look bigger than in NBI.

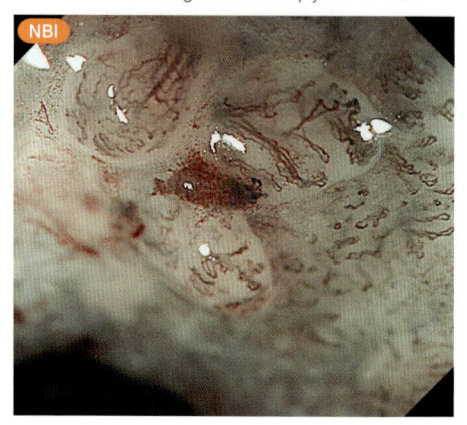

NBI observation (high magnification): In the granular elevations, the extension and tortuosity of dilated vessels stand out noticeably from the surrounding area. However, as the loop structure is only barely distinguishable, the lesion is diagnosed as B1 of the JES (the Japan Esophageal Society) Classification.

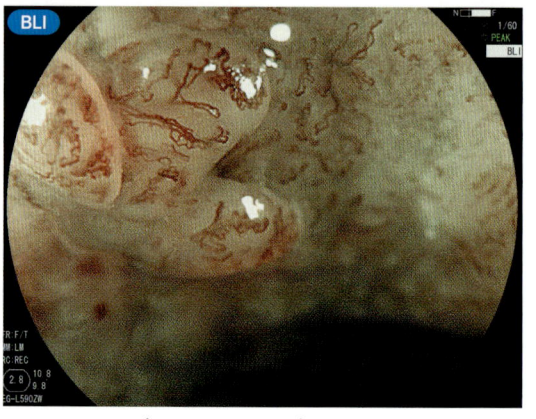

BLI observation (high magnification): As in NBI, dilated vessels maintaining the loop structures are observed. Both imaging methods show similar vascular morphology.

Endoscopic photos (left row)
 Endoscope : GIF-H260Z (Olympus)　Light source : EVIS LUCERA ELITE (Olympus)
 NBI setup : Structure enhancement B8, color mode 1
Endoscopic photos (right row)
 Endoscope : EG-L590ZW (Fujifilm)　Light source : LASEREO (Fujifilm)
 BLI setup : Structure enhancement A6, color enhancement C1

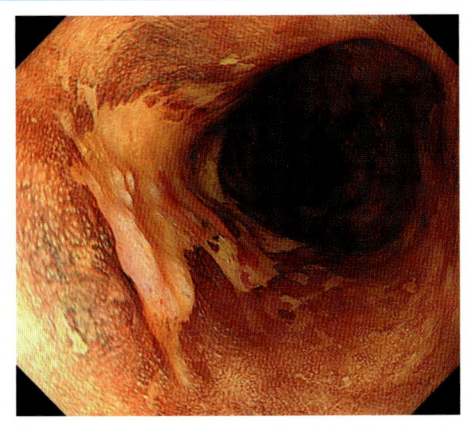

Observation after iodine staining (ELITE) : A well-demarcated iodine-unstained area is observed. The proximal side of the lesion presents a pink color.

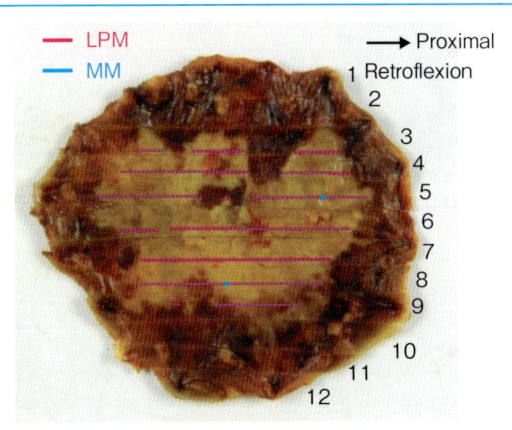

ESD-resected specimen : Granular elevations are observed on the proximal side of the unstained area.

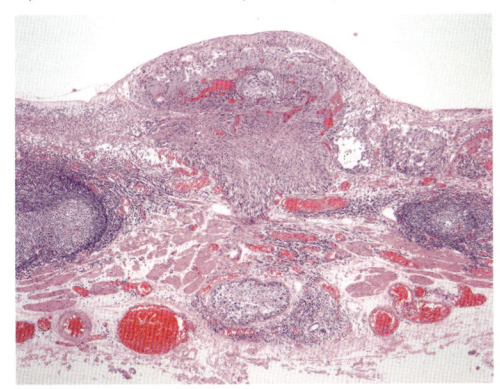

— LPM
— MM
→ Proximal
1 Retroflexion

Histopathological image (section 5) : As the squamous epithelial carcinoma is infiltrated as far as the muscularis mucosa, the invasion depth is diagnosed as T1a-MM (M3). The tumor cell nests observed in the submucosal layer is diagnosed as intraductal development.

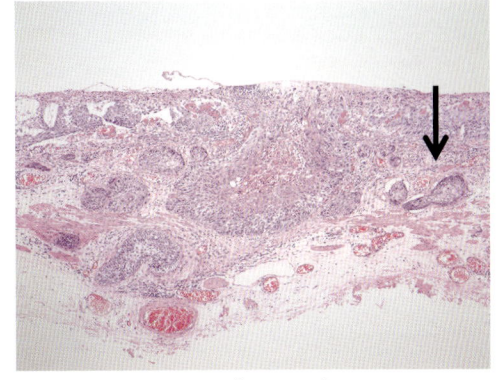

Histopathological image (section 8) : Infiltration in the muscularis mucosa is observed in a small area, and lymph node invasion is observed in the area indicated by the arrow on the right side of the infiltration. The histopathological diagnosis is : squamous cell carcinoma, 25 mm×20 mm, T1a-MM, INFa, ly1, v0, pHM0, pVM0.

Comment

The endoscopic photos obtained by NBI and BLI of this lesion are shown side-by-side. The low-magnification images are slightly different, but the intraepithelial papillary capillary loops (IPCLs) in the lesion look similar in the high-magnification images. Although BLI and NBI employ different mechanisms and systems to enhance images, both systems show vessels with about the same depth. In this case, infiltration into MM to SM1 was suspected in the granular elevations on the proximal side of the lesion as both NBI and BLI magnifying observation showed that the loop structures were maintained. Preoperative diagnosis of the lesion identified the vessels as B1 vessels according to the JES Classification. The invasion depth was cT1a-LPM.

▶**Observation tips** Brightness in the far-view field has been improved relative to previous systems in both the newly introduced ELITE system's NBI (Olympus) and LASEREO's BLI-bright mode (Fujifilm). As these improvements have made it easier to comprehend the overall image of the superficial esophageal carcinoma, they can be regarded as modalities supporting the diagnosis of both the presence and the extent of lesions. Like NBI, the BLI modes are useful for observation of microvessels in the mucosal superficial layer, but it should be noted that excessive structure enhancement can cause noise interference in the image when high magnification is used.

(Abe, S., Yoshinaga, S., Kushima, R.)

Case 20 Type 0-IIc superficial esophageal cancer
—Comparison of NBI/BLI observations

Male in 60s |Purpose| Detailed examination of esophageal cancer
|Location| Right wall of lower thoracic esophagus |Macroscopic type| 0-IIc

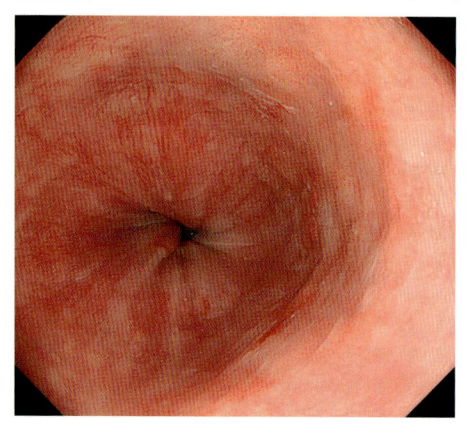

WLI observation (ELITE): Slightly reddish rough mucosa without normal vascular pattern is observed on the right-side wall of the lower thoracic esophagus.

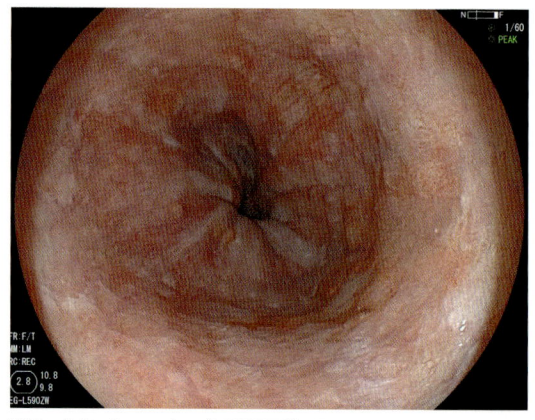

White-light observation (LASEREO): The redness of the lesion is quite noticeable and the normal mucosa intercalated on the posterior wall side of its center can be seen more clearly than with the ELITE.

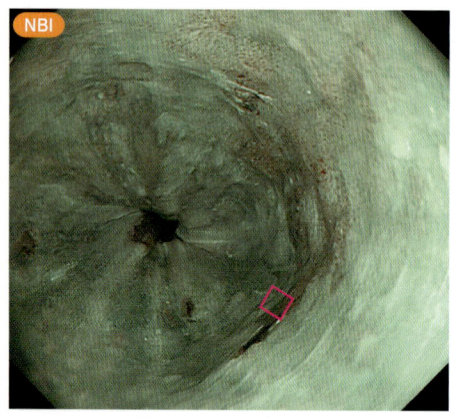

NBI observation (non-magnifying): The lesion appears as a brownish area.

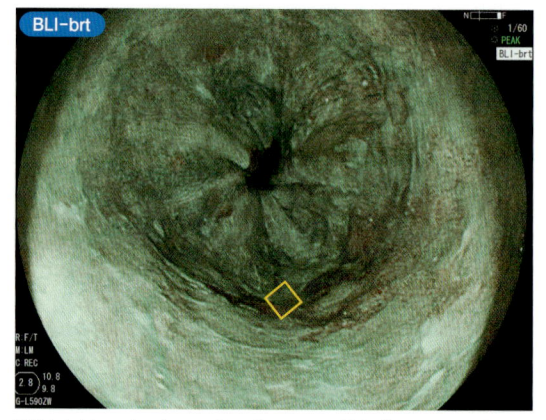

BLI-bright mode observation (non-magnifying): As with NBI, the lesion appears as a brownish area, but the contrast between the neoplastic and non-neoplastic areas is clearer than with the NBI.

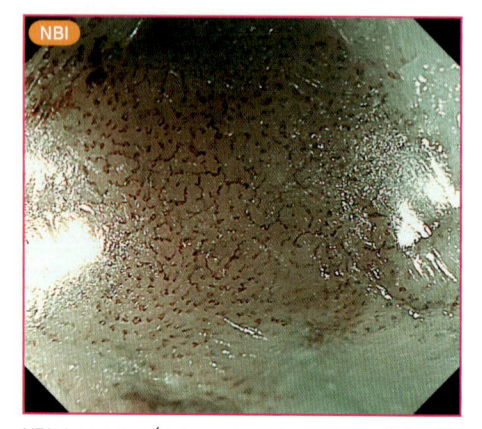

NBI observation (red square section on the posterior side of the distal side of lesion, with high magnification): Dot-shaped dilated vessels are observed and some of them form meshed structures. However, as the atypism is not so strong and the loop structures are maintained, the vessels are diagnosed as B1 vessels according to the JES (the Japan Esophageal Society) Classification. The margins of the vessels are imaged more sharply by NBI than BLI.

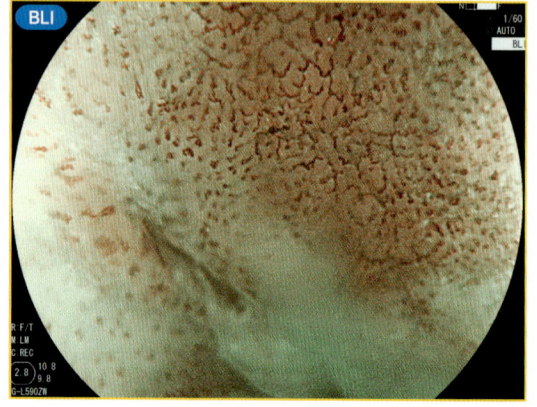

BLI observation (same region as the NBI observation): As with NBI, dilated vessels with loop structures maintained are observed. The vessels appear larger than in NBI observation.

Endoscopic photos（left row）
　Endoscope：GIF-H260Z（Olympus）　　Light source：EVIS LUCERA ELITE（Olympus）
　NBI setup：Structure enhancement B8, color mode 1
Endoscopic photos（right row）
　Endoscope：EG-L590ZW（Fujifilm）　　Light source：LASEREO（Fujifilm）
　BLI setup：BLI—Structure enhancement A4, color enhancement C1；BLI-bright—structure enhancement A4, color enhancement C1

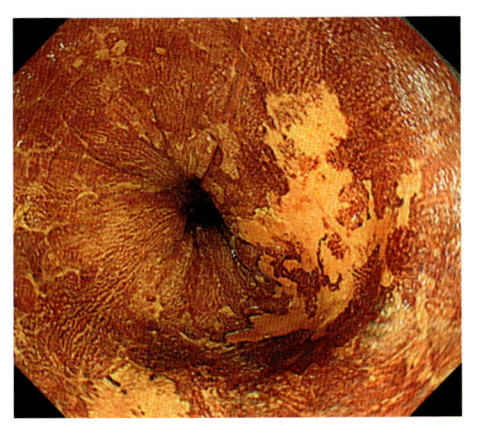

Observation after iodine staining（ELITE）：A well-demarcated iodine-unstained area is observed. The area on the posterior side is more densely stained than the center area where normal mucosa is probably intercalated.

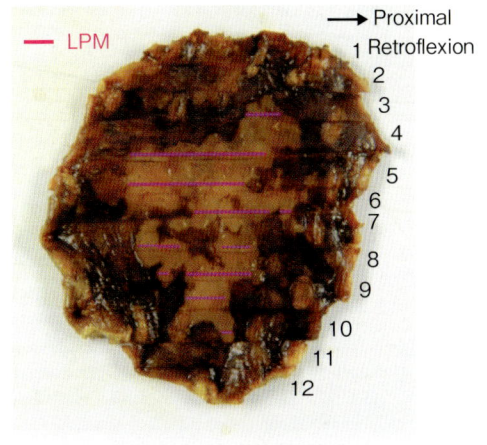

ESD-resected specimen：Squamous cell carcinoma is observed in the same location as the iodine-unstained area.

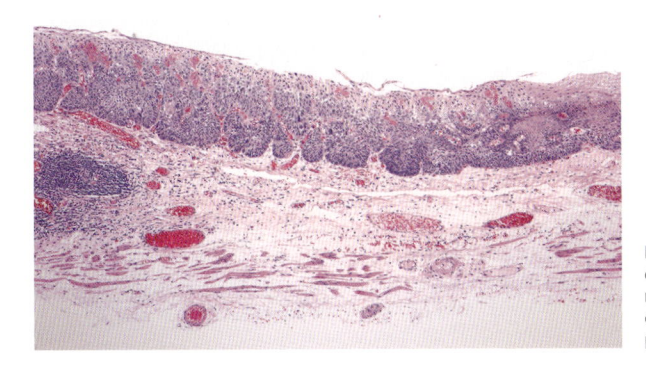

Histopathological image（section 9）：The squamous cell carcinoma is infiltrated as far as the lamina propria mucosa. Histopathological diagnosis：Squamous cell carcinoma, 18 mm×15 mm, T1a-LPM, INFa, ly0, v0, pHM0, pVM0.

Comment

Under white-light observation, this case looked like a shallow depressed lesion without height irregularities or findings suggesting invasion to M3 or lower. In NBI and BLI observation, B1 vessels according to the JES Classification were observed, but were not accompanied by an avascular area. Based on the above findings, the preoperative diagnosis determined that the invasion depth is cT1a-LPM. This lesion was subjected to an ESD.

▶**Observation tips**　Before NBI/BLI magnifying observation, the lesion should be rinsed with Gascon solution and then observed under white light in order to examine the regions where factors related to invasion depth diagnosis such as surface irregularities and reddening are noticeable, while increasing the magnification gradually. The black hood should be attached in magnifying observation to maintain the optimum distance.
In high-magnification observation, manipulate the endoscope so that the region of interest comes in the 12 o'clock direction of the image. Try to view the lesion from the front by adjusting the amount of air and maintaining the optimum distance with upward angulation. Be careful not to manipulate the endoscope forcibly, as this could cause bleeding and make subsequent magnifying observation difficult.

（Abe, S., Yoshinaga, S., Kushima, R.）

Case 21 Type 0-Ⅱc superficial esophageal carcinoma

Female in 70s **Purpose** Detailed examination of esophageal lesion **Location** Mid-thoracic esophagus
Macroscopic type 0-Ⅱc

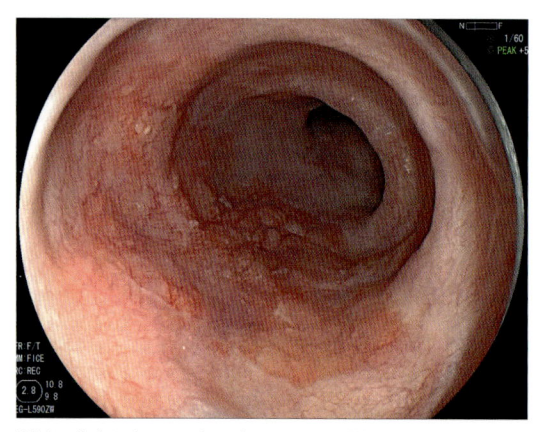

White-light observation shows a roughly semi-circumferential, erythematous, irregularly shaped, depressed lesion. The demarcation on the distal side can also be observed from the far view.

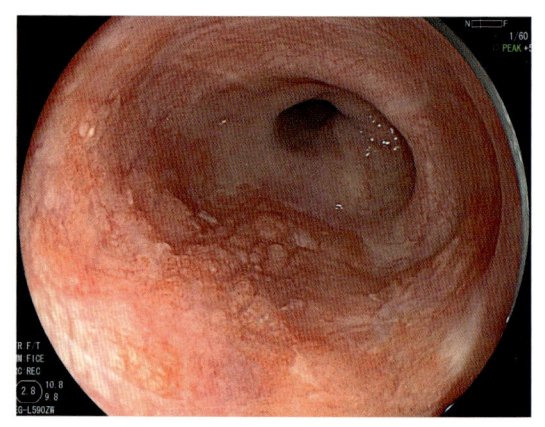

When the endoscope is advanced slightly toward the distal direction, the distal demarcation can be recognized more clearly.

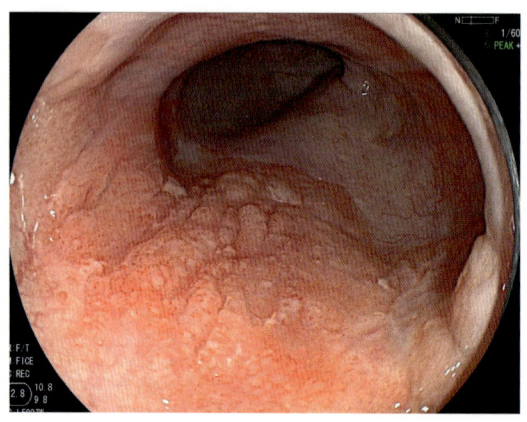

Advancing the endoscope further produces a three dimensional image of the surface height irregularities inside the lesion.

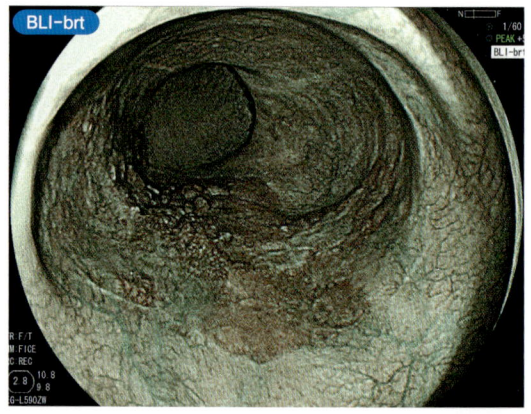

BLI-bright mode non-magnifying observation shows the lesion as a brownish area. The color tone change on the demarcation is more clearly.

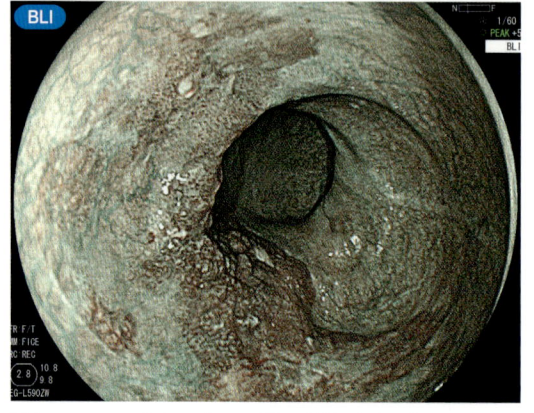

BLI non-magnifying observation : The lesion is represented as a brownish area and the demarcation in the 9 to 10 o'clock direction can be seen more clearly than under white-light observation. The surface irregularities are also shown more clearly.

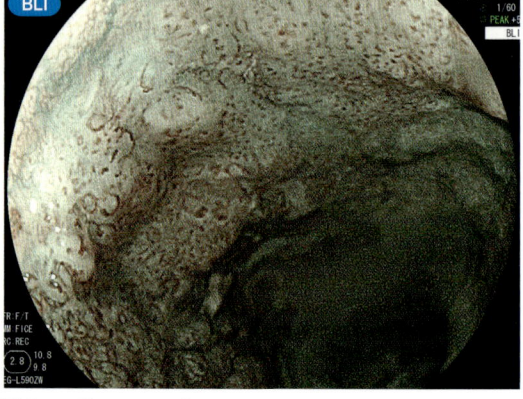

BLI medium-magnification observation : The lesion demarcation is clear and the proliferation of irregular vessels with irregular arrangement is observed.

Endoscope：EG-L590ZW（Fujifilm）　Light source：LASEREO（Fujifilm）
BLI setup：BLI—Structure enhancement A8, color enhancement C1；BLI-bright—structure enhancement A8, color enhancement C1

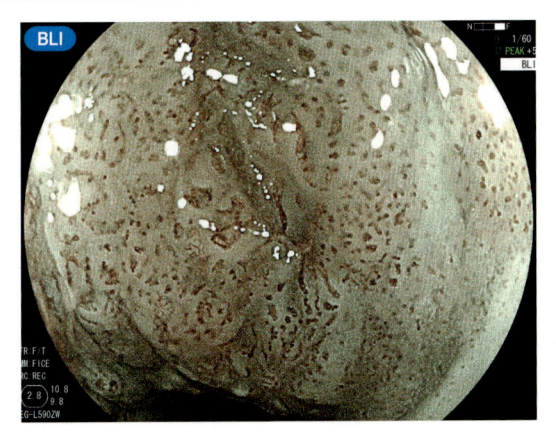

BLI magnifying observation：Under magnifying observation of the central area of the lesion irregularly arranged IPCLs with irregular diameters and tortuosity are observed. As the loop formation is maintained, the vessels are diagnosed as B1 according to the JES (The Japan Esophageal Society) Classification.

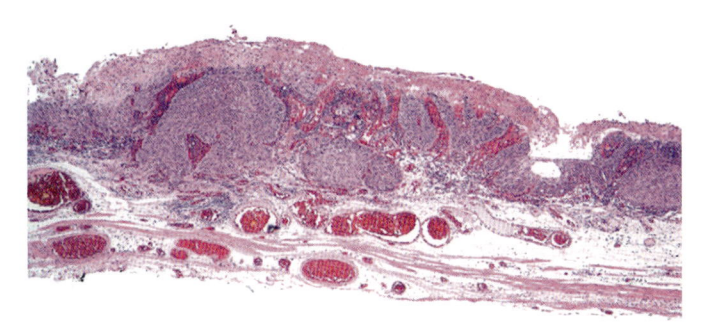

Pathological findings after ESD：Atypical squamous cells with chromatin growth have infiltrated and grown in the form of a sheet as far as the LPM. The pathological diagnosis is：squamous cell carcinoma, pT1a-LPM, ly0, v0, pHM0, pVM0.

Comment

The lesion has a rough semi-circumferential shape and extends toward the distal side. However, as the BLI-bright mode can offer a universally bright field of view, it is relatively easy to interpret the overall image including the distal demarcation of the lesion. Non-magnifying observation led to the suspicion of MM invasion due to the noticeable elevation components in the depression, but BLI magnifying observation showed that the invasion was within the LPM. According to the pathological findings after ESD, the lesion was a tumor that seemed to be growing toward the upper side of the mucosal layer. The histopathologically identified invasion depth was LPM.

▶Observation tips In both the white-light and BLI-bright modes, non-magnifying observation provides a universally bright field of view that makes it easy to find the lesion by the strong contrast between the surrounding normal mucosa and the lesion. With BLI observation, the brownish area is contrasted clearly from the color tone of the surrounding mucosa. We used medium magnification to confirm the lesion demarcation, and high magnification to diagnose the invasion depth in the region with strong height irregularities in the center of the lesion. The BLI-bright mode seems to be useful for overall evaluation of the lesion by its relatively bright narrow-band imaging, while the BLI mode magnification observation seems to be useful for invasion depth diagnosis.

(Yamamoto, F., Miyahara, R., Goto, H.)

Case 22 Barrett's esophagus

Female in 80s **Purpose** Surveillance of Barrett's esophagus **Location** Esophagogastric junction

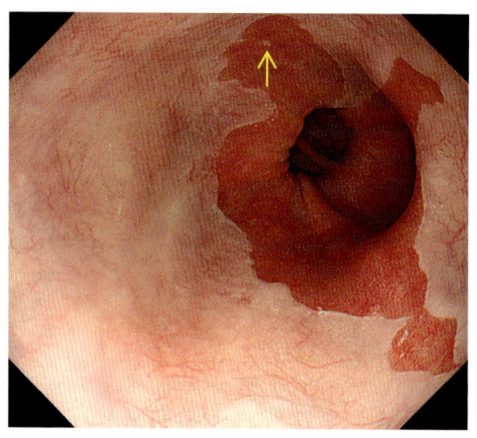

WLI observation: A columnar epithelium with a maximum length of 3 cm is continuously extended from the esophagogastric junction, so the lesion can be diagnosed as a short segment Barrett's esophagus (SSBE : C0, M3). A small squamous epithelial island is observed in the 12 o'clock direction (arrow). Light white turbid area is observed on the esophageal squamous epithelium on the proximal side of the SSBE.

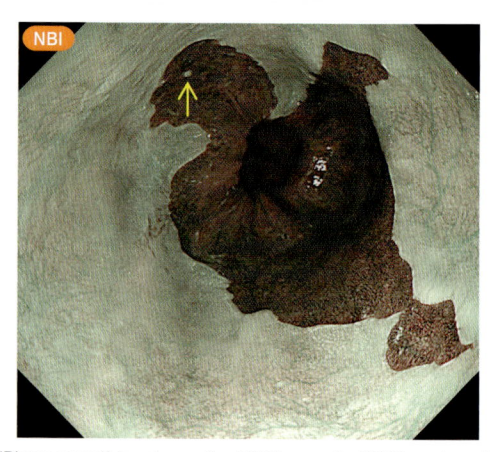

NBI non-magnifying observation: NBI images the SSBE as a brownish area extending from the stomach and improves the visibility of the small squamous island in the 12 o'clock direction.

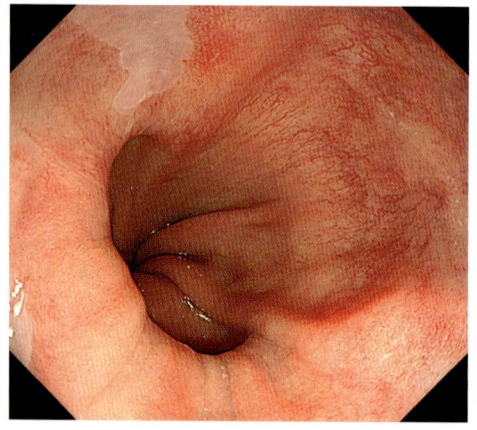

WLI observation: The lower end of the palisade vessels in the lower esophagus and the upper end of the gastric folds are observed.

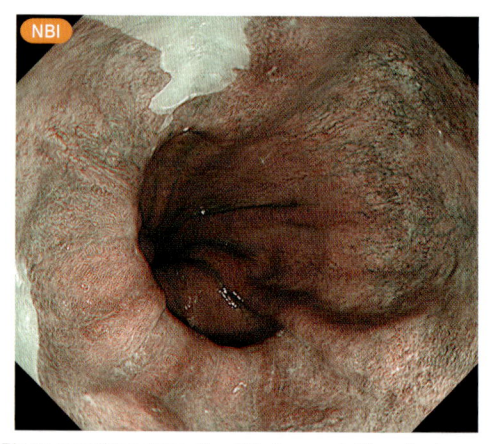

NBI non-magnifying observation: The lower end of the palisade vessels in the lower esophagus and the oral margin of the gastric folds can be seen but are not as clear as under WLI observation.

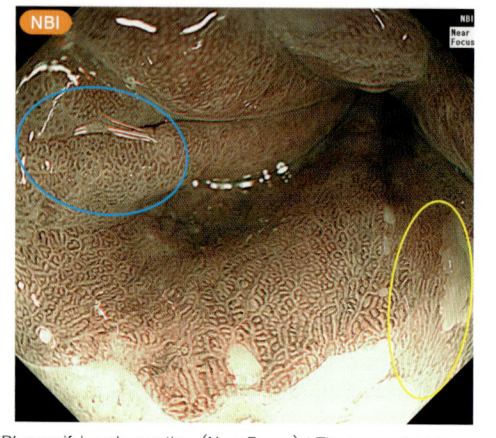

NBI magnifying observation (Near Focus): The mucosal patterns are visible in a broad area (4 o'clock direction : long straight [inside the yellow ellipse] ; 5-7 o'clock direction : round or oval ; 9 o'clock direction : villous or cerebriform [inside the blue ellipse]).

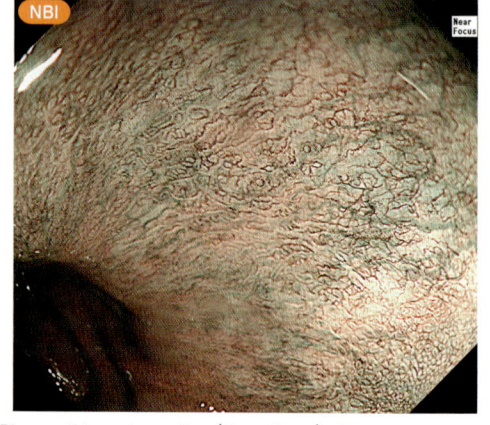

NBI magnifying observation (Near Focus): Flat mucosa with no mucosal pattern is observed and dendritically-branched, slightly tortuous vessels can also be seen. As there is no clear regionality and it can be diagnosed that there is no neoplastic change.

Endoscope：GIF-HQ290（Olympus）　Light source：EVIS LUCERA ELITE（Olympus）
NBI setup：Structure enhancement A7, color mode 1

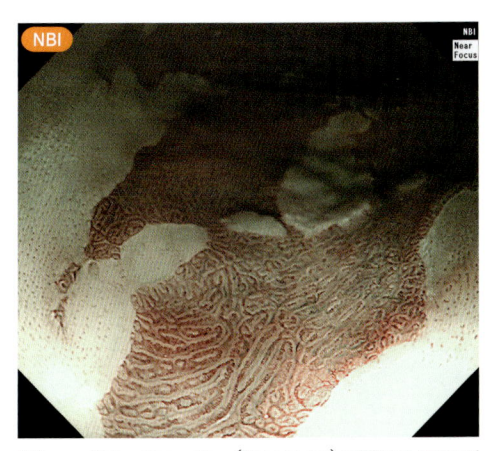

NBI magnifying observation（Near Focus）：Different mucosal patterns with shapes ranging from circular to linear shapes can be seen, together with white margins so-called as 'white zone'. DNA-spiral like formed vessels that several vessels are entangled with one another are running along the mucosal patterns.

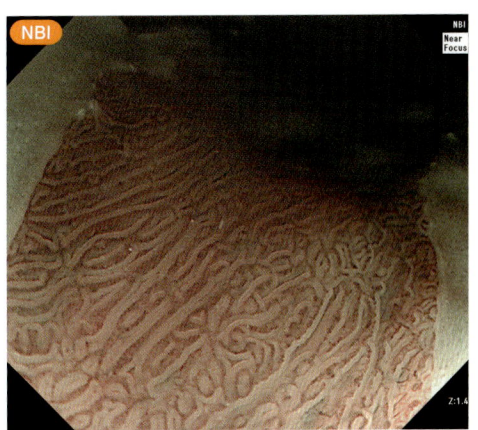

NBI magnifying observation（Near Focus＋1.4×electronic zoom）：The electronic zoom can magnify the vascular structures but cannot clearly visualize details such as the morphology of each vessel.

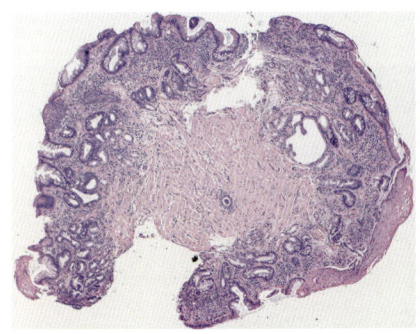

Histological findings：The biopsy tissue specimen presents a mix of glandular and squamous epithelia. The glandular epithelium has specialized intestinal metaplasia with goblet cells.

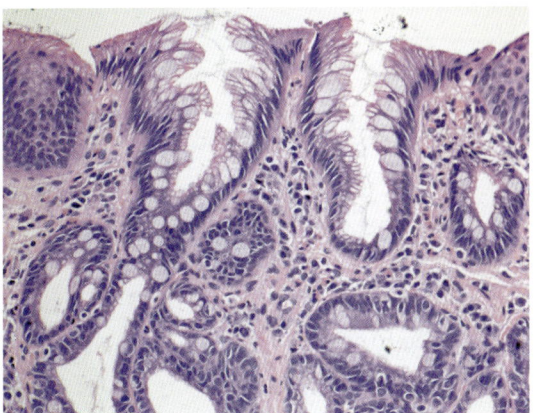

Comment

The important thing when diagnosing the presence of Barrett's esophagus is to observe the lower end of the palisade vessels in the lower esophagus and the upper end of the gastric folds. Conventional WLI will be useful for this purpose than NBI. The clinical significance of endoscopic observation of Barrett's esophagus is that it has the potential to be predispose to the development of adenocarcinoma and is early detection of the carcinoma. The neoplastic lesions (dysplasia/adenocarcinoma) generated on Barrett's esophagus are often hard to find with WLI observation, and the usefulness of magnifying observation combined with NBI has been demonstrated. The new HQ290 dual focus endoscope with moderate magnification power has a large depth of focus, so it can clearly image mucosal patterns across a wide area in the field of view. This allows endoscopists to quickly check abnormalities in the surface structure of the entire Barrett's esophagus with a single push of the button. The magnification level of the HQ290 is 'half zoom'（max. 45×）but it seems sufficient for observing the surface structures. However, when an abnormal surface structure is found, magnification has to be increased in order to check for any abnormality in the microvascular structures by increasing the magnification. This can be done with the HQ290 by using its electronic zooming capability in combination with the optical zoom. Nevertheless, its microvascular imaging capability is somewhat insufficient as mentioned above. Therefore, in the detailed preoperative examination including diagnosis of the horizontal extent of Barrett's adenocarcinoma, it is recommended to use the 'full zoom'（approx. 90×）of the H260Z magnifying endoscope.

（Goda, K., Dobashi, A., Tajiri, H.）

Case 23 Barrett's esophagus

Case 1 Male in 60s **Purpose** Routine endoscopic examination

BLI setup : Structure enhancement A8, color enhancement C1

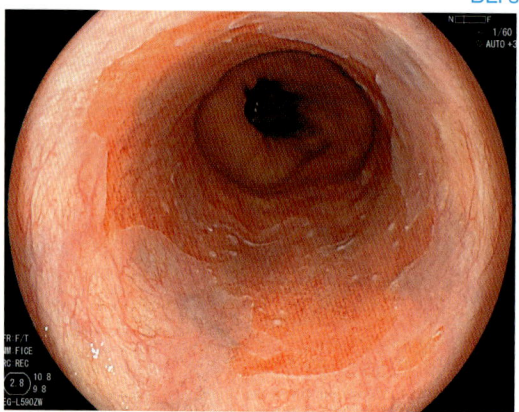

White light observation : A circumferential columnar epithelium extends from the upper end of gastric folds toward the proximal side.

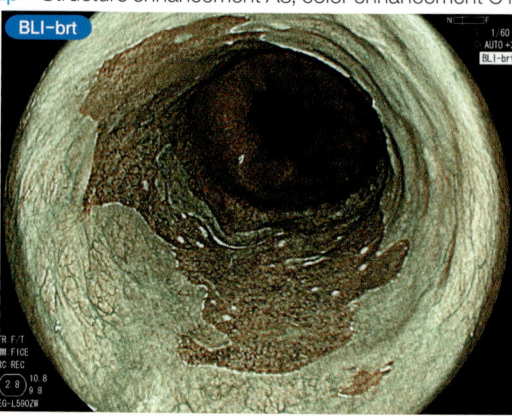

BLI-bright mode non-magnifying observation : The demarcation with the esophageal mucosa is clarified, making it easier to recognize the whitish squamous epithelial island in the columnar epithelium.

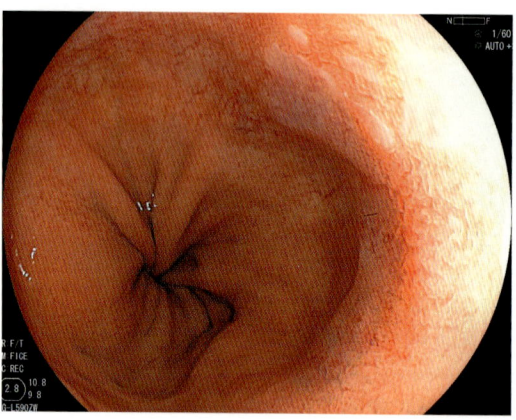

The lower ends of the palisade vessels and the terminal portion on the proximal side of the gastric mucosal folds are visible.

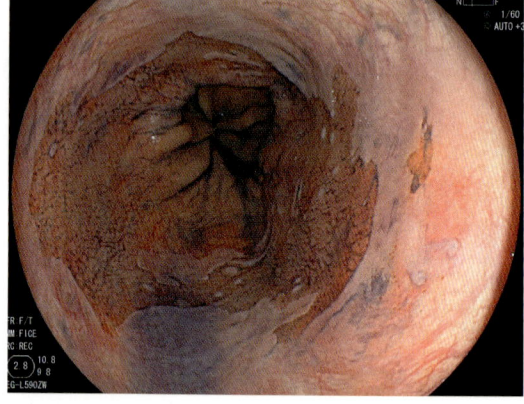

Indigo carmine dye spraying chromoendoscopy : The mucosal structures inside the columnar epithelium can be seen clearly.

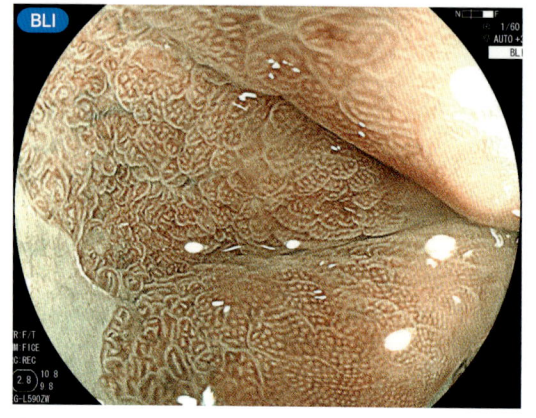

BLI medium-magnification observation : The microstructures of the villous mucosa can be seen clearly.

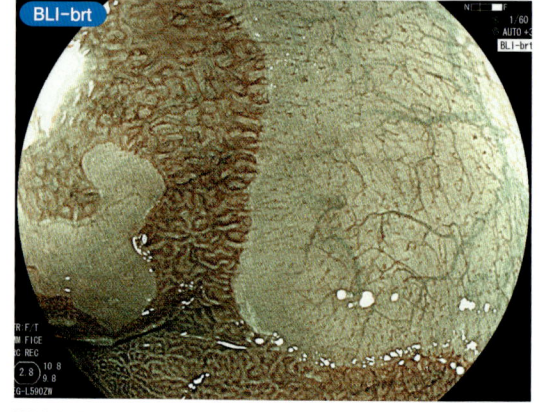

BLI-bright mode medium-magnification observation : Brownish microvessels with well-arranged organization are observed.

Endoscope: EG-L590ZW (Fujifilm)　Light source: LASEREO (Fujifilm).
BLI setup: Specified for each case

Case 2　Female in 70s　*Purpose*　Screening

BLI setup: Structure enhancement B8, color enhancement C1

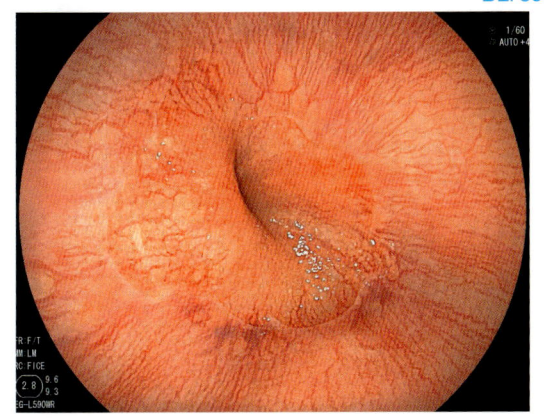

White-light observation: Barrett's mucosa that extends like a tongue is observed.

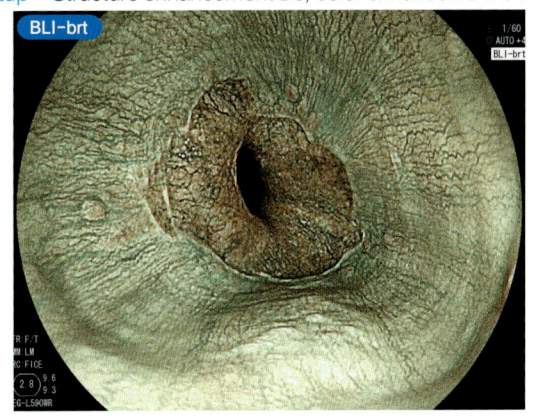

BLI-bright mode observation: The palisade vessels in the Barrett's mucosa are more visible.

Comment

Identification of the esophagogastric junction is important for the diagnosis of Barrett's esophagus. White-light observation is able to image the palisade vessels clearly by its high overall brightness. In BLI observation, the columnar epithelium is rendered brownish, making the squamous epithelial islands clearly recognizable by their whitish color. Magnifying observation is useful for checking the columnar epithelium and differentiating the neoplastic lesion because it clarifies the surface mucosal structure.

▶**Observation tips** Having the patient take a deep breath expands the lower esophagus and facilitates observation because it makes the intrathoracic pressure negative and displaces the esophagogastric junction toward the proximal side. For diagnosis of Barrett's esophagus, it is important to identify the esophagogastric junction based on the finding of palisade vessels while the esophagus has been expanded as described above.

(Yamamoto, F., Miyahara, R., Goto, H.)

Case 24 Barrett's esophageal adenocarcinoma

Female in 80s **Purpose** Preoperative endoscopy of esophageal adenocarcinoma
Location Middle esophagus (35 cm from incisors) **Macroscopic type** 0-IIc

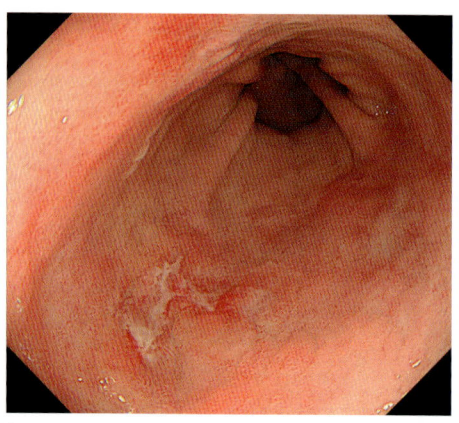

WLI observation: A lesion with a map-shaped white-coat attached is seen in a circumferential, 14-cm long segment of Barrett's esophagus (LSBE). The demarcation is unclear and the margins are erythematous.

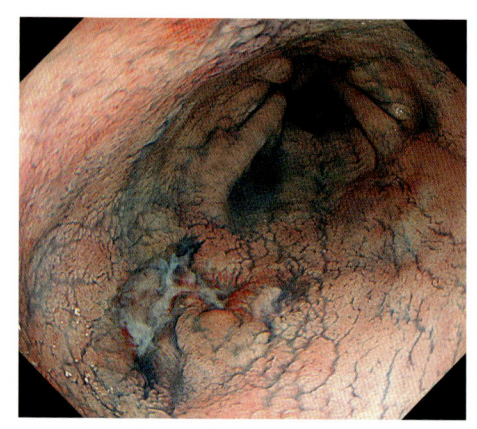

Indigo carmine chromoendoscopy: Dye spraying clarifies the demarcation on the left to distal side of the lesion. The accumulation of dye indicates that the lesion is slightly depressed.

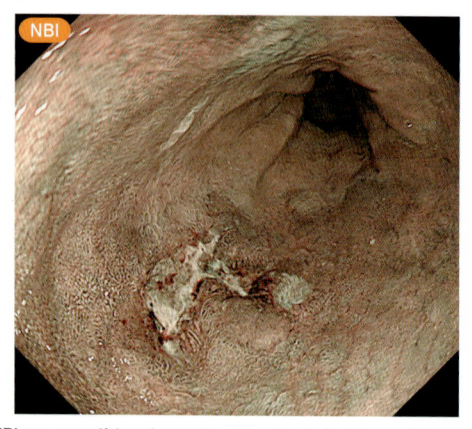

NBI non-magnifying observation: The attached white-coat is imaged in white and the regions including where blood is attached are shown in a brownish color tone.

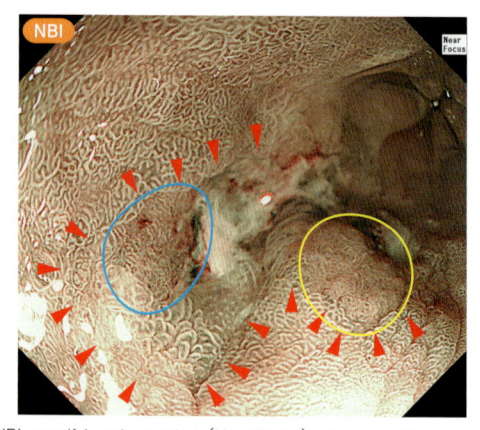

NBI magnifying observation (Near Focus): The magnified image of the proximal margin shows that the lesion has mucosal patterns that are slightly smaller (left side [inside the blue ellipse]) or less visible (right side [inside the yellow ellipse]) than the surrounding area. The demarcation of the lesion is imaged relatively clearly (arrowheads).

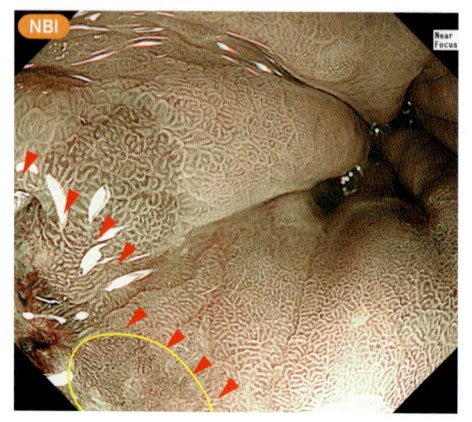

NBI magnifying observation (Near Focus): The distal demarcation of the lesion is also clearly recognizable (arrowheads). The mucosal patterns visible inside the lesion are congested with blood (left side) or smaller in size (right side [inside the yellow ellipse]) compared to the mucosal patterns in the surrounding normal area.

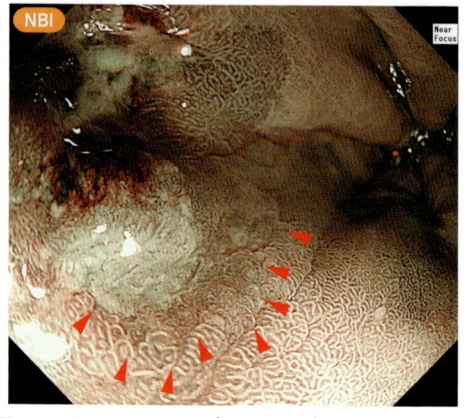

NBI magnifying observation (Near Focus): A well-demarcated depression with a brownish color tone is observed on the marginal area of erosion to which white coated is attached. The mucosal patterns are smaller or less visible than the white-marginated mucosal patterns in the surrounding area. No white-marginated mucosal pattern is clearly observed in the lesion.

92

Endoscope：GIF-HQ290（Olympus）　Light source：EVIS LUCERA ELITE（Olympus）
NBI setup：Structure enhancement A7, color mode 1

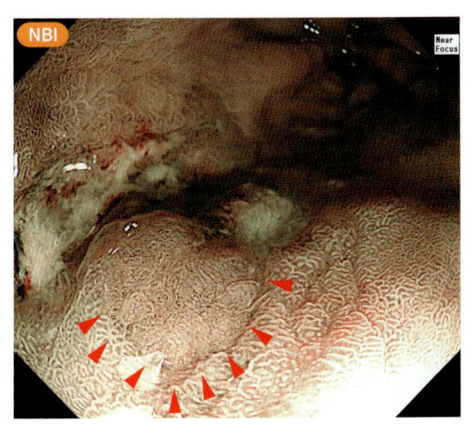

NBI magnifying observation (Near Focus)：The demarcation is clearly visible (arrowheads), while margins of mucosal patterns inside the lesion are less visible than the surrounding area. The mucosal patterns inside the lesion are complex and dense.

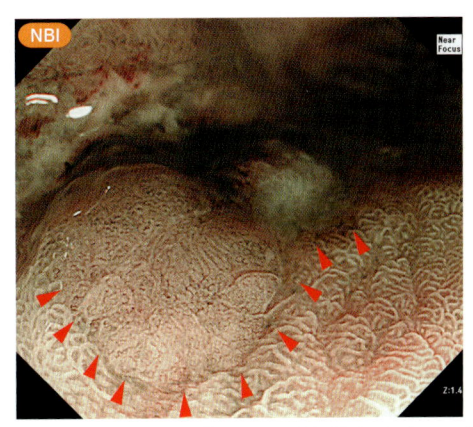

NBI magnifying observation (Near Focus＋1.4×electronic zoom)：Applying the electronic zoom can clearly images the mucosal patterns as well as the proliferation of abnormal microvessels with irregular branching and changes in caliber.

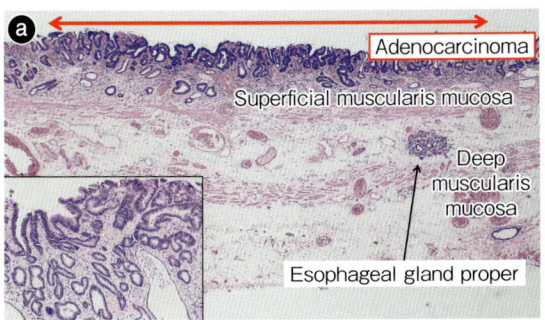

Histological findings：Dense presence of atypical glands localized in the mucosal layer is observed (a). The atypical grade corresponded to a well-differentiated adenocarcinoma with distinct glandular lumen (figure inserted in (a)). The double layer structure of muscularis mucosae and the proper esophageal gland are observed immediately below the carcinoma. Moderately to poorly differentiated adenocarcinoma (b) and mild lymphatic invasion, ly1 (figure inserted in (b)) are also observed.
Final histological diagnosis：20×12 mm, 0-Ⅱc, differentiated (well to moderately＞poorly), ly1, v0, negative margin.

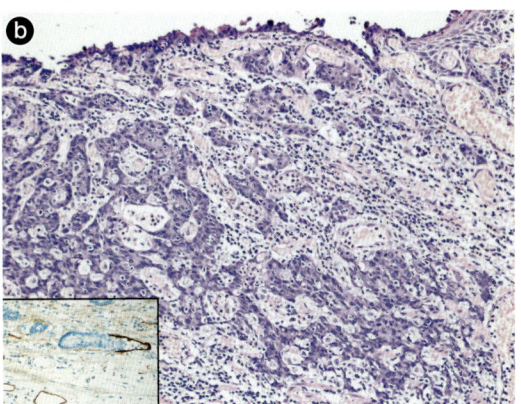

Comment

The lesion is a tubular adenocarcinoma developed in an LSBE. Since Barrett's esophagus is caused by gastroesophageal reflux disease, benign inflammatory changes such as erosion and ulcers are important lesions which should be differentiated from dysplasia or carcinoma lesions. The key points to diagnosis this lesion as a carcinoma include the following：①with WLI endoscopy or indigo carmine chromoendoscopy, the lesion should be recognized as a localized depressed lesion；②with NBI magnifying observation, the circumferential demarcation should be visible and the lesion should contain small, less visible mucosal patterns and abnormal microvessels. As only focal presence of poorly-differentiated adenocarcinoma components is found in the eroded portion and its margins, it is hard to point them out in preoperative endoscopy. Since this case is accompanied with a poorly differentiated carcinoma and the lymphatic invasion is positive, it should be subjected to an additional surgical resection. However, considering the absence of a metastatic lesion in the chest and abdominal computed tomography, the age, the comorbid chronic lung disease and the requests of the patient and her family, this case is currently under close follow-up. No recurrence has been occurred in these three years after ESD.

(Goda, K., Dobashi, A., Tajiri, H.)

Case 25 Barrett's esophageal adenocarcinoma

Male aged 75　*Purpose*　Follow-up of Barrett's esophagus　*Location*　Lower thoracic esophagus

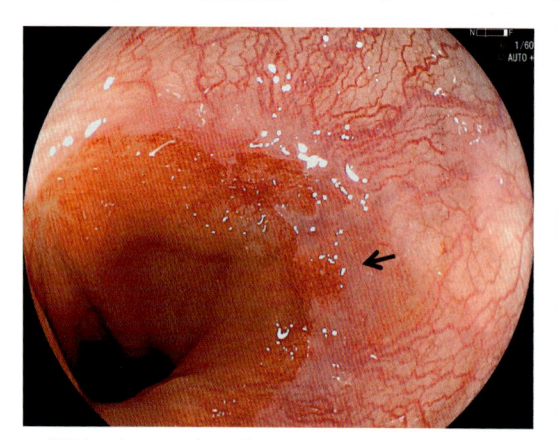

WLI observation image : Squamocolumnar junction (SCJ) 40 cm, hiatus 42 cm. In addition to the findings of an esophageal hiatus hernia and the SSBE in the region from the right wall to the posterior wall, an erythematous area of about 4 mm is observed in the 3 o'clock direction from the SCJ (arrow).

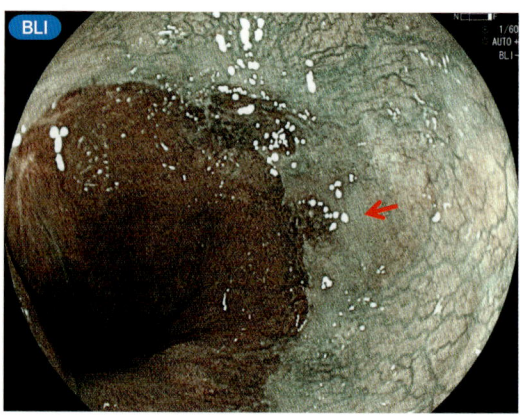

BLI-combined observation (arrow)

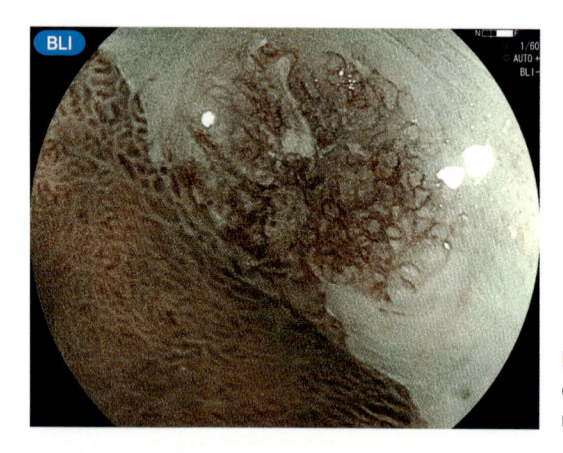

BLI low-magnification observation : The lesion contains irregular glandular groove patterns and microvessels with a mesh-like arrangement.

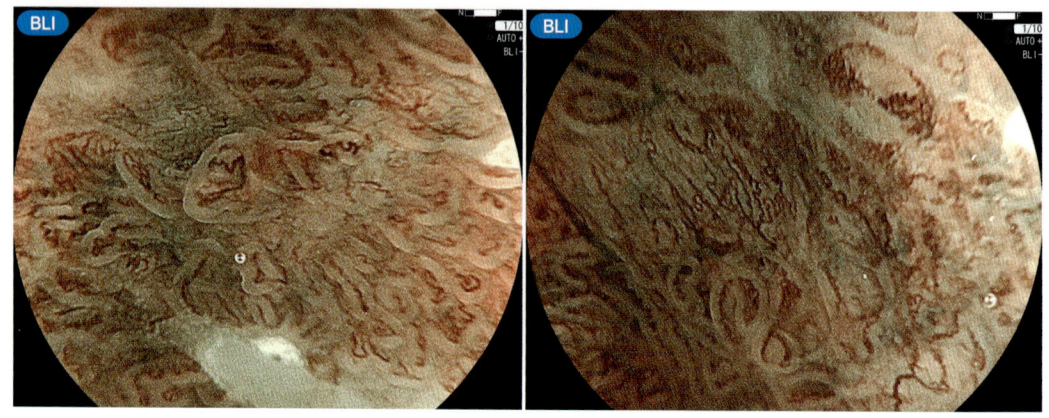

BLI high-magnification observation : Aggregation of irregular, poorly arranged glandular grooves are observed with abnormal microvessels inside.

Endoscope : EG-L590ZW (Fujifilm)　Light source : LASEREO (Fujifilm)
BLI setup : Structure enhancement B8, color enhancement 1

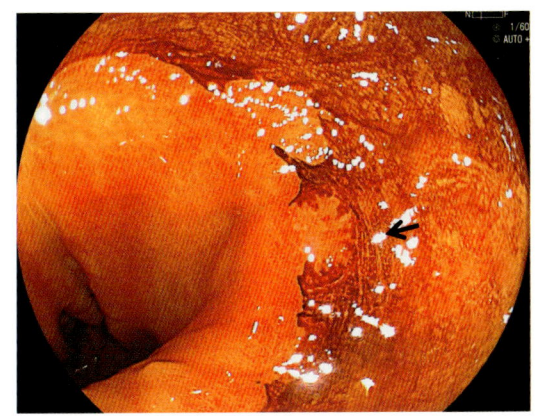

Under iodine staining, the lesion presented as an unstained area of 4 mm with irregular margins (arrow)

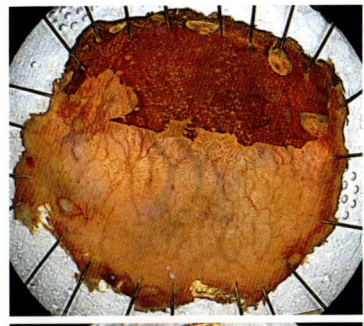

Freshly resected specimen Iodine-stained image

Construction

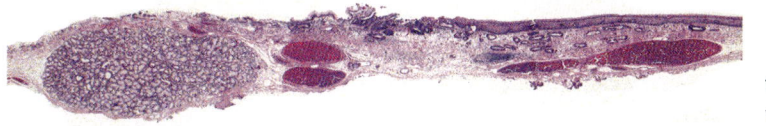

tub1-tub2, pT1a-LPM, ly0, v0, INFb, 8×8 mm.

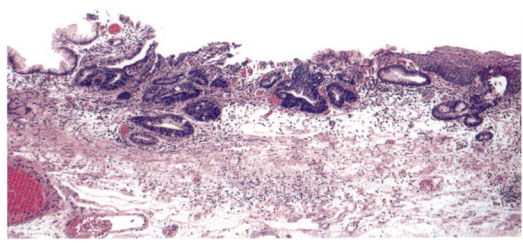

An adenocarcinoma invading the LPM is observed in the vicinity of the SCJ.

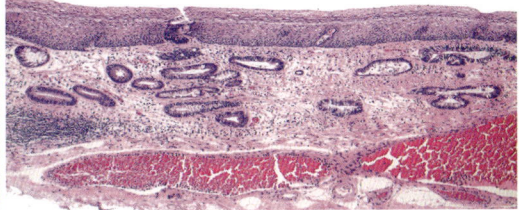

The LPM below the squamous epithelium on the proximal side presents development of atypical gland ducts.

Comment

This lesion is a small Barrett's esophageal adenocarcinoma generated from SSBE. It was located in white-light observation because the endoscopist noticed slight reddening and irregular morphology of the margins, though the region otherwise appeared no different than the surrounding Barrett's epithelia, particularly from Barrett's mucosa located in the 1 o'clock direction. Diagnosis of the portion exposed on the inner cavity is easy but, on the proximal side, the lesion has penetrated below the squamous epithelium and at 8 mm is twice as large as the exposed portion. This means that when ESD is performed on this lesion, the dissecting line on the proximal side should be set for a wide area.

▶Observation tips BLI magnifying observation shows that the lesion is composed of abnormal vessels in a fine network pattern and atypical gland ducts even under low magnification. When atypical gland ducts develop toward the proximal direction, the gland duct orifices can sometimes be recognized as irregularly arranged pores on the squamous epithelium. In this case, however, diagnosis based on the above is impossible also due to the effects of biopsy.

(Arima, M.)

Stomach and Duodenum

See page 4 for explanation of abbreviations.

Stomach and Duodenum

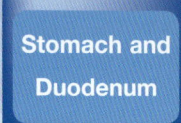

General Theory : How to Observe These Regions with NBI or BLI

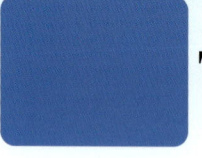

Tips on NBI Observation

■ Introduction

Recent developments in endoscopic technology have led to the combination of innovative new image enhancement systems such as NBI with conventional white light imaging. NBI magnifying observation facilitates clear observation of microstructures and microvascular architecture on the mucosal surface, helping make possible the establishment of more sophisticated endoscopic diagnoses[1)-3)]. In conventional NBI magnifying endoscopy, the observation depth is from 1.5 to 3 mm, so the endoscope has to be approached very closely to the lesion. As it takes some time to get accustomed to manipulating the lever used to control magnification, this system was not considered especially helpful in screenings. In response, Olympus Medical Systems Corporation developed a new and improved system—EVIS LUCERA ELITE. Launched in November 2012, and soon followed by the GIF-HQ290 endoscope in January 2013, EVIS LUCERA ELITE features high image quality that surpasses that of conventional HDTV quality and a simplified one-touch two-step focus switching system. Thanks to the improved ease of use and enhanced image quality, Olympus expects these products to stimulate rapid dissemination of NBI magnifying observation.

In this section, the authors summarize new NBI observation in the gastric and duodenal regions using the GIF-HQ290 and the EVIS LUCERA ELITE system.

■ I. Screening diagnosis

Since NBI irradiates light by filtering out the components outside the narrow band, it is significantly less bright than WLI and has been considered unsuitable for screening diagnosis of gastric lesions. Although brightness has been almost doubled in the new NBI system and far-point observation is now possible, NBI is still not as bright as WLI. Nevertheless, it seems to be sufficient. Even in the stomach, which has a wide lumen, NBI proved bright enough to enable screening observation of lesions from the normal observation distance (**Fig. 1a-c**). It is also bright enough for use in the duodenum, though duodenal observation does become difficult when bile is present, leading to some degree of instability (**Figs. 2 & 3**). It would be helpful if objective achievements concerning the effectiveness of the screening of lesions in the stomach and duodenum are reported in the future.

■ II. NBI magnification observation

In conventional NBI magnifying endoscopy, it was necessary to attach a distal hood to the endoscope. In addition, when maximum magnification was used, it was also necessary to approach the endoscope as close as 2 mm to the lesion. As the distal

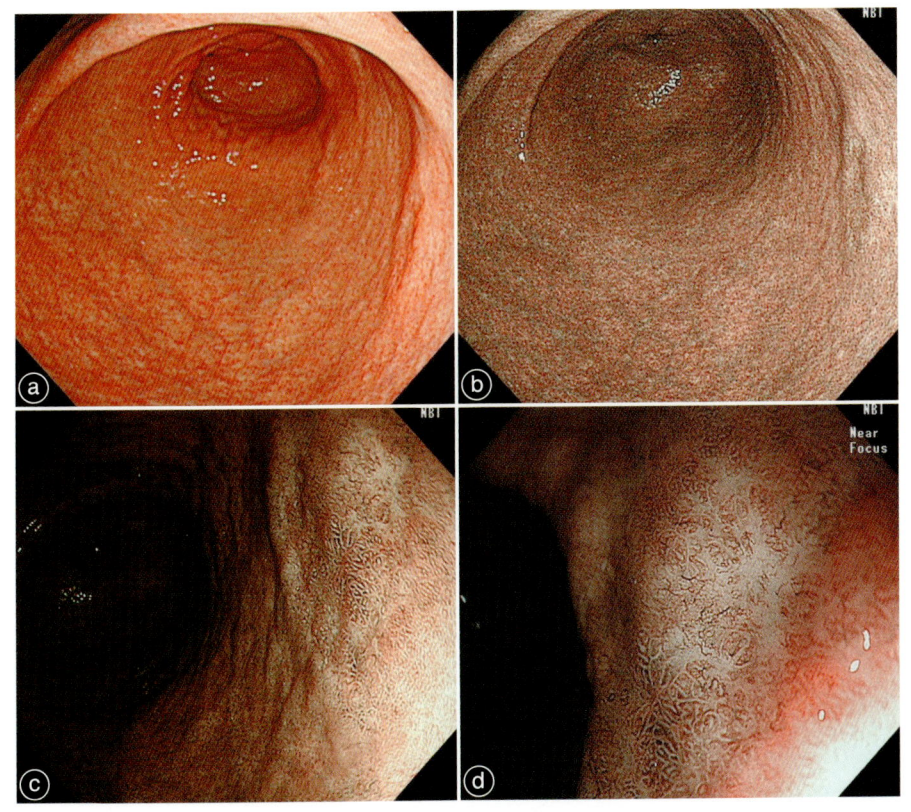

Fig. 1 Endoscopic images of Undifferentiated Depressed Early Gastric Carcinoma
a：Normal WLI observation（far view）　b：NBI non-magnifying observation（far view）
c：NBI non-magnifying observation（near view）　d：NBI Near Focus observation

A 0-Ⅱc lesion with a size of 15 mm is recognized on the posterior wall of the gastric angulus. NBI non-magnifying observation can provide an overview of the entire antrum from the far view, but normal WLI observation provides superior visibility. In the near view, NBI non-magnifying observation can clearly image the lesion. In NBI Near Focus observation, the microvessels in the depressed surface present a corkscrew pattern.

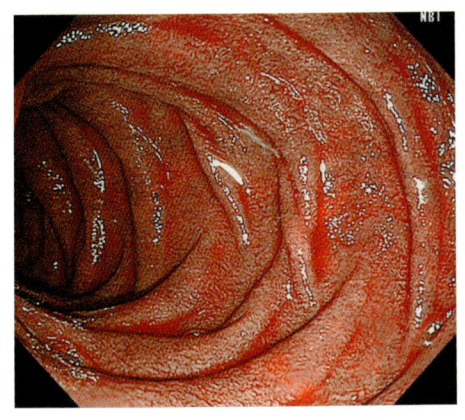

Fig. 2 NBI Non-Magnifying Observation of Normal Duodenal Mucosa (in the presence of bile)

The mucosal structures are almost impossible to see when bile is present.

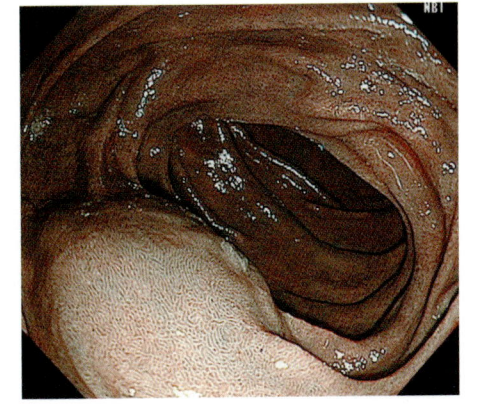

Fig. 3 NBI Non-Magnifying Observation of Duodenal Submucosal Tumor (in the absence of bile)

The mucosal structures can be imaged clearly when there is no bile.

hood increased the endoscope's diameter and effective manipulation of the magnification lever took practice, magnification observation proved to be unsuitable for screening. There were other problems, as well. For example, reducing the field of view to 75° made it hard to orient the scope towards the region of interest unless the magnification was increased very slowly. One of the biggest problems was the fact that contact with a lesion could easily occur. If this resulted in bleeding, which was quite likely since gastric carcinomas tend to bleed easily, subsequent NBI observation would be extremely difficult.

With the new EVIS LUCERA ELITE system, the problems associated with NBI observation have been largely solved thanks to the Dual Focus function, which combines a Normal Focus mode suitable for mid to far view and a Near Focus mode for close-up observation. As the depth of field in the Near Focus mode is 3 to 7 mm, detailed observation of a lesion is now possible without any risk of touching it with the endoscope. The distal hood is no longer necessary and the focus mode can be switched with one-touch operation. The field of view is maintained at 140° even in the Near Focus mode, enabling observation with a wide view field. Orientation in magnifying observation is also much easier than it was with the previous system (**Fig. 1d**), making the new system suitable for routine screenings as well as for detailed preoperative examinations. When a lesion with potential to become carcinomatous is found in WLI observation, move the endoscope close to the lesion, switch the focus mode to Near Focus with one-touch operation and start NBI observation. This method is expected to reduce unnecessary biopsies.

In actual observation, first use the Normal Focus mode to observe the far view ; then move the endoscope toward the lesion so that you can observe it in the near view. When the extent and overall view of the lesion have been identified, switch the focus mode to Near Focus for NBI magnifying observation. You can also use the electronic zoom if there are regions to be magnified. Keep in mind that, unlike in conventional magnifying observation, observation in the Near Focus mode can be affected by respiratory fluctuation because the distal end of the endoscope is not in contact with the gastric wall. This is particularly noticeable when the electronic zoom is used in the Near Focus mode. One way to minimize respiratory fluctuation is to ask the patient to hold their breath. Another point to keep in mind is that the maximum magnification of the optical zoom of the HQ290 is about 45x, which is roughly half that of the H260Z. Consequently, in some cases, you may not be able to observe the microvascular architecture in the mucosal surface layer in detail with the HQ290. Where diagnosis is difficult and you need to make more detailed observation, we recommend that you use the Q240Z or H260Z.

III. Recommended image enhancement settings

The appearance of the microstructures and microvascular morphology observed with NBI magnifying endoscopy are affected by the image enhancement settings, making it important to maintain consistent settings to ensure reliable observation results. This makes observations under constant setting conditions another key points in observation.

The EVIS LUCERA ELITE system has two image enhancement modes : contour enhancement and structure enhancement.

Contour enhancement is an image processing function that emphasizes the edges of subjects by means of mathematical differentiation. While the previous EVIS LUCERA SPECTRUM system only offered LOW, HIGH and OFF, the new EVIS LUCERA ELITE system lets you choose from 8 settings : E0 to E8 (E0=OFF). Contour enhancement is based on the principle that enhancing contours increases sharpness, thus making it

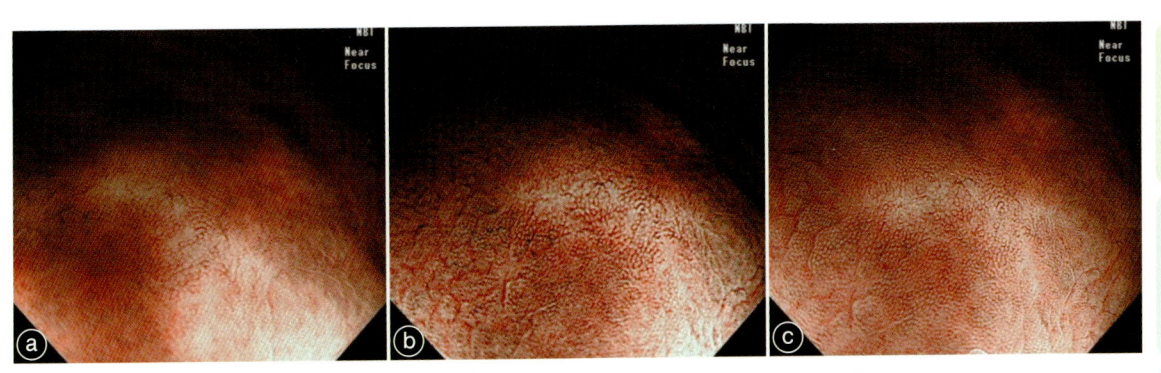

Fig. 4 NBI Near Focus Observation of Gastric Ulcer Scar
a：E8 mode   b：A8 mode   c：B8 mode

In the E8 mode, noise is also enhanced so the contrast is less clear. In the A8 mode, microvessels appear larger, making it more difficult to recognize mucosal microstructures in regions with densely clustered microvessels. In the B8 mode, both the microvessels and the mucosal microstructures are recognizable.

possible to diagnose the presence of lesions in the mid to far views. However, when contour enhancement is used in the stomach, noise is enhanced as well as the contours, so the visibility is not as good as with structure enhancement (**Fig. 4a**).

Structure enhancement is a digital image enhancement function. It enhances only the video frequency components useful to clarify changes in the structures displayed in the image such as the mucosal patterns and vascular directions. Structure enhancement has two modes—A and B—and the degree of enhancement can be set independently in each mode from 0 to 8 (0=OFF). The A mode is used to enhance relatively coarse patterns or observe rough mucosal structures in high contrast. In the gastroduodenal region, it is usually used in combination with WLI. The B mode is used to enhance finer patterns or observe small changes in mucosal structures or microvascular directions. In the gastroduodenal region, it is usually used in combination with NBI magnifying observation. In fact, as the A mode enhances microvessels in such a way that they appear excessively large, it can make it harder to see mucosal microstructures as they will be hidden when there is a dense cluster of microvessels which may appear as an undifferentiated mass (**Fig. 4b**). It is up to you which mode you use, but at our hospital we prefer to use B8 mode in the NBI magnifying observation (**Fig. 4c**).

Three color modes are available. In conventional practice, color mode 1 is usually used in the esophagus and stomach, color mode 2 in the stomach, and color mode 3 in the colon. This is the same with the EVIS LUCERA ELITE system.

IV. Findings on normal gastroduodenal mucosa

The normal mucosa in the gastric fundic gland region and that in the pyloric gland region have different surface microstructures and microvascular architecture. In the fundic region, the crypt is perpendicular to the mucosa so the ducts present a white circular shape while the microvessels surround the ducts with a meshed pattern (**Fig. 5**). In the pyloric region, the crypt is oblique with respect to the mucosa, so the ducts present an arc-like shape and microvessels are recognized as open coiled loops (**Fig. 6**). It has been reported that the surface microstructures and microvascular architecture tend to be irregular or disappear in neoplastic lesions[1,2].

The normal duodenal mucosa presents regular villous architecture. As observation of the crypts is difficult because these are hidden by the villus, observation of the

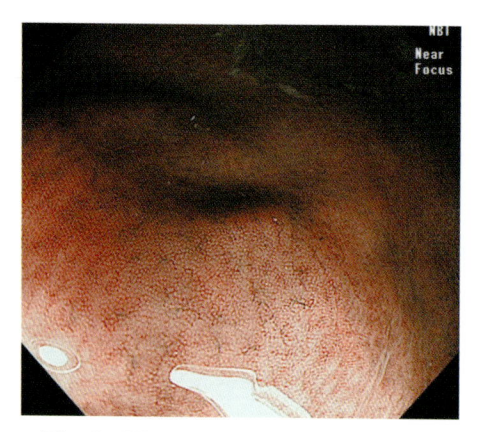

Fig. 5 NBI Near Focus Observation of Normal Mucosa in Fundic Gland Region

The gland ducts present a white circular shape and microvessels present a mesh pattern surrounding the gland ducts.

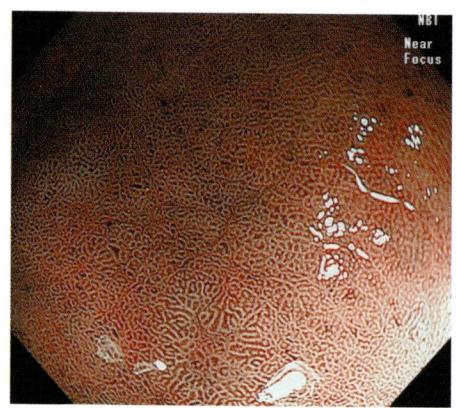

Fig. 6 NBI Near Focus Observation of Normal Mucosa in Gastric Pyloric Gland

The gland ducts present an arc-like shape, and microvessels present a coil-like open loop.

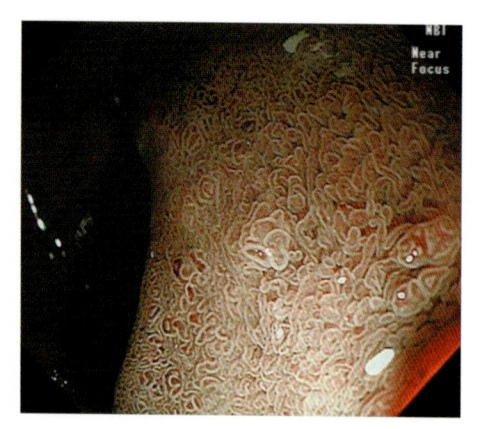

Fig. 7 NBI Near Focus Observation of Normal Duodenal Mucosa

The duodenal mucosa presents regularly arranged villous architecture.

morphology of villus is more important in the duodenum (**Fig. 7**). With neoplastic lesions, the villous morphology disappears and irregular mucosal microstructures and microvascular architecture are observed in its place[4].

Conclusion

Endoscopic diagnosis based on NBI magnifying observation is being established, but its application has thus far been limited to detailed preoperative examinations. The introduction of the EVIS LUCERA ELITE system will expand the use of NBI magnifying observation from this limited area to screenings. NBI Near Focus observation can not only be expected to reduce unnecessary biopsies, but will also help considerably in early detection of lesions in cases with a high risk of carcinogenesis such as chronic gastritis cases.

References

1) Nakayoshi, T., Tajiri, H., Matsuda, K. et al. : Magnifying endoscopy combined with narrow band imaging system for early gastric cancer : correlation of vascular pattern with histopathology. Endoscopy 2004 ; 36 (12) : 1080-1084
2) Yao, K., Anagnostopoulos, GK. and Ragunath, K. : Magnifying endoscopy for diagnosing and delineating early gastric cancer. Endoscopy 2009 ; 41 (5) : 462-467
3) Ezoe, Y., Muto, M., Uedo, N. et al. : Magnifying narrowband imaging is more accurate than conventional white-light imaging in diagnosis of gastric mucosal cancer. Gastroenterology 2011 ; 141 (6) : 2017-2025
4) Yoshimura. N., Goda, K., Tajiri, H. et al. : Endoscopic features of nonampullary duodenal tumors with narrow-band imaging. Hepatogastroenterology 2010 ; 57 (99-100) : 462-467

(Mochizuki, S., Fujishiro, M., Koike, K.)

Stomach and Duodenum

General Theory : How to Observe These Regions with NBI or BLI

Tips on BLI Observation

■ Introduction

Conventional endoscopy systems use white light from a xenon light source for illumination. LASEREO (Fujifilm), a new-generation endoscopy system, is the world's first to use laser light for illumination. Based on a narrow-band imaging method called BLI (Blue Laser Imaging), which generates illumination using two types of laser combined with phosphor, this new system is able to image microvessels in the mucosal surface layer and the mucosal surface structures in high contrast by taking advantage of the light absorbance characteristics of hemoglobin and the light scattering characteristics of mucosa. The LASEREO series currently includes the VP-4450HD processor, the LL-4450 laser light source, the L590 series dedicated endoscopes (including the EG-L590ZW gastrointestinal magnifying endoscope, the EG-L590WR general-purpose gastrointestinal endoscope, the EC-L590ZW magnifying colonoscope and the EC-L590ZWM general-purpose colonoscope) (as of August 2013).

Until now, the illumination used to capture endoscopic images has been the white light from a xenon light source. Using laser illumination instead makes it possible to obtain endoscopic images quite different in appearance from conventional ones. Although the LASEREO system has only recently begun to be applied clinically, we will offer some tips on using BLI that have been gleaned from its use so far.

■ I. Characteristics of the LASEREO system

The LASEREO light source incorporates two lasers with different wavelengths and is able to provide a range of illumination from white light imaging to BLI by changing the light emission intensities of the two lasers. The white light laser (450 nm±10 nm) is used to obtain white light with a wide spectral wavelength for normal observation by causing phosphor to emit the light. The BLI laser for narrow-band imaging (410 nm±10 nm) emits light with a shorter wavelength that is easily absorbed by blood vessels and resistant to scattering inside the mucosa. Like NBI, this improves the contrast of the microvascular architecture and fine mucosal patterns on the mucosal surface layer. The clinical significance of BLI observation is similar to NBI observation[1,2], and it is capable of finding the brownish area that indicates a neoplastic lesion on the squamous epithelial mucosa, as well as the light blue crest (LBC) that indicates an intestinal metaplasia of the gastric mucosa.

The optical zoom function is motorized. Information on the approximate location of the lens is displayed and the shutter speed that is interlocked with the lens location is increased. Deterioration-free magnification up to 135× on a 19-inch monitor is possible with optical zoom, and magnification up to 270× can be obtained by using it in combination with the electronic zoom.

When the resolution of the EC-L590ZW was measured independently using a resolution chart (negative) (**Fig. 1**) (**Table**), we were able to resolve a thin line equivalent to 4.9 μm (6-5 in the chart) at full magnification (130×) in white-light observation. With full magnification (130×) in BLI observation, resolution is as high as 5.5 μm, which is regarded as suitable for observation of microvessels on the mucosal surface.

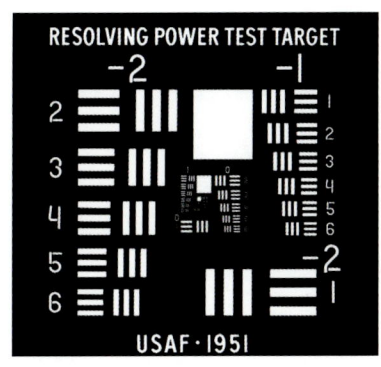

Fig. 1 Resolution Chart (Negative)

Table Resolution of the EC-L590ZW Obtained from the Resolution Chart

Magnification	Structure enhancement	White light	BLI	BLI-bright
Normal		4-3		
	A0		4-1	4-1
	B0		4-1	4-2
40×		4-6		
	A0		4-5	4-6
	B0		4-5	4-6
70×		6-3		
	A0		6-2	6-2
	B0		6-3	6-2
130×		6-5		
	A0		6-4	6-3
	B0		6-4	6-3

II. How to use the BLI and BLI-bright modes

Narrow-band imaging is available in two modes: BLI and BLI-bright. In the BLI mode features, the ratio of BLI laser light is increased in order to maximize the contrast of microvessels on the mucosal surface layer. The BLI-bright mode combines BLI laser light with white-light laser light, providing an optimum balance between the two that enables the observer to benefit from improvements in both image brightness and vascular imaging contrast. The illumination radiated in the BLI mode is comprised almost entirely of short-wavelength components, making it suitable for observing surface structures and microvessels using mid to high magnification, while the BLI-bright mode has a slightly higher white-light component; its high brightness is suitable for non-magnifying observation of the far view or for low- to mid-magnification observation (**Figs. 2 & 3**).

The authors interviewed endoscopists experienced in the use of BLI and asked them to describe the appropriate uses of the BLI and BLI-bright modes. Most reported that in routine observation of the laryngopharynx and esophagus, they would switch to the BLI-bright mode during endoscope insertion and use white-light imaging for endoscope withdrawal. In routine observation of the stomach, some said they did not use the BLI mode because it was not bright enough, while others reported using the BLI-bright mode in about half of all examinations they performed. While use of the BLI mode in magnifying observation is standard, many considered high magnification observation in the BLI-bright mode to be of comparable quality to that in the BLI mode. It was also found that in order to maintain brightness in the BLI mode, the shutter speed was normally set to 1/100, whereas in the BLI-bright mode, image quality can be maintained with higher shutter speeds, meaning that shutter speed can be increased to 1/200 when necessary without compromising image quality.

III. Setting the structure enhancement

Endoscopy covers a broad range of observation targets, from the background mucosa to microlesions. In magnifying observation, it is also necessary to observe the microstructures and microvessels in the superficial mucosa. To deal with various observation conditions and targets, the structure enhancement of BLI provides two enhancement modes with different enhanced frequency bands, the A mode and the B mode. Each mode has nine enhancement

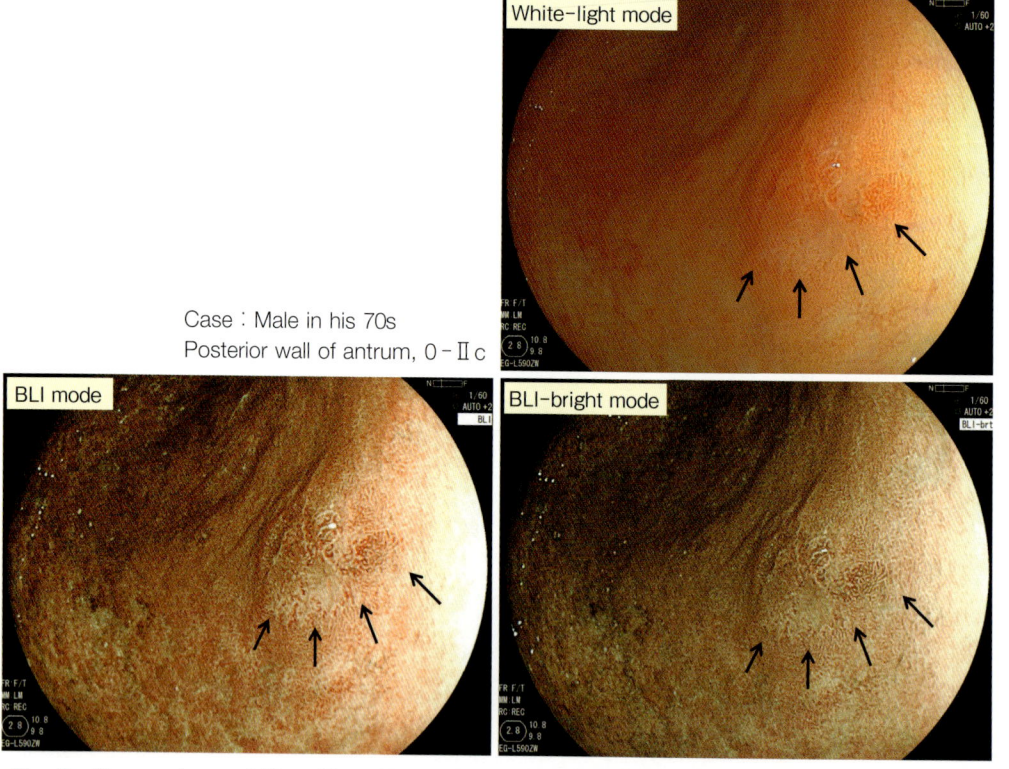

Case : Male in his 70s
Posterior wall of antrum, 0 - Ⅱ c

Fig. 2　Comparison of Non-Magnifying Observation between BLI and BLI-bright Modes

steps from 0 to 8 (A0 to A8 and B0 to B8). The A mode is designed to enhance lower frequency bands than the B mode and is therefore considered best for structure enhancement in colonoscopies, while the B mode is designed to enhance only thin lines, making it more suitable for microvascular observation (**Fig. 4**).

In fact, general opinion has it that there is not much difference between the A and B modes. Many endoscopists say that they utilize the capabilities of both settings. For example, prior to endoscopic observation of the stomach, structure enhancement is set to B8 and B6 of the B mode so that they can be switched on the front panel as required. Usually B6 is used, as B8's stronger image enhancement often results in more noticeable noise such as graininess or glittering.

Ⅳ. Setting the color enhancement

Lesions in the gastrointestinal tracts can cause variations in mucosal epithelium and vascular densities that cause a similarly wide variation in the reproduced color tones. To obtain the best lesion imaging effects in different regions, BLI provides three color tones : C1, which was originally intended for the esophagus ; C2 for the stomach ; and C3 for the colon (**Fig. 5**). Furthermore, the BLI-bright mode provides an additional color tone that closely resembles white-light imaging, called "no color enhancement". The color tone becomes increasingly green as the tone is stepped up from C1 to C2 and C3. Many endoscopists employ C1, which has a strong brownish tone similar to NBI, in upper gastrointestinal observations, and C2 in the lower gastrointestinal observations.

Ⅴ. Features of BLI observation

The laser light source has some features not available with conventional xenon light sources, which include a monochromatic property thanks to the very narrow wavelength band,

<a>

BLI mode   BLI-bright mode

<b>

BLI mode   BLI-bright mode

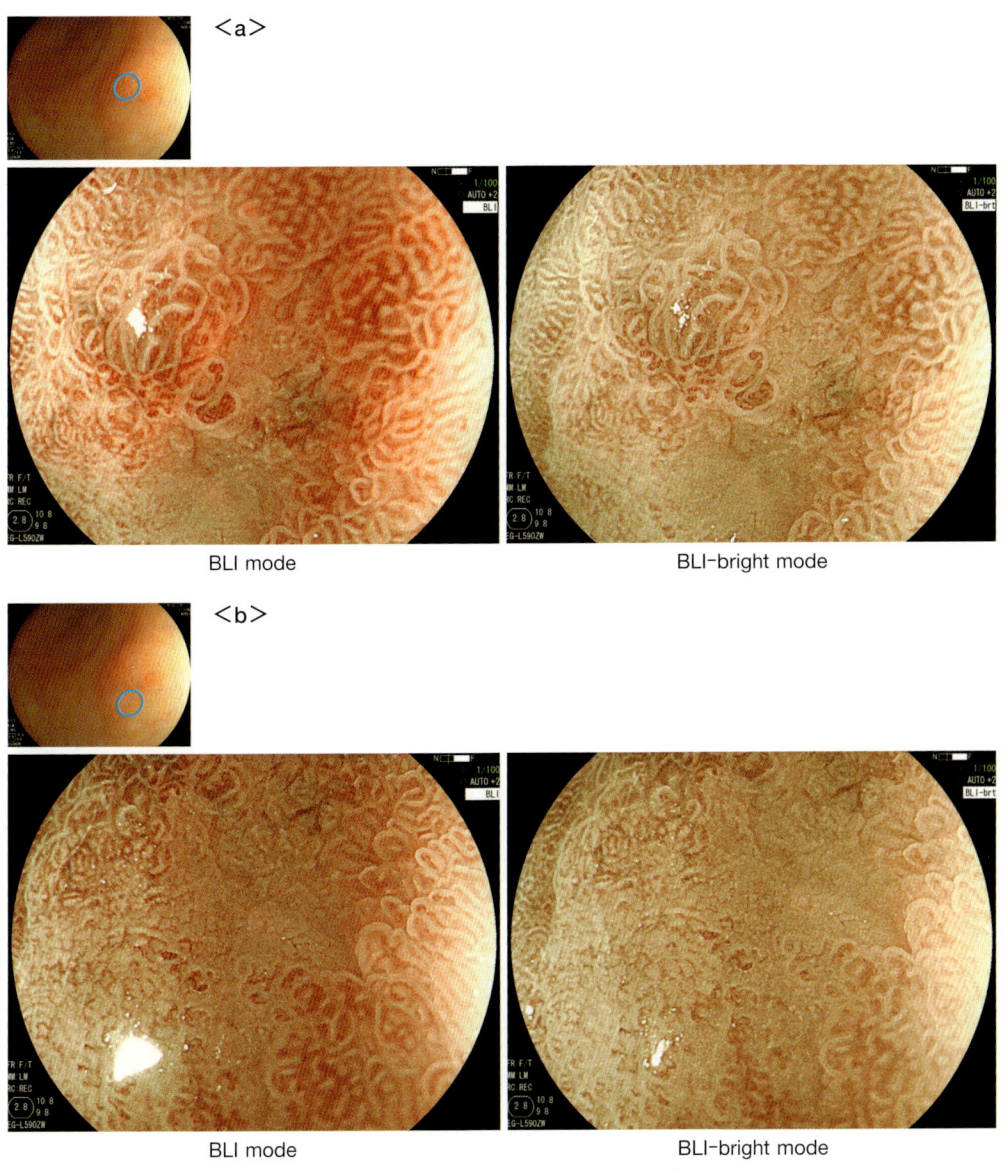

Fig. 3   Comparison of Magnifying Observation between BLI and BLI-bright Modes
(same case as Fig. 2)

directivity that does not cause scattering or expansion of light, and economy thanks to the compact size, light weight, low power consumption and long service life. These features lead to certain differences between BLI observation and NBI observation. Instead of producing narrow-band light by using a filter like the NBI system, the BLI system can emit narrow-band light directly so that bright images can be obtained even from a far view, the light source does not need to be replaced, and the low power consumption helps reduce the running cost.

Many endoscopists also found focus adjustment easy with the BLI system. Though when considered from a photographic standpoint, the images lack depth and do not clearly represent surface irregularities ; they offer an improved view of surface microstructures and make it possible to observe microvessels at a deeper location. On the other hand, the clear

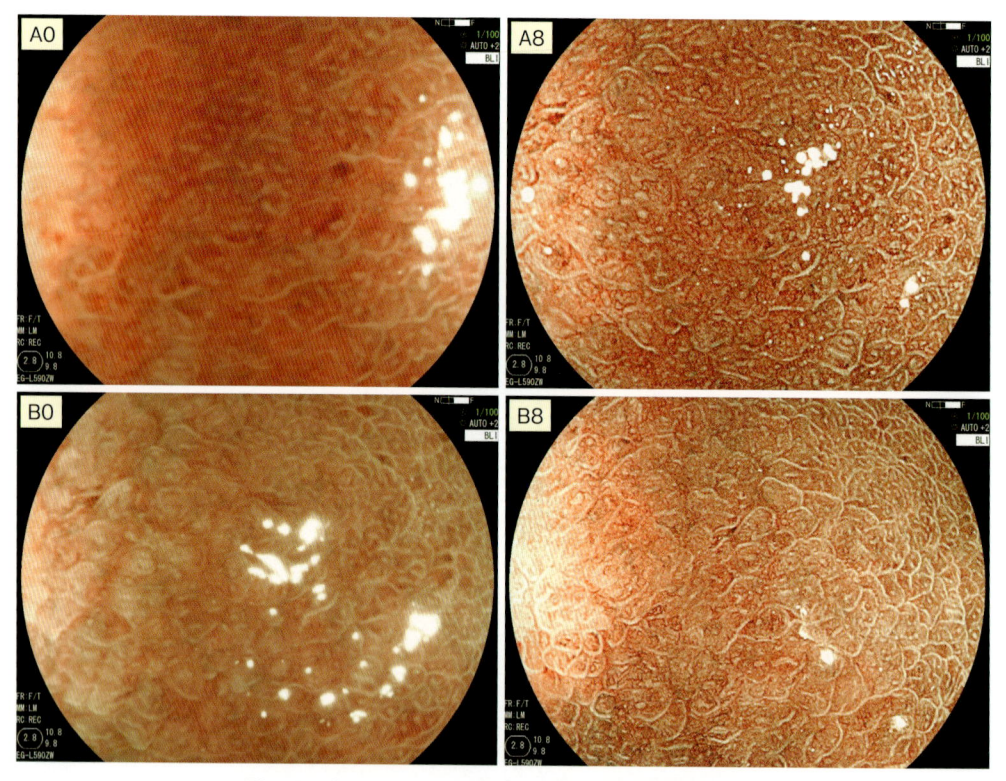

Fig. 4 Comparison of Structure Enhancement

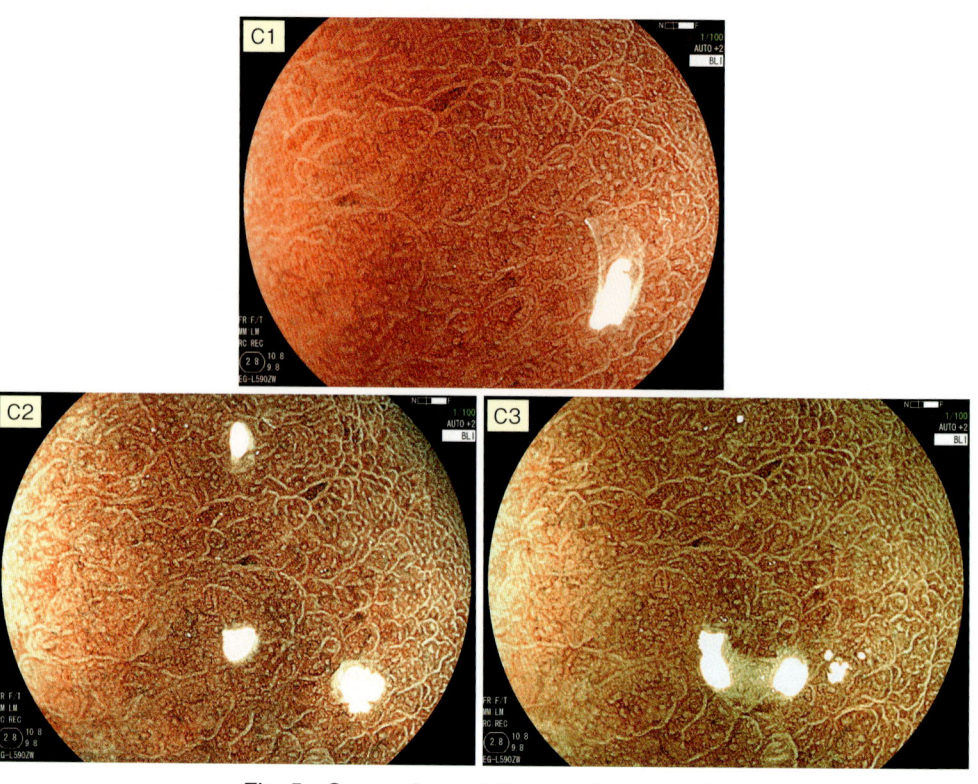

Fig. 5 Comparison of Color Enhancement

108

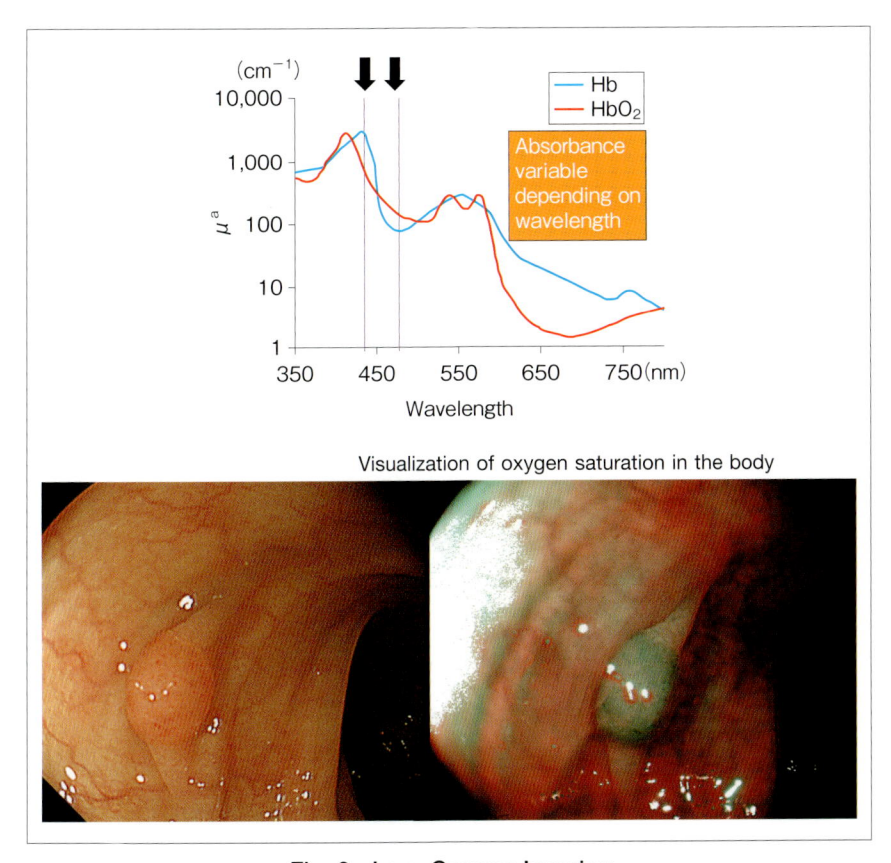

Fig. 6 Low-Oxygen Imaging
Two kinds of laser light (↓↓) for low-oxygen imaging are irradiated in the living body.

view of microvessels makes identification of demarcations difficult in some cases.

Conclusion

The LASEREO system has been designed to incorporate laser light with any wavelength, so it can be developed into a new endoscopic diagnosis system by creating observation modes for specific functionality, as well as for specific target tissue and target molecules. At this time, a low-oxygen imaging system has been put to practical use, which visualizes the oxygen saturation in the living body by irradiating the laser light specialized for low-oxygen imaging in the body (**Fig. 6**).

References
1) Yoshida, N., Hisabe, T., Inada, Y. et al. : The ability of a novel blue laser imaging system for the diagnosis of invasion depth of colorectal neoplasms. J. Gastroenterol. 2013 Mar 15. [Epub ahead of print]
2) Yoshida, N., Yagi, N., Inada, Y. et al. : Ability of a novel blue laser imaging system for the diagnosis of colorectal polyps. Dig. Endosc. 2013 Jun 3. [Epub ahead of print]

(Kato, M., Ono, S., Yagi, N., Yoshida, S.)

Case 26 Chronic gastritis

Case 1 Female in her 30s **Purpose** General checkup *H. pylori* negative case

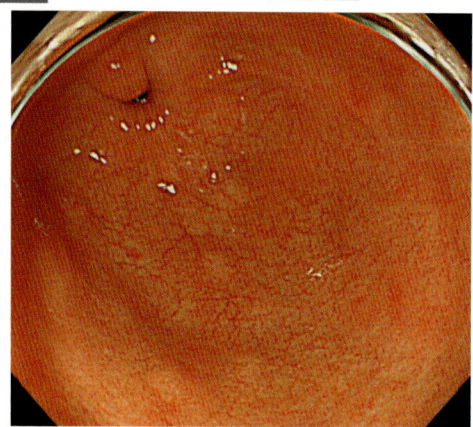

Endoscopic image of antrum: The mucosa has no surface irregularities and light erythematous erosion is observed. Blood vessels are visible in the region close to the pyloric ring. This is a typical endoscopic image of an antrum of an *H. pylori* negative case. [Quoted from Reference 1)]

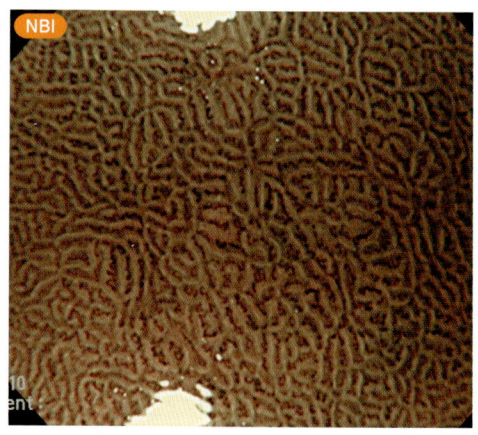

NBI magnifying observation of antrum: A tubular pattern is formed by white zones, and vessels look as if they are enclosed inside it. This is a typical magnifying endoscopic image of the antrum of an *H. pylori* negative case. [Quoted from Reference 1)]

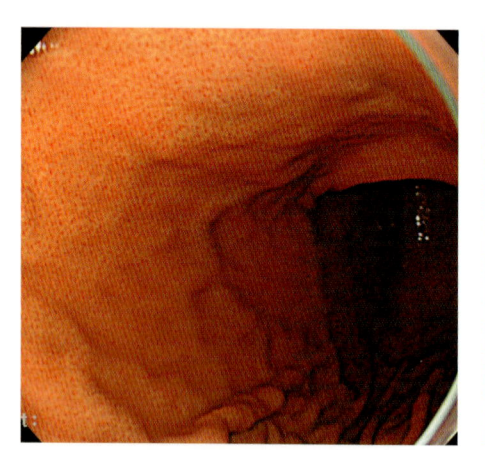

Endoscopic image of gastric body: The branched vessels observed with atrophic mucosa are not observed here. Collecting venules that look like dots are observed on the whole gastric body. This is a typical endoscopic image of the gastric body of an *H. pylori* negative case.

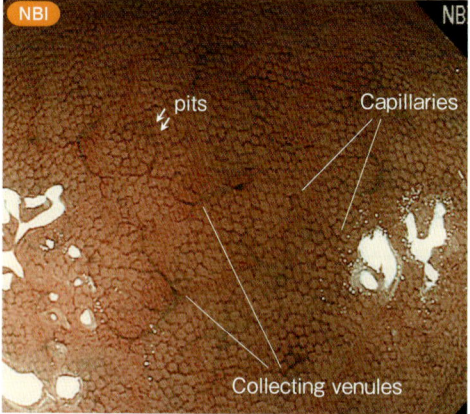

Magnifying observation of gastric body: Capillaries forming a network are observed around the collecting venules, and circular gland pits are observed in the network. This is a typical magnifying endoscopic image of the gastric body of an *H. pylori* negative case. [Quoted from Reference 1)]

Reference
1) Yagi, K. and Ajioka, Y. : Magnification Endoscopic Diagnosis of Stomach (in Japanese, title translated). 2010, Igaku-Shoin, Ltd., Tokyo.
2) Uedo, N. et al. : Endoscopy 2006 ; 38 : 819-824

Endoscope：GIF-H260Z（Olympus）　Light source：EVIS LUCERA SPECTRUM（Olympus）
NBI setup：Structure enhancement A8, color mode 3

Case 2　Male in his 50 s　*Purpose*　Epigastric discomfort　*H. pylori* positive case

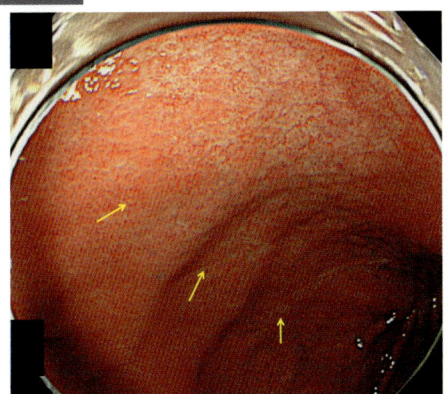

Endoscopic image of anterior wall of body：The yellow arrows indicate the gland boundary. The region below the yellow arrows（greater curvature side）indicates fundic gland mucosa, while the region above them（lesser curvature side）is atrophic mucosa ; pseudopyloric glands mucosa or intestinal metaplasia.

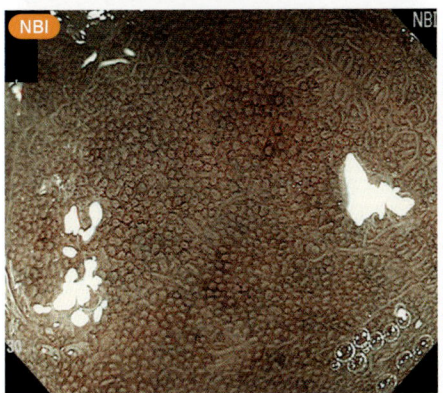

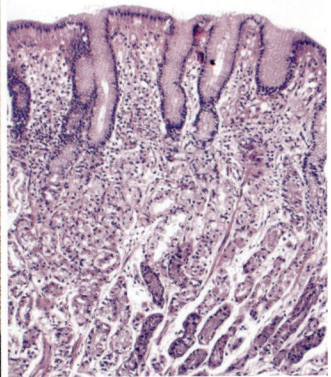

Left：NBI magnifying observation of non-atrophic region. Circular pits are observed accompanied by size irregularities and irregular morphology. It is a magnified image of the fundic gland mucosa accompanied with inflammation. [Quoted from Reference 1)]
Right：Biopsy tissue observation of the left image. The gastric fundic gland is still there, but infiltration of inflammatory cells is observed from neck zone to subepithelial region. [Quoted from Reference 1)]

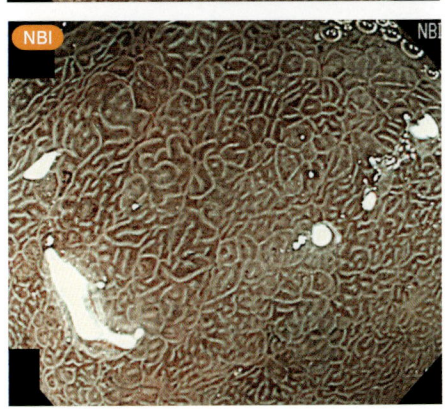

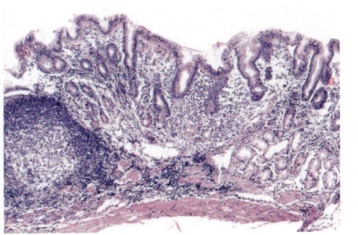

Left：NBI magnifying observation of atrophic region. A tubular pattern by the white zone is observed but no circular pits like those observed in the non-atrophic region can be identified. Light blue materials are observed on the margin of the white zone. These are what is called the light blue crests（LBCs）and is coincident with the brush border of the intestinal metaplasia[2]. [Quoted from Reference 1)]
Right：Biopsy tissue observation of the left image. Infiltration of inflammatory cells is observed. The fundic gland has disappeared, and the pseudopyloric glands are observed instead. It is the histologic image of an atrophic mucosa. [Quoted from Reference 1)]

Comment

Chronic gastritis cases are caused by *H. pylori* or the autoimmune mechanism, but the overwhelming majority of cases in Japan are due to *H, pylori*. To understand the findings accompanying chronic gastritis, it is necessary to understand the normal *H. pylori*-negative stomach. The body region and the proximal side of the antrum consist of fundic gland mucosa, which is recognized as collecting venules in endoscopic observation. The distal side of the antrum consists of pyloric gland mucosa. The crypt epithelium of the fundic gland mucosa presents circular pits, while that of the pyloric gland mucosa presents a tubular pattern. Continuous infection of *H. pylori* causes an inflammation, makes the fundic gland atrophic, transforms it into a pseudopyloric gland metaplasia and eventually produces intestinal metaplasia. This is the chronic gastritis induced by *H. pylori*.

（Yagi, K., Nozawa, Y., Nakamura, A.）

Case 27 Chronic gastritis

Male in his 60s | Purpose | Detailed observation of background mucosa of a patient undergoing endoscopic treatment for early gastric carcinoma | Location | Posterior wall of the antrum

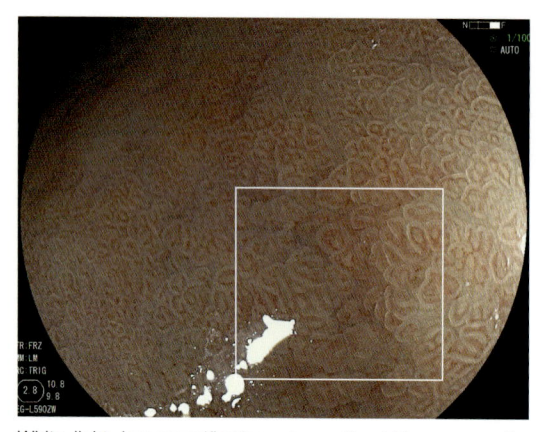

White-light low-magnification observation: Mucosa on the posterior wall of the antrum of an *H. pylori* positive case subjected to endoscopic treatment of early gastric carcinoma.

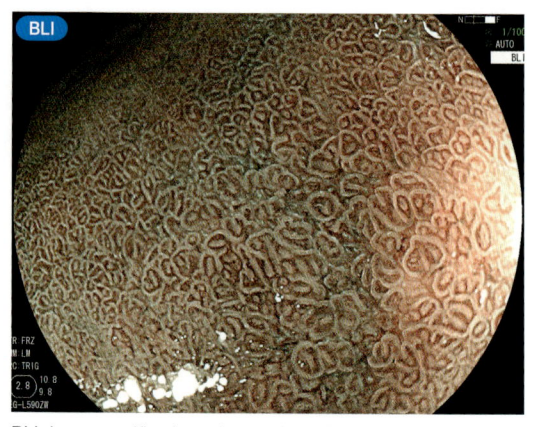

BLI low-magnification observation: From the center to the bottom of the image, strip-shaped mucosa that seems to have a light blue crest (LBC) is observed.

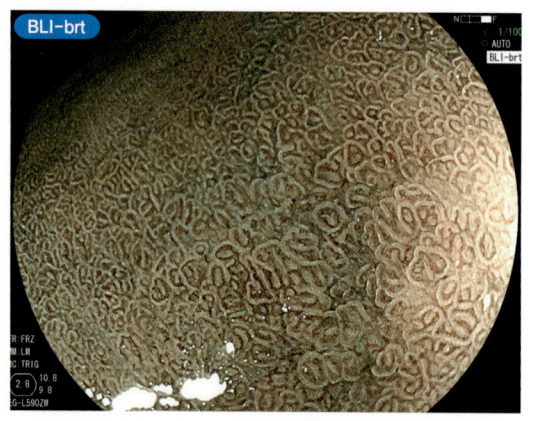

BLI-bright low-magnification observation.

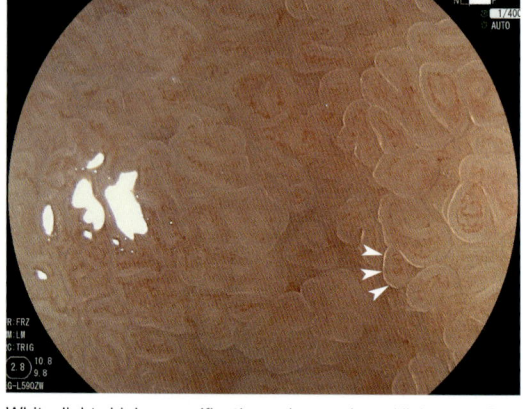

White-light high-magnification observation: High-magnification image of the area inside the white square in the white-light low-magnification image. On the right part of the image, a white edge formed by back-scattered light generated by a tangential projection of light on the surface of the crypt epithelium can be seen (white arrowheads).

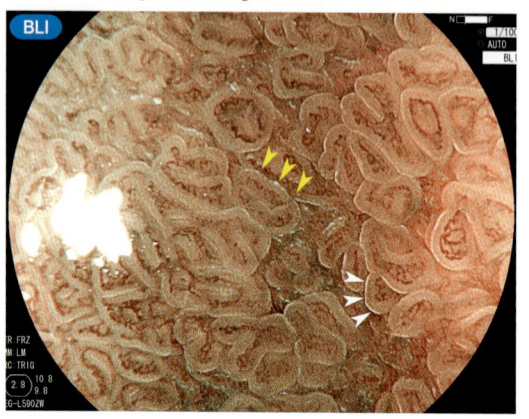

BLI high-magnification observation: Light blue edges (LBCs, indicated by yellow arrowheads), which are hard to see with white-light observation, are observed in the BLI mode on the surface of the marginal crypt epithelium of the intestinal metaplasia in the center of the image. While the edge formed by the back-scattered light from the margin of the crypt epithelium (white arrowheads) has a whitish color, regular margin and even thickness, the LBCs have a light bluish color, slightly irregular margin and irregular thickness.

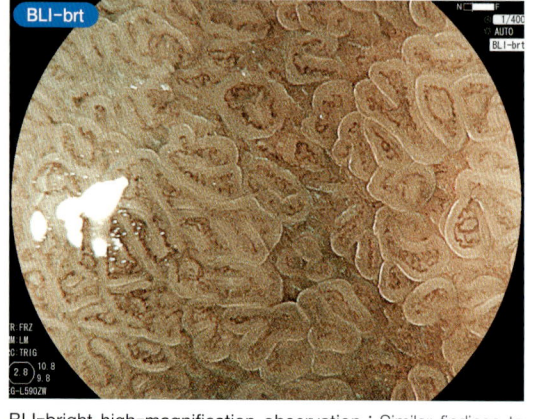

BLI-bright high-magnification observation: Similar findings to those found in BLI high-magnification observation are identified but they do not look as sharp.

Endoscope : EG-L590ZW (Fujifilm)   Light source : LASEREO (Fujifilm)
BLI setup : Structure enhancement A6, color enhancement C1

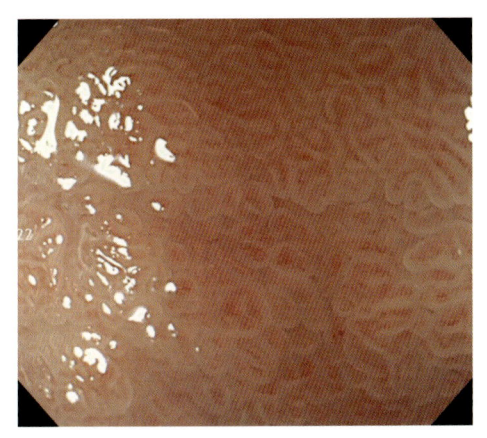

WLI magnifying observation images of the same case in almost the same region, obtained using the EVIS GIF-H260Z and the CV-290 processor (LUCERA ELITE).

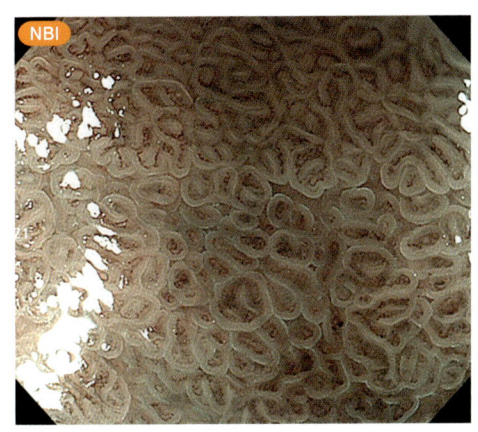

NBI magnifying observation : LBCs are found on the surface of the marginal crypt epithelium of the intestinal metaplasia in the center to the bottom of the image.

Comment

These are endoscopic images of intestinal metaplasia with chronic atrophic gastritis observed in an *H. pylori* positive case. The intestinal metaplasia is distributed in a patchy or diffuse way on the gastric mucosa and often presents a ridged or papillary surface structure. When illuminated with narrow-band light with a short wavelength, light blue edges (light blue crests) are produced on the surface of the crypt epithelium. This is believed to be produced by strong reflection of the short-wavelength light by the microvilli (brush border) on the surface of the intestinal metaplasia.

In the NBI image, the white edges formed by the convergence of back-scattered light produced light projected tangentially on the surface of the marginal crypt epithelium are whitish (white arrowheads) because the light is composed of the both 400 to 430 nm and 525 to 555 nm wavelengths. The LBCs, on the other hand, are imaged in cyan (yellow arrowheads)—the color produced by the stronger reflection of the 400 to 430 nm light (assigned to Green and Blue color channels) (**Figure**). The LBCs are not uniformly thin lines and can be differentiated by their relatively irregular margins and uneven thickness.

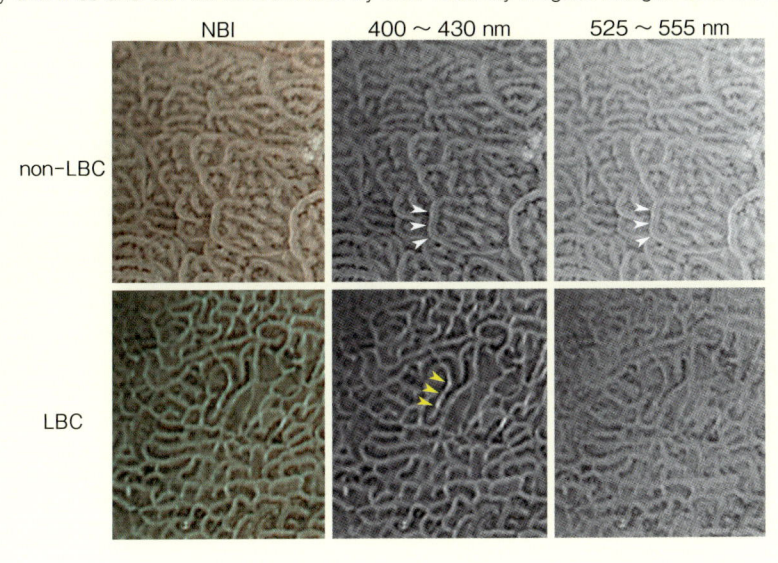

Figure

(Uedo, N.)

Case 28 Gastric adenoma

Male in his 60s | **Purpose** Follow-up of adenoma in another region
Location Lesser curvature of gastric angle | **Macroscopic type** Surface elevation

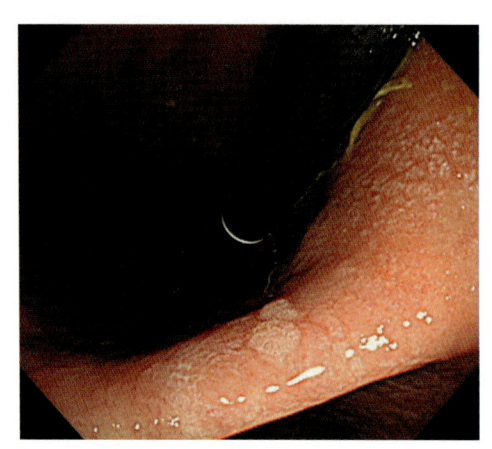

WLI non-magnifying observation: A white elevated lesion with a 5-mm diameter is observed on the lesser curvature of the gastric angle. The lesion has different properties from the normal mucosa but presents a regular surface structure.

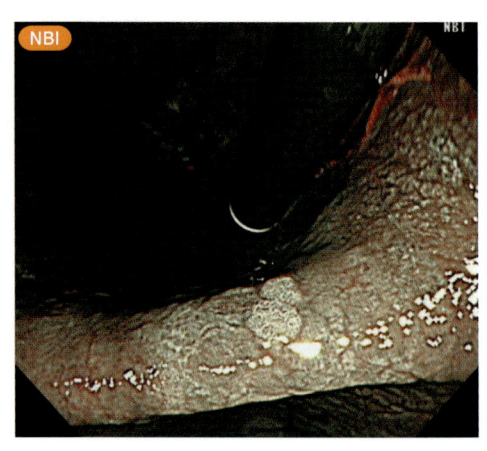

NBI observation of the same region: Surface structure can be observed more easily in NBI image than in WLI image, NBI image shows that this lesion has different surface structure from the normal mucosa with clear demarcation.

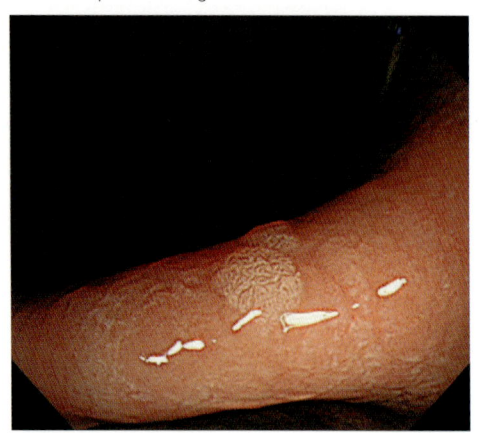

WLI non-magnifying observation: Even though an endoscope does not have magnifying function, the regular surface microstructures can be observed by approaching the lesion and adjusting the focus correctly.

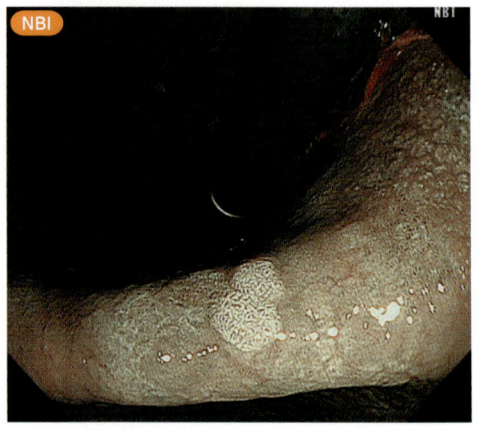

NBI non-magnifying close-up observation: The surface microstructures can be observed more clearly than WLI.

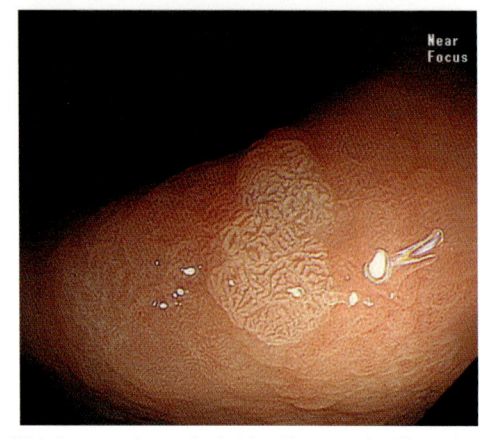

WLI close-up observation in Near Focus mode: The surface microstructures can be observed more clearly than the non-magnifying observation.

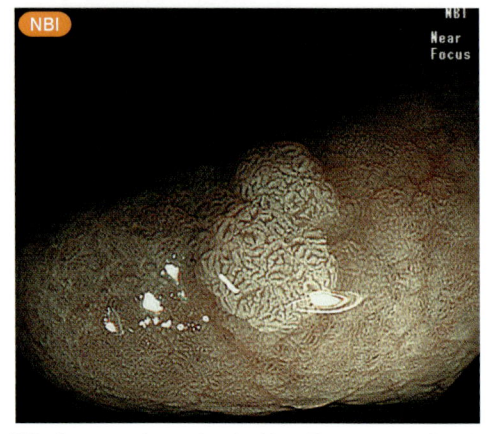

NBI close-up observation in Near Focus mode: Regular surface microstructures can be observed. The microvessels are not recognizable due to the white opaque substance (WOS), but the regular structures of the WOS can be observed.

> Endoscope : GIF-HQ290 (Olympus)　　Light source : EVIS LUCERA ELITE (Olympus)
> NBI setup : Structure enhancement B8 (A8 used partially in far view), WLI A8, color mode 1

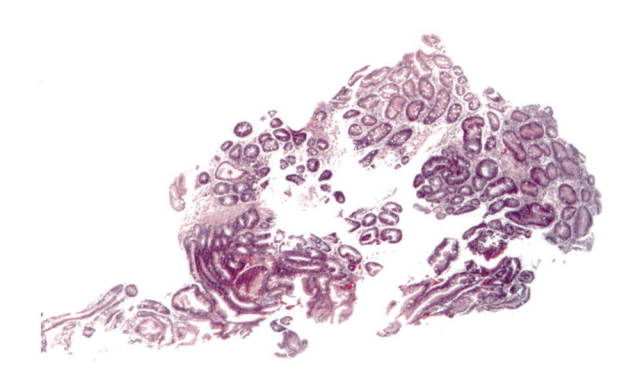

As a result of biopsy, the lesion is diagnosed as a tubular adenoma with mild atypia.

Comment

The endoscopic diagnosis is made using the EVIS LUCERA ELITE system and the GIF-HQ290 endoscope. The non-magnifying observations using WLI and NBI represents this whitish flat elevated lesion respectively as a normal mucosa and a region with obvious color tone alteration. The surface microstructures can be viewed roughly even with the non-magnifying close-up observations, but the use of NBI and the Near Focus mode makes them more clearly observable. The lesion can be recognized as a structurally changed region with clear demarcation from the normal mucosa. Although microvessels cannot be recognized due to the WOS, the WOS has a regular structure so the lesion is diagnosed endoscopically as an adenoma. After the biopsy, it is diagnosed as a tubular adenoma with mild atypia. As the atypia is actually mild and the result is not contradictory to the endoscopic diagnosis, the lesion is put to follow-up observation.

▶**Observation tips** With this system, even microstructures can be recognized clearly by the close-up observation in the Near Focus mode. When the endoscope is approached to the target lesion, the focus is lost at a certain distance. By switching the observation mode to the Near Focus mode at that distance, a well-focused close-up image can be obtained and the microstructures can be observed.

(Kodashima, S.)

Case 29 Gastric adenoma

Male in his 60s   Purpose Detailed observation of gastric lesion
Location Posterior wall of greater curvature of antrum   Macroscopic type 0-IIa

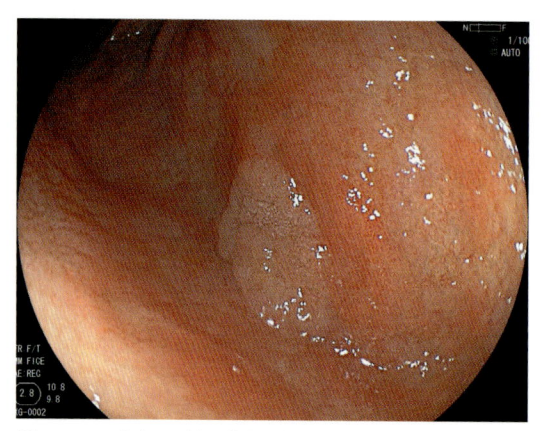

Non-magnifying white-light observation : A flat elevated lesion of less than 10 mm with a regular surface is observed in the greater curvature of the antrum.

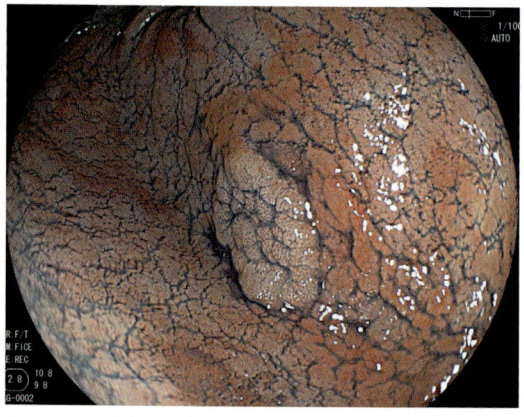

Non-magnifying chromoendoscopy : Indigo carmine spraying clarifies the surface structures of the lesion, showing that it is a well-demarcated lesion with surface irregularities.

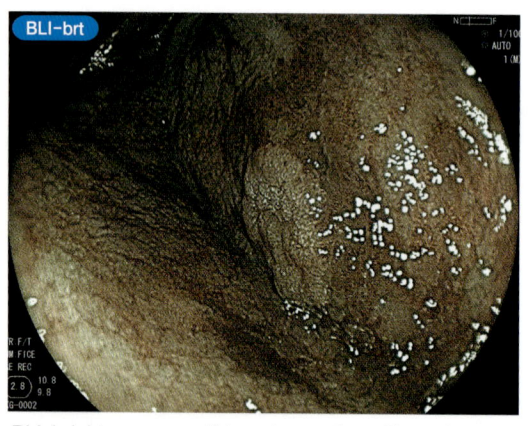

BLI-bright non-magnifying observation : The color tone of the lesion is enhanced and clarified.

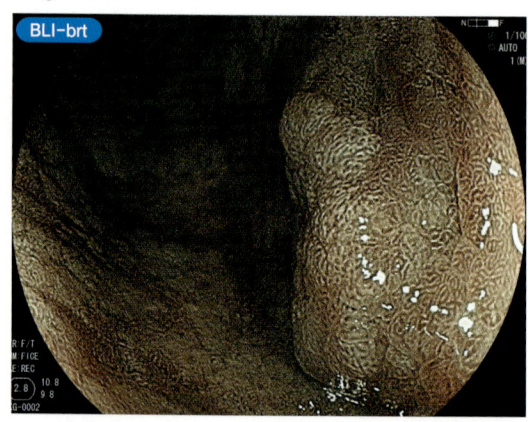

BLI-bright low-magnification observation.

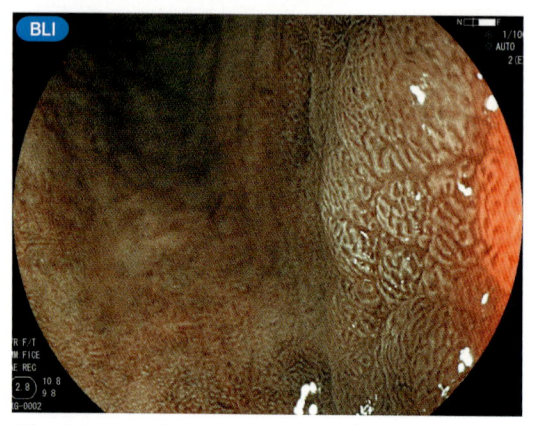

BLI high-magnification observation (greater curvature on the distal side) : The presence of WOS (white opaque substance) obscures the subepithelial microvascular architecture. When the WOS is utilized as an alternative optical sign, the WOS shows well-organized and symmetrical distribution with a regular reticular pattern.

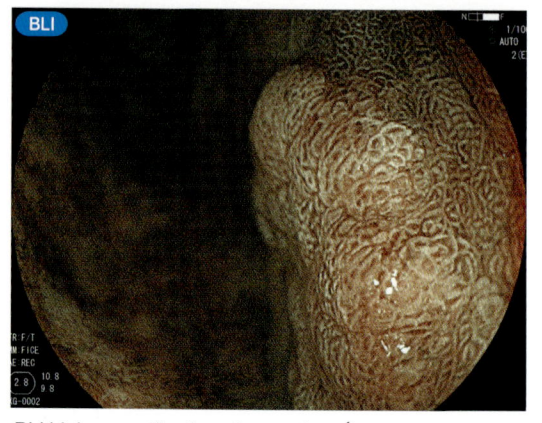

BLI high-magnification observation (lesser curvature on the proximal side) : A clear demarcation line is observed in the margin.

> Endoscope：Prototype（EG-L590ZW equivalent）（Fujifilm）　　Light source：LASEREO（Fujifilm）
> BLI setup：BLI—Structure enhancement A6, color enhancement C1 ; BLI-bright—Structure enhancement B8, color enhancement C1

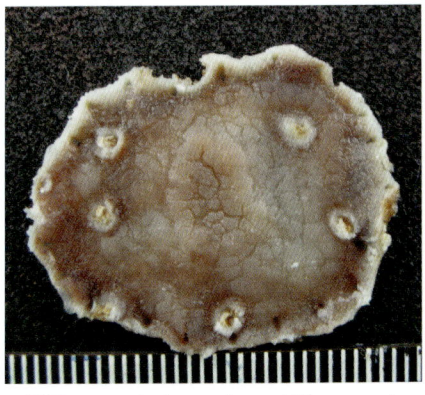

Loupe image

ESD resected specimen：The specimen is 30×25 mm and has an adenoma lesion of 8×6 mm.

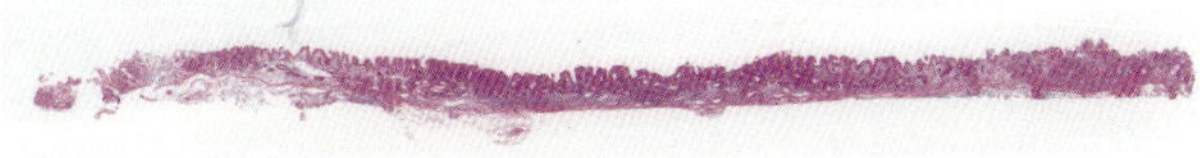

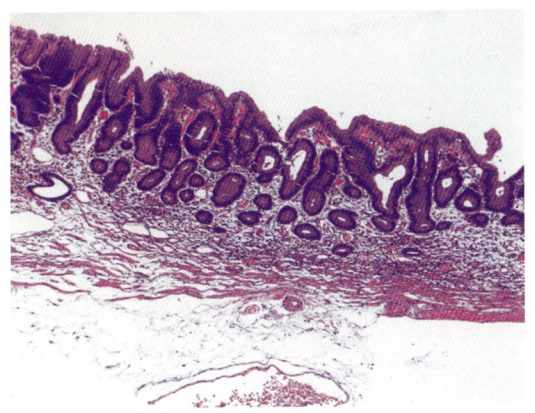

Low-magnification image：Tubular adenoma of stomach, moderate atypia, HM0, VM0.

Comment

In this case, because the WOS obscures the subepithelial microvascular architecture, the microvascular pattern could not be visualized, making it impossible to evaluate the microvascular architecture. In cases like this, the WOS should be utilized as an alternative optical sign. When this case was observed with 100× magnification, it was found that the WOS showed well-organized and symmetrical distribution with a regular reticular pattern. Many of the WOS found on adenomas are well-organized with symmetrical distribution in a dense regular reticular/maze-like/speckled pattern. With BLI magnifying observation, magnification of about 100× is possible by moving the indicator in the top right bar by 2 gradations from the maximum optical magnification (5/7 of the sale).

▶**Observation tips** With BLI, an image containing the information required for diagnosis can be obtained at about 100× magnification, which is slightly lower than the maximum optical magnification. With some adenoma cases, the microvascular pattern cannot be visualized because of the presence of the WOS. In such cases, the morphology of the WOS could be an alternative optical sign.

(Yoshida, S.)

Case 30 Differential diagnosis of adenoma and gastric carcinoma

Female in her 80s **Purpose** Detailed observation of gastric lesion
Location Lesser curvature of lower gastric body **Macroscopic type** 0-Ⅱa

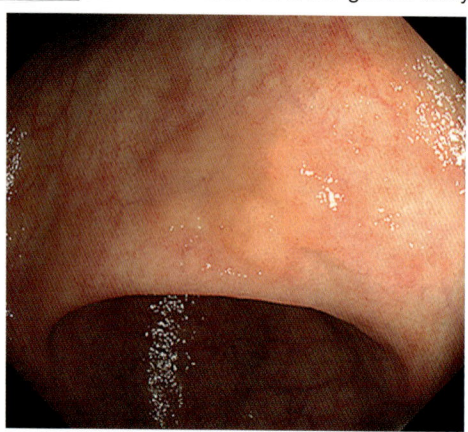

Normal WLI observation : A discolored flat elevated lesion with a diameter of 15 mm is observed on the lesser curvature of the lower gastric body.

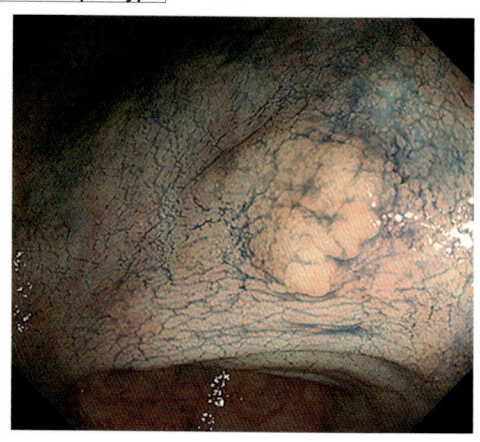

Indigo carmine-sprayed observation : When indigo carmine is sprayed, granular changes in various sizes are observed on the surface.

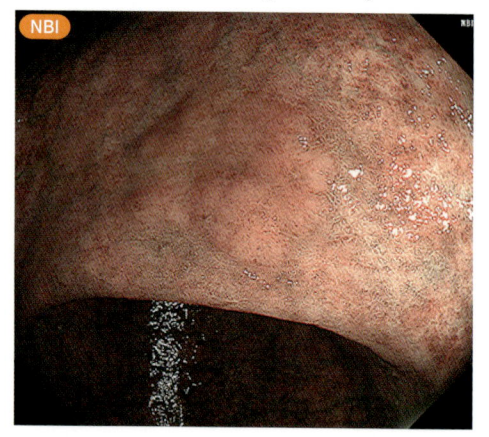

NBI non-magnifying observation : The brightness is maintained so overall observation is possible.

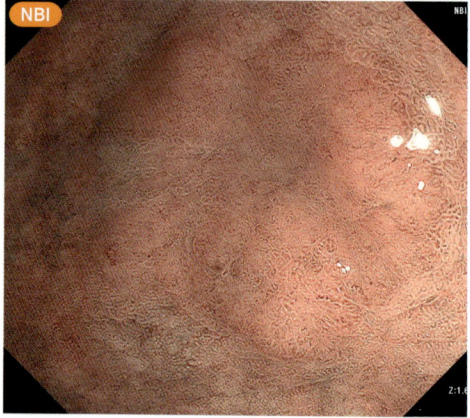

NBI electronic zoom (1.6×) observation : Irregularities in the mucosal surface structures are observed. A demarcation line is observed around the region due to the difference in the surface structures of the surrounding mucosa.

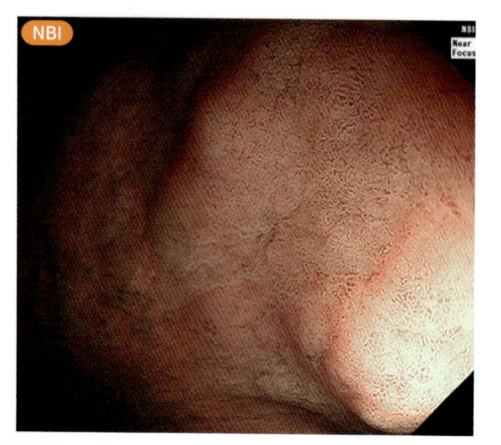

NBI Near Focus observation of the center of the lesion : Irregularities are observed in the mucosal surface structures and vascular structures.

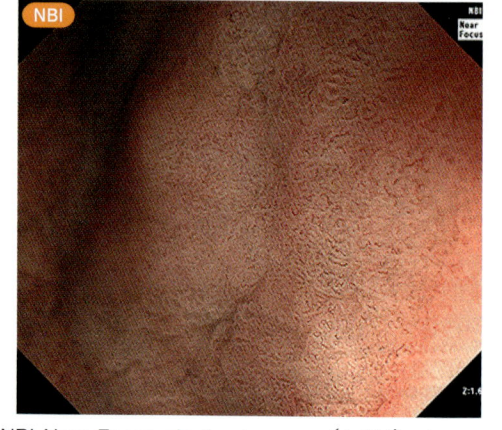

NBI Near Focus electronic zoom (1.6×) observation : Crypt marginal epithelium with irregular morphology and irregular arrangement are observed.

Endoscope：GIF-HQ290（Olympus）　Light source：EVIS LUCERA ELITE（Olympus）
NBI setup：Structure enhancement B8, color mode 1

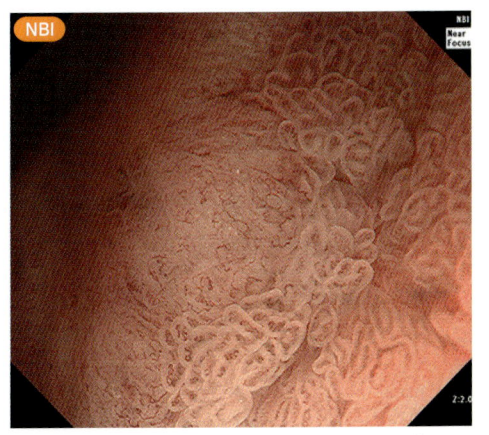

NBI Near Focus electronic zoom（2.0×）observation of the margin of lesion：microvessels with irregular shapes and diameters are observed together with the demarcation line.

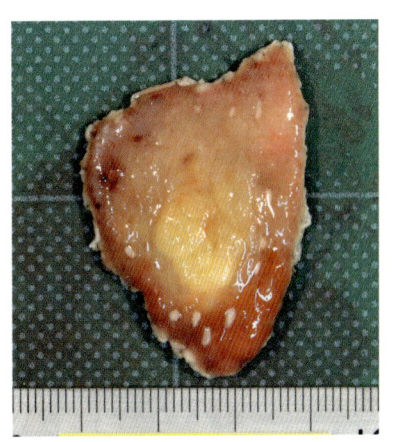

ESD resected specimen（after formalin fixation）.

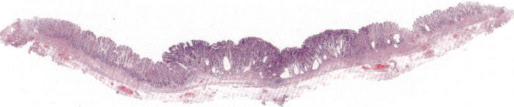

Magnified histological image：The pathological diagnosis results are：well-differentiated adenocarcinoma, 0-Ⅱa, 16×11 mm, tub1, pT1a, UL（−）, ly（−）, v（−）, HM0, VM0.

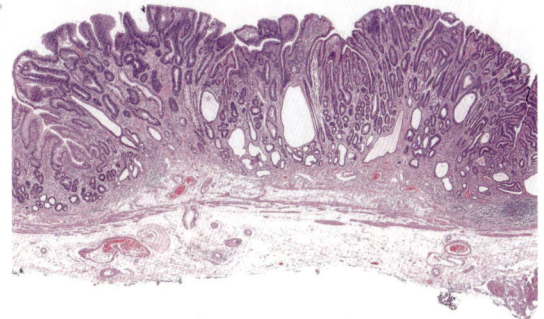

Pathological low-magnification observation：A well-differentiated adenocarcinoma presenting a branched tubular structure is recognized.

Comment

In WLI or indigo carmine sprayed observation, it is sometimes difficult to differentiate between a gastric carcinoma and adenocarcinoma with a flat elevated lesion with a low height and discoloration. Evaluation of the surface and vascular structures using NBI magnifying observation is useful for the benign/malignant differentiation.

▶Observation tips This case was subjected to NBI magnifying observation in the Near Focus mode. The results—including recognition of ductal structures with irregular morphology and arrangement and microvessels with irregular diameters and shapes—led to a diagnosis of differentiated gastric carcinoma. An appropriate combination of electronic and optical zoom enables more detailed observation of surface and vascular structures. In extent analysis, NBI electronic zoom observation is useful thanks to its surface structure observation capability and wide visible range. NBI magnifying observation in the Near Focus mode also has a wide visible range and is considered useful for extent diagnosis.

（Suzuki, A., Yasuda, K.）

Case 31 Differential diagnosis of erosion and early gastric carcinoma

Female in her 80s | **Purpose** Detailed observation of gastric lesion | **Location** Posterior wall of cardia
Macroscopic type 0-IIc

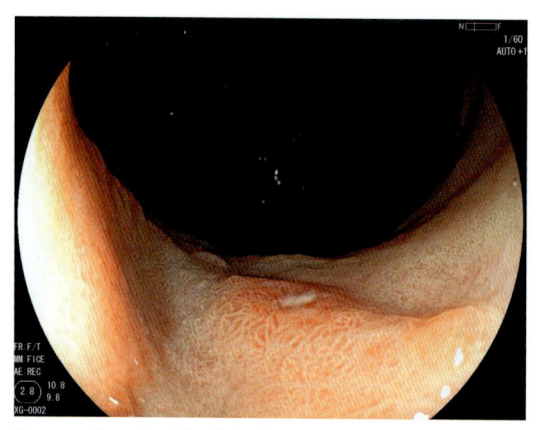

Conventional white-light image : A 5-mm erythematous lesion with shallow erosion can be seen on the posterior wall of gastric cardia.

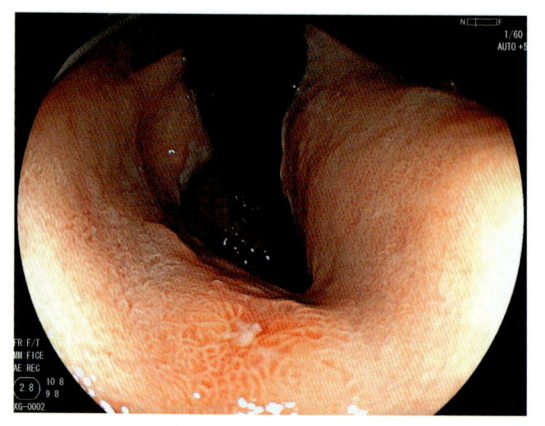

Inverse view of the same region : An irregular slightly depressed area is observed on the anterior side of the erosion.

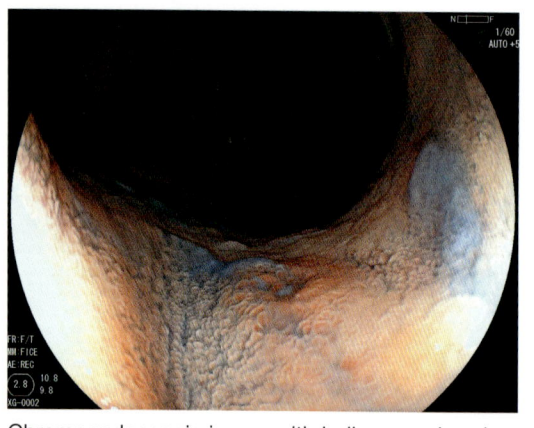

Chromoendoscopic image with indigo carmine dye

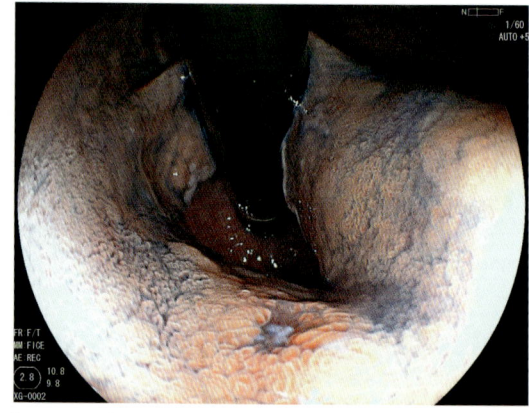

Inverse view of chromoendoscopic image : Indigo carmine dye has enhanced the image on the left.

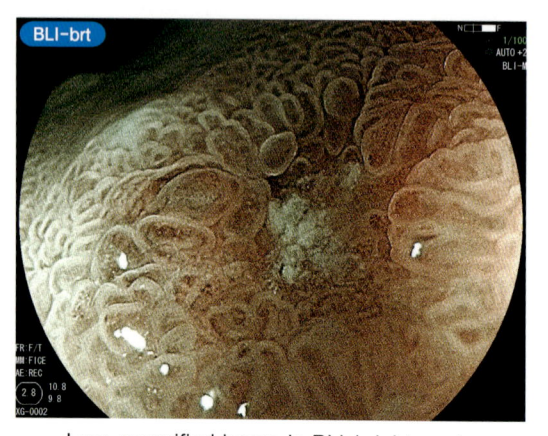

Low-magnified image in BLI-bright mode

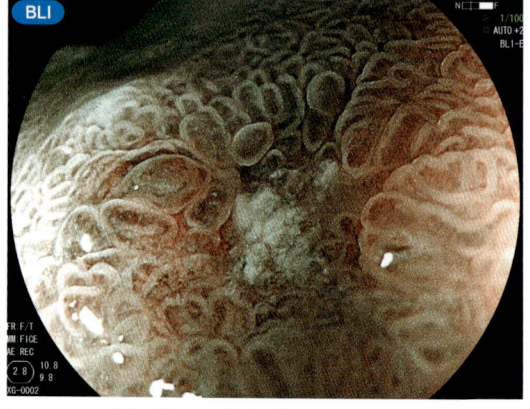

Low-magnified image in BLI mode : The microstructures are irregularly enlarged or unclear in the margin of the anterior side of the erosion. From the posterior to the distal side, no irregularities can be seen in the microstructures.

Endoscope : Prototype (EG-L590ZW equivalent) (Fujifilm)　　Light source : LASEREO (Fujifilm)
BLI setup : Structure enhancement A6, color enhancement C1

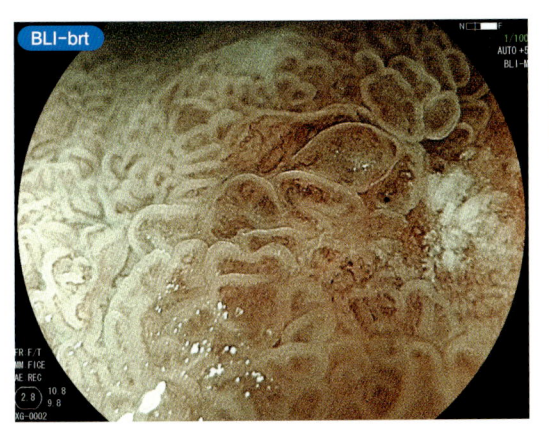

High-magnified image in BLI-bright mode

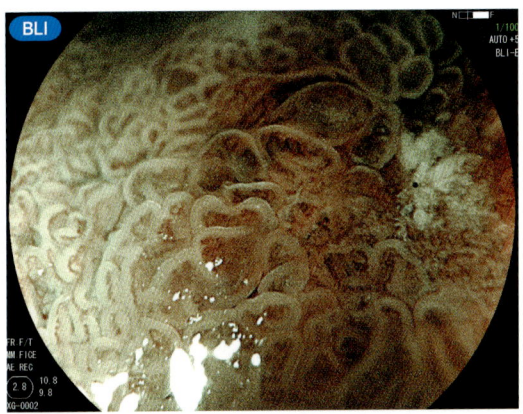

High-magnified image in BLI mode : irregularly arranged large and small microstructures can be seen. Dilated irregular microvessels are occasionally observed inside them. In the vicinity of the erosion, the microstructures are absent and only irregular microvessels can be seen.

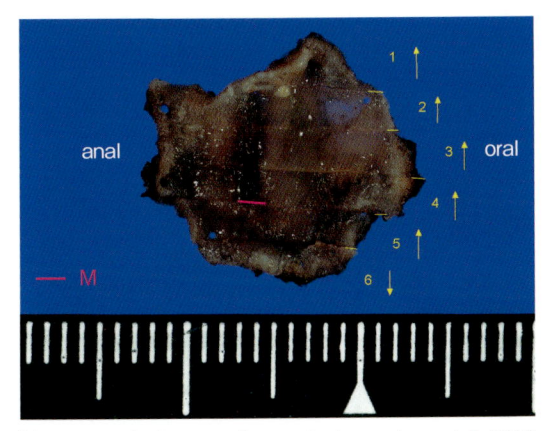

Macroscopic image of resected specimen : A 6×3 mm Ⅱc lesion on 15×13 mm resected specimen. Carcinoma cells are observed only on the anterior wall side of the depressed lesion.

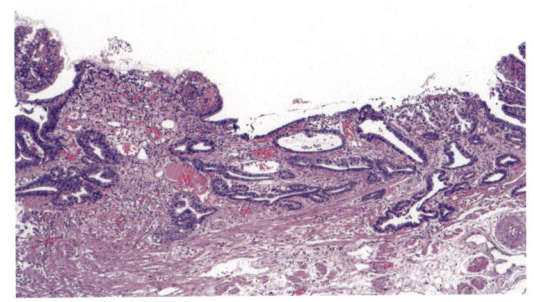

Histological image (hematoxylin-eosin, original magnification : 40×) : Carcinoma cells forming incompleted glandular ducts are observed in the lamina propria. Tubular adenocarcinoma (tub2>1), pT1a, UL (−), ly (−), v (−), HM0, VM0.

Comment

This is a micro-carcinoma case and differentiation from a benign micro-erosion is important. Erosions of such a small size are often eliminated from biopsy targets in actual clinical practice. The characteristics of carcinoma in this case were observed only on the anterior wall side in magnified images with BLI, where the carcinoma cells had invaded.

▶Observation tips　The margin of a benign erosion is often surrounded by regular microstructures, as seen in the region from the distal side to the posterior wall side of this case. On the other hand, microstructures with irregular shapes and irregular arrangement are observed in the neoplastic region on the anterior side. The microvascular image is not clear due to congestion ; therefore, this lesion can be diagnosed based on the microstructure abnormalities described above. High-magnified images with BLI mode are sometimes too dark, so medium magnification is often useful for diagnosis.

(Ono, S.)

Case 32 **Diagnosis of extent of early gastric cancer**

Male in his 40s *Purpose* Screening *Location* Lesser curvature side of antrum *Macroscopic type* 0-Ⅱa

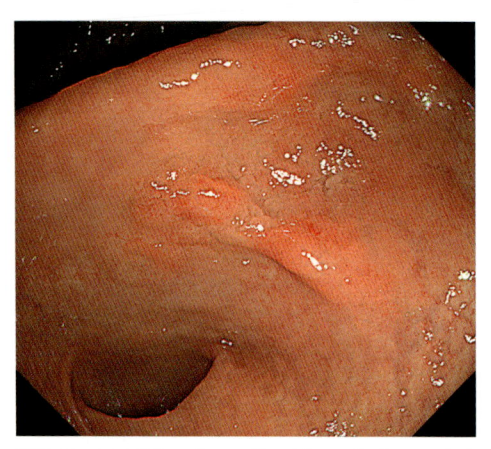

WLI non-magnifying observation : A poorly demarcated, erythematic flat elevated lesion is observed on the lesser curvature side of the antrum. The elevated lesion is accompanied with height irregularities inside.

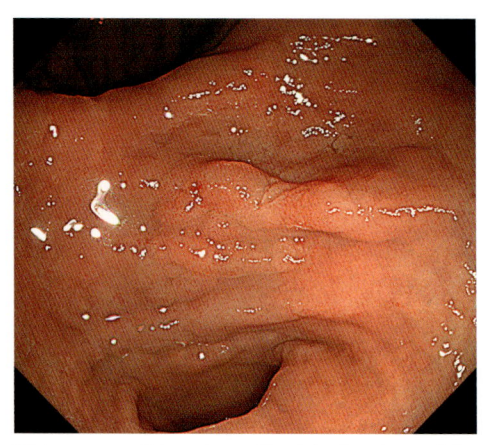

WLI non-magnifying observation : As the shape of the lesion changes easily when the insufflation amount is reduced, its invasion depth is considered intraepithelial.

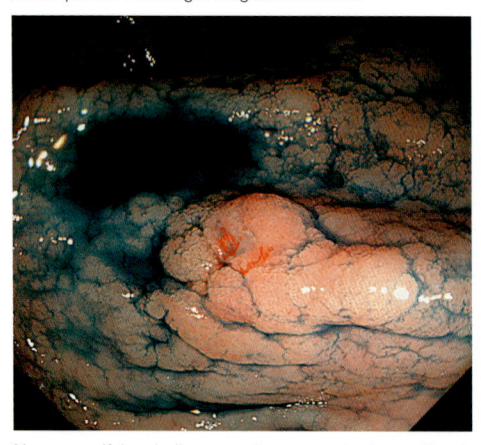

Non-magnifying indigo carmine spayed observation : Indigo carmine spraying makes it easy to detct the lesion.

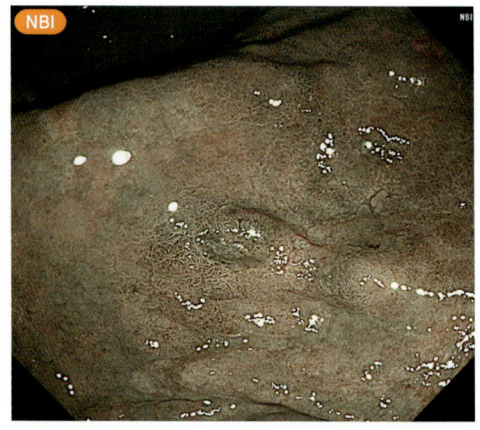

NBI non-magnifying observation : NBI shows a region in which the dense and pale colors are mixed compared to the background. It is also accompanied with surface irregularities.

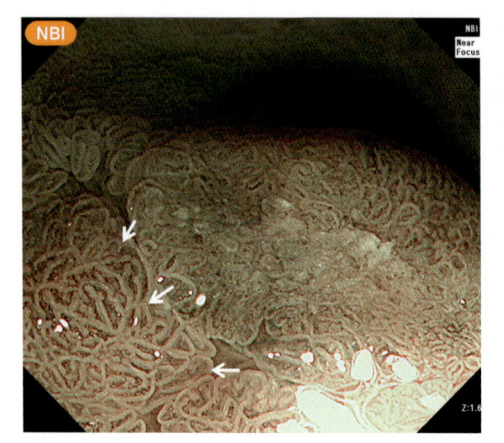

NBI magnifying observation (Near Focus+1.6×electronic zoom) : Compared to the background mucosa (white arrows), the surface structure of the lesion is irregular.

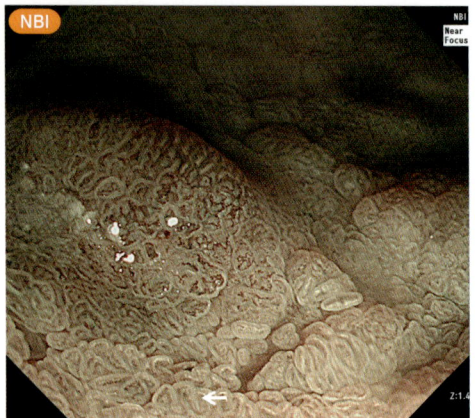

NBI magnifying observation (Near Focus+1.4×electronic zoom) : Compared to the background mucosa (white arrow), the lesion presents more proliferation of atypical vessels with bending, tortuosity and dilation inside.

Endoscope: GIF-HQ290 (Olympus)　Light source: EVIS LUCERA ELITE (Olympus)
NBI setup: Structure enhancement B8, color mode 2

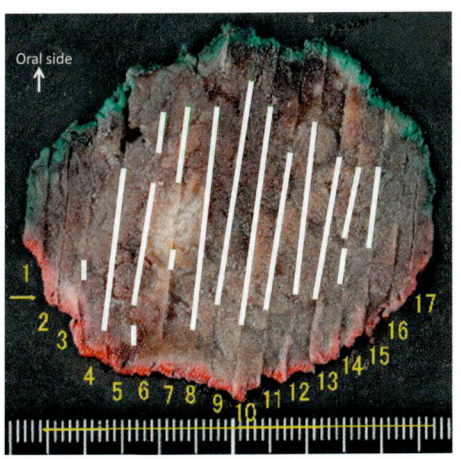

Resected specimen (ESD).
Early gastric cancer, tubular adenocarcinoma, well differentiated (tub1).
pT1a/pM, ly (−), v (−), pHM0, pVM0 0 Ⅱa, 41×34 mm, Less, M.

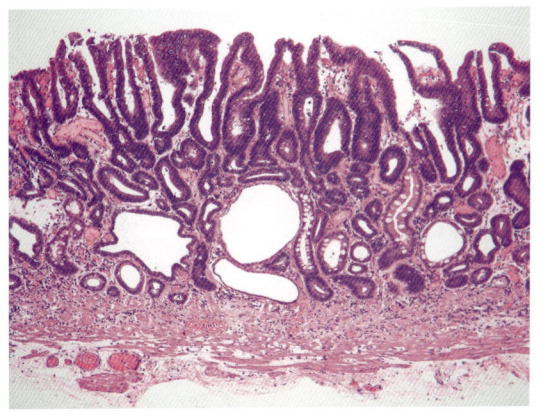

Tubular adenocarcinoma, well differentiated (tub1)

Comment

This is a 0-Ⅱa case of early gastric cancer on the lesser curvature side of the anterior wall. WLI non-magnifying observation shows the background mucosa as a whitish smooth mucosa without surface irregularities, while presenting the lesion as a poorly demarcated region accompanied with surface irregularities, in which erythematous and whitish areas are mixed. The demarcation is hard to distinguish with NBI non-magnifying observation, but easy to look clearly with NBI magnifying observation. The surface structures of the lesion show the size irregularities and the fusion tendency, and proliferation of atypical vessels with bending, tortuosity and dilation is observed. The fact that the atypical vessels form a mesh-like morphology suggests that the lesion is tub1. The indigo carmine spraying make it easy to detect the lesion as an unstained region. The fact that the shape of the lesion can be changed easily by decreasing the amount of insufflation suggests that the invasion depth of the lesion is intraepithelial.

▶**Observation tips** NBI non-magnifying observation is sometimes ineffective in the diagnosis of early gastric cancer, but magnifying observation is often effective in the diagnosis of differentiated gastric cancer. If atypical vessels and irregular surface structures (size irregularities and fusion tendency) are observed in a well-demarcated region, the lesion can be diagnosed as a cancer. The vessels of differentiated gastric cancer are mesh-like pattern. Now, the diagnosis of invasion depth with magnifying endoscopy is not established. The endoscopic findings of intraepithelial are low elevated lesion, shallow depressed lesion and easy to change the shape of the lesion.

(Morita, S., Muto, M.)

Case 33 Diagnosis of extent of early gastric carcinoma

Male in his 60s Purpose Detailed observation of gastric lesion
Location Greater curvature of antrum Macroscopic type 0 - Ⅱc

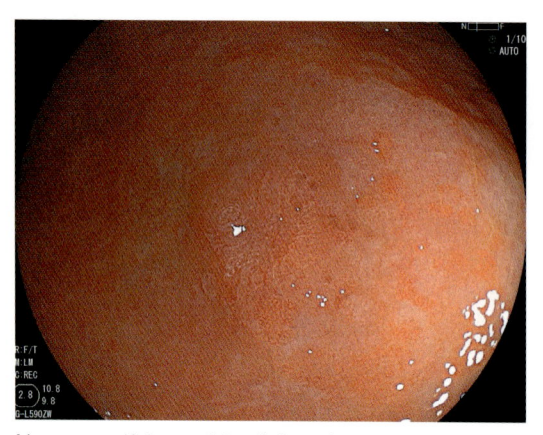

Non-magnifying white-light observation: A reddened slightly depressed lesion less than 10 mm in diameter on the greater curvature of the gastric antrum.

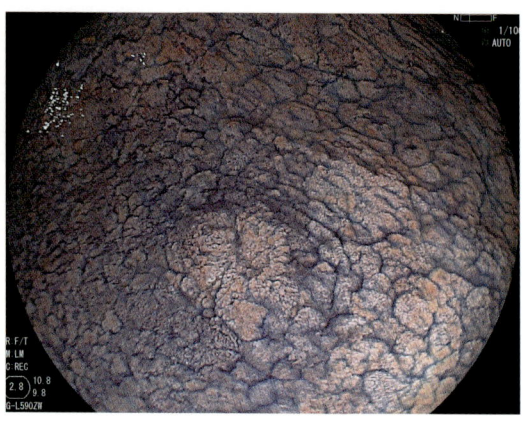

Non-magnifying chromoendoscopy: Indigo carmine spraying clarifies the demarcation of the depression, accentuating the distinction between the depression and the marginal elevations. The demarcation line is slightly irregular.

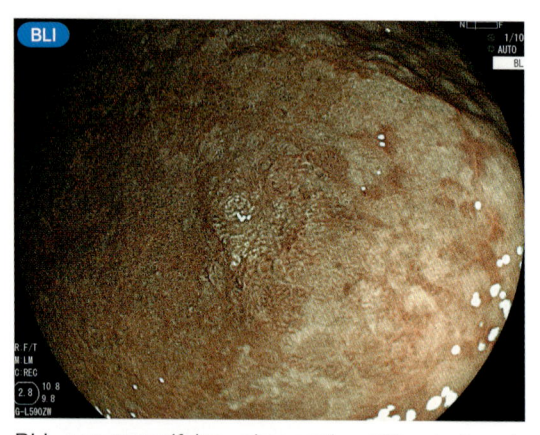

BLI non-magnifying observation: The lesion is imaged more clearly.

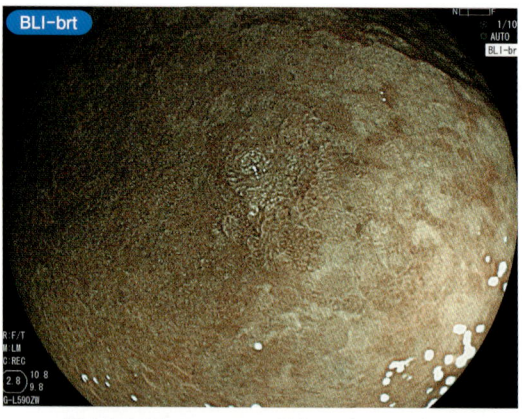

BLI-bright non-magnifying observation.

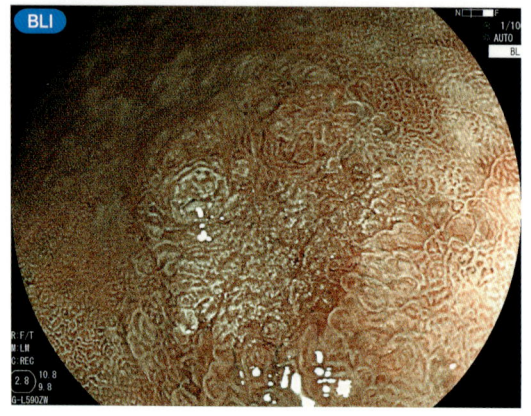

BLI low-magnification observation: Irregular microsurface structure is observed in the depressed part of the lesion. WOS (white opaque substance) is recognized on the anterior wall side.

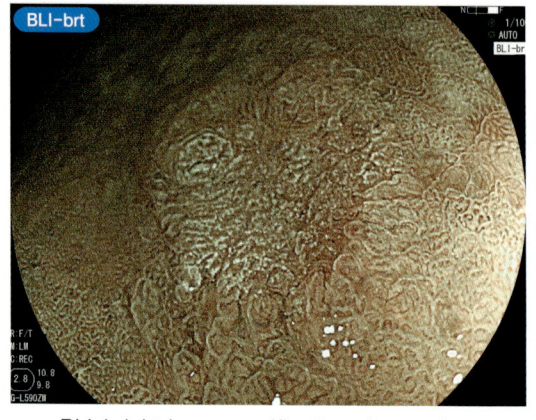

BLI-bright low-magnification observation.

Endoscope：EG-L590ZW（Fujifilm）　　Light source：LASEREO（Fujifilm）
BLI setup：BLI—Structure enhancement B8, color enhancement C1；BLI-bright—Structure enhancement B8, color enhancement C1

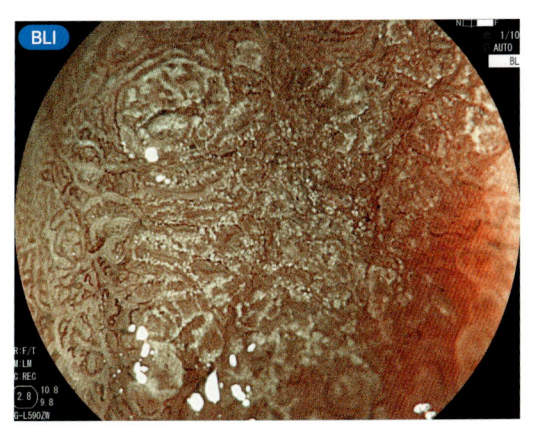

BLI high-magnification observation（anterior wall side）：Irregular WOS can be seen.

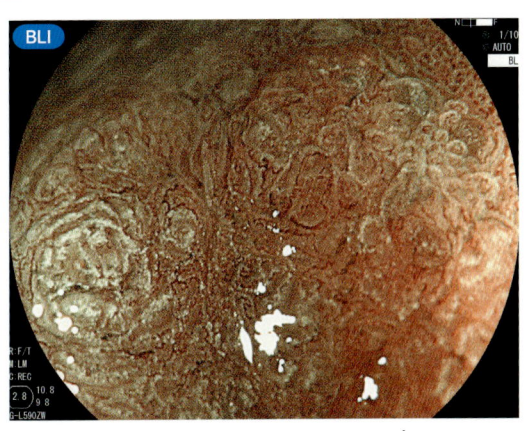

BLI high-magnification observation（posterior wall side）：Irregular microsurface structure and irregular microvascular architecture.

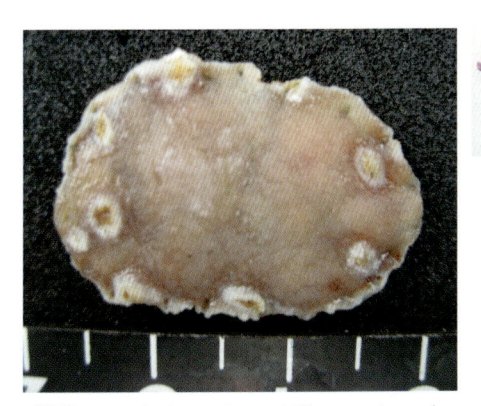

ESD-resected specimen：The specimen is 25×18 mm and has a Ⅱc lesion of 10×5 mm.

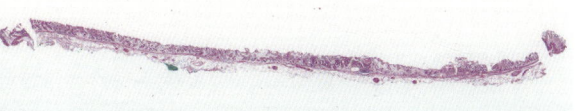

Loupe image

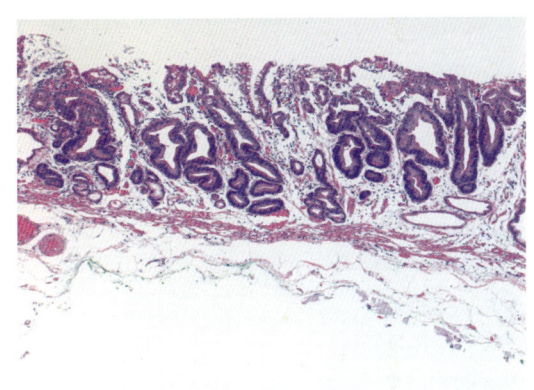

Low-magnification observation：Adenocarcinoma in stomach, tub1, pT1a, UL（−）, ly（−）, v（−）, HM0, VM0.

Comment

A depressed differentiated carcinoma is typically observed as a spiny depression accompanied with an irregular margin. BLI allows us to observe these characteristics more clearly. High magnification of around 100× shows a demarcation line, as well as irregular microvascular architecture with various shapes. An irregular arrangement of marginal crypt epithelia（MCE）is observed inside the microsurface structure. In the lesion where WOS is present, the subepithelial microvascular architecture is obscured due to the diverse shapes of the irregular WOS. In this case, the diagnosis should be made by utilizing the WOS as an alternative optical sign.

▶Observation tips　Evaluation of BLI magnifying observation images requires analysis of both the microsurface structure and microvascular architecture. When both can be observed as in this case, be sure to take a look at both of them. If the microvascular architecture is obscured due to the WOS, take a look at the microsurface structure.

(Yoshida, S.)

Case 34 Diagnosis of extent of early gastric carcinoma

Male in his 50s **Purpose** Detailed observation of gastric lesion found in general checkup
Location Lesser curvature of mid body **Macroscopic type** 0-Ⅱc

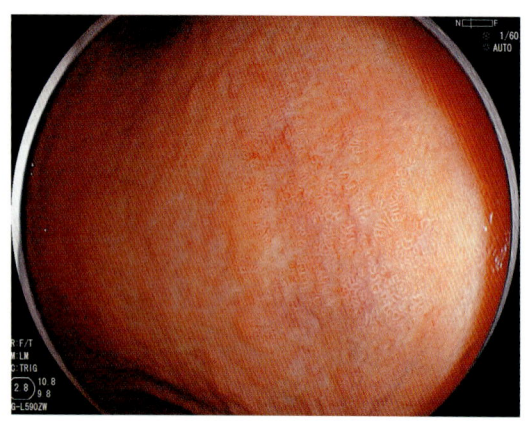

Non-magnifying observation with White-light: A poorly demarcated, discolored depressed lesion is recognized in the lesser curvature on the middle part of the gastric body. Irregular mucosa seems to extend on the posterior wall side of the discolored mucosa.

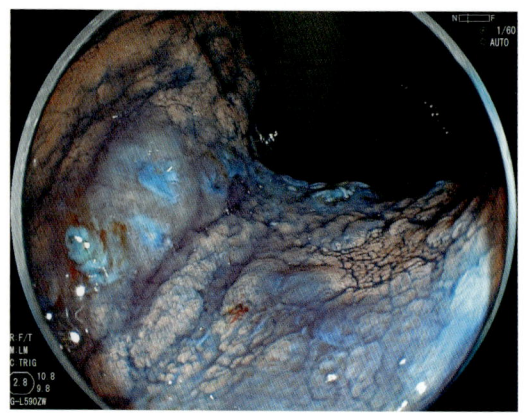

Non-magnifying observation with Indigo carmine-sprayed: Dye spraying makes the discolored mucosa on the anterior wall side less clear, but makes the irregular mucosal patterns on the posterior side clearer. Overall, the extent of the lesion is hard to diagnose.

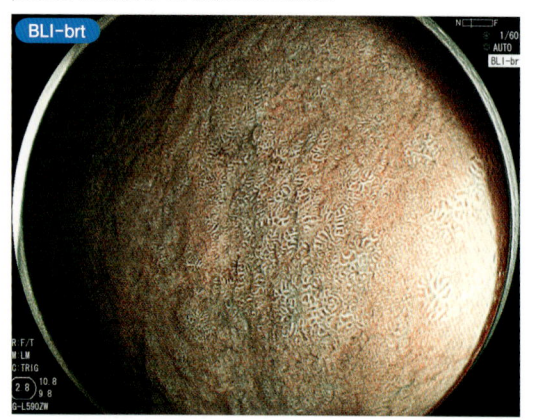

Low-magnifying observation with BLI-bright mode: The entire lesion is observed as a depression with fine mucosal patterns from a relatively far view.

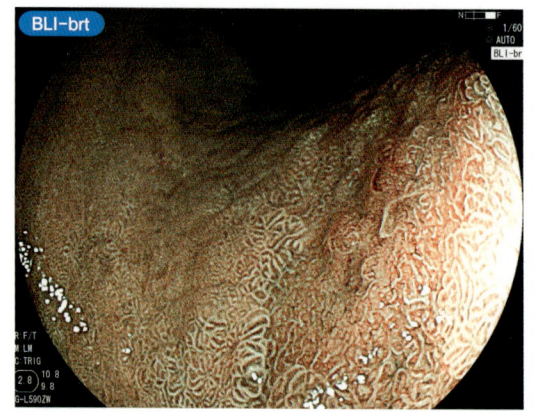

Middle-magnifying observation with BLI-bright mode: The demarcation with the depression on the lesser curvature side and the granular nodes on the lesion center are observed clearly. The mucosal patterns on the lesser curvature side of the depression are slightly enlarged.

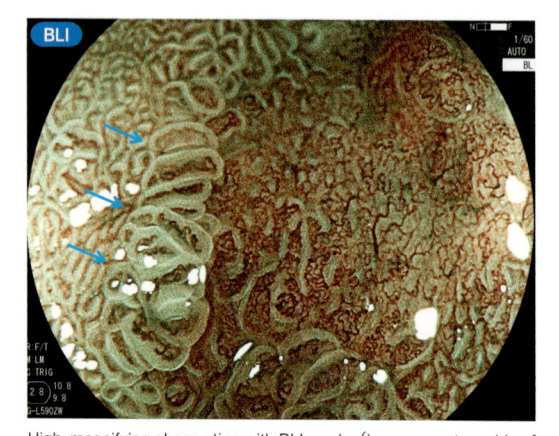

High-magnifying observation with BLI mode (lesser curvature side of lesion): On the margin on the lesser curvature side, irregular enlargement of fine duct gland structures is observed (the blue arrows indicate the pathological invasion extent).

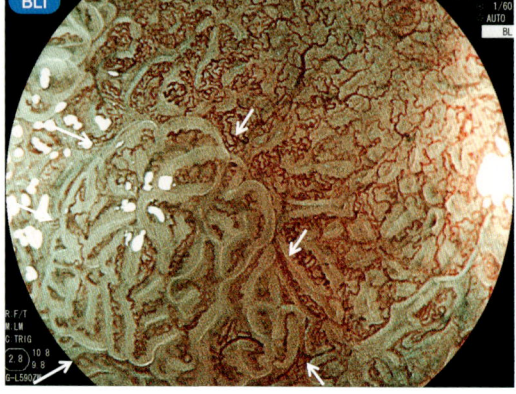

High-magnifying observation with BLI mode (distal side of lesion): In the center of the depression, the fine mucosal patterns have disappeared and the microvessels present corkscrew patterns. With the granules on the distal lesser curvature, the fine ductal structures are enlarged irregularly (the white arrows indicate invasion of carcinoma in the mucosa).

Endoscope : EG-L590ZW (Fujifilm)　　Light source : LASEREO (Fujifilm)
BLI setup : BLI—Structure enhancement A6, color enhancement C2 ; BLI-bright—Structure enhancement A6, color enhancement C2

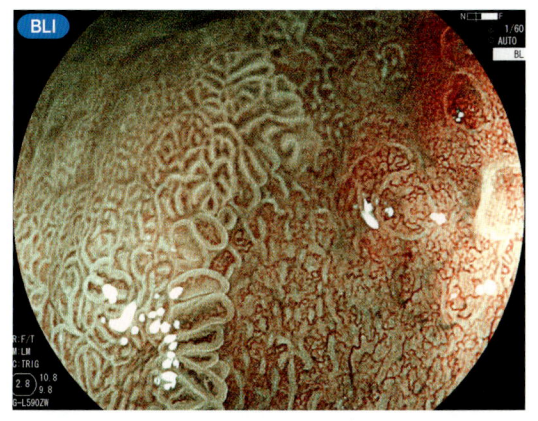

High-magnifying observation with BLI mode (center of proximal side of lesion) : With the nodes in the lesion center (right of the image), irregularly dilated microvessels are observed inside the ductal structures that have become unclear.

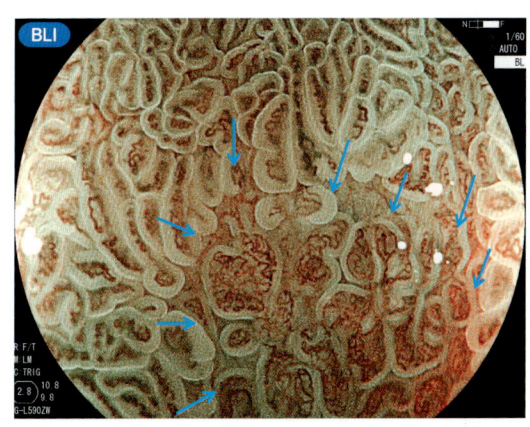

High-magnifying observation with BLI mode (proximal side of lesion) : Irregular arrangement of ductal structures of various sizes is observed together with irregularly dilated microvessels inside (the blue arrows indicate the pathological invasion extent).

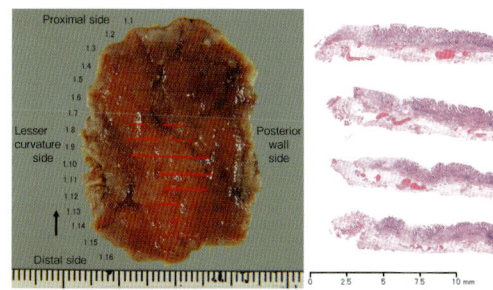

Left : Mapping of ESD-resected specimen
Right : Loupe images of sections in the resected specimen : Adenocarcinoma mucocellulare, sig≫tub2, type 0-Ⅱc, 19×11 mm, depth m, ly (−), v (−), pHM0, pVM0 (inside red rectangle)

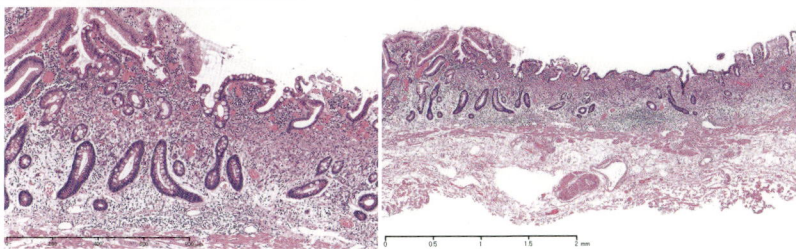

Left : High-magnification image. The crypt epithelium is not cancerous but proliferation of signet-ring cells are found in the mucosa immediately below. Tubular structures can be seen that are fused as if holding hands with each other.
Right : Low-magnification image. The tumor is localized in the mucosa and no clear vascular invasion is observed.

Comment

Histopathologically, the lesion is a depressed early gastric carcinoma localized in the mucosa with a diameter of 19 ×11 mm and sig≫tub2. Identification of the lesion extent is difficult with white light imaging or indigo carmine spraying, but, thanks to its far-view observation capability, the BLI-bright mode can observe the whole lesion as a depression presenting fine mucosal patterns. In BLI high-magnification observation, microvessels with irregular corkscrew patterns can be seen. These allow the lesion to be diagnosed as an undifferentiated early gastric carcinoma. In addition, the irregular enlargement of fine ductal structures with irregularly dilated microvessels inside make possible accurate identification of the extent of the carcinoma, including the invasion depth of the carcinoma below the mucosal epithelium.

▶Observation tips　Enlargement or de-clarification of the lesion margin or the fine mucosal patterns in the depressed area often indicate invasion of cancer cells (signet-ring cells with this case) below the normal crypt epithelium. Because BLI is excellent at imaging microvessels, as well as at finding ductal structures, it can definitely be considered a good tool for obtaining information on the layer immediately below the mucosa.

(Yagi, N.)

Case 35 Type 0-IIc differentiated early gastric carcinoma
—Comparison between H260Z/LUCERA and HQ290/ELITE

Male in his 50s | **Purpose** Detailed examination of depressed lesion on the anterior wall of the gastric body, detected during upper GI endoscopy performed as part of standard health check
Location Anterior wall of lower body | **Macroscopic type** 0-IIc

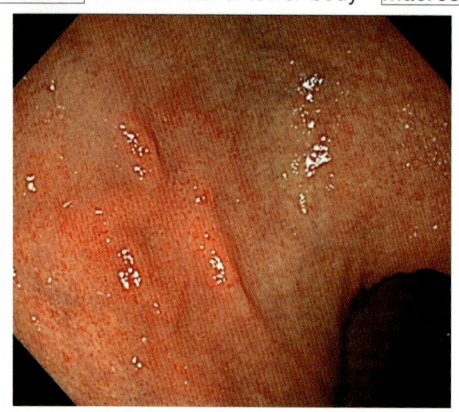

HQ290 (structure enhancement A5): In normal WLI observation, a shallow depressed 25-mm lesion is recognized on the anterior wall of the lower body. The lesion is slightly erythematous compared to the background mucosa and the mural extension of the lesion is good.

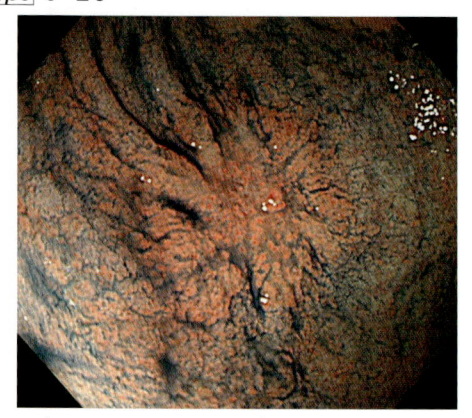

HQ290 (structure enhancement A5): In normal WLI observation with indigo carmine spraying, the extent of the spiny lesion and the marginal elevation are imaged more clearly. The convergence of folds oriented toward the minor elevation in the center of the depression is a change believed to have occurred post-biopsy.

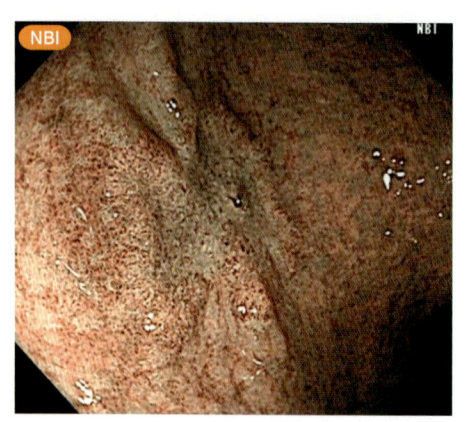

NBI normal observation (without magnifying): HQ290 (structure enhancement A7). The extent of the lesion can be seen more clearly in NBI normal observation than in WLI observation.

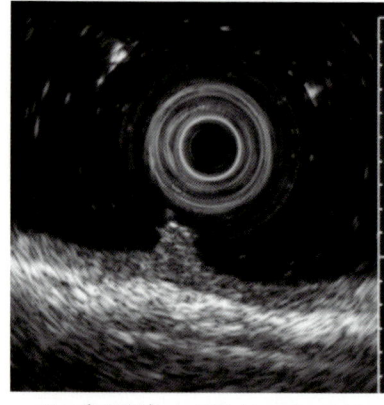

EUS observation (20 MHz): In EUS, low-echo regions indicating the presence of a lesion are present in the first and second layers, allowing us to classify the lesion as an intramucosal carcinoma.

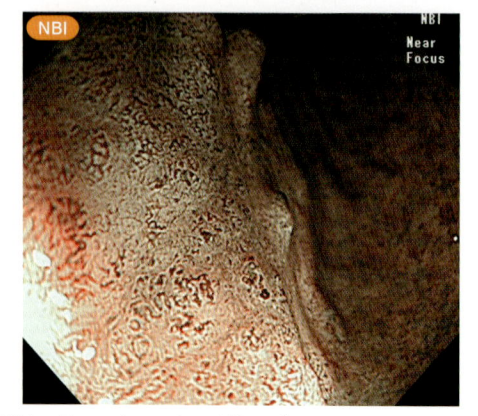

NBI Near Focus observation: HQ290 (structure enhancement A7). On the greater curvature on the proximal side of the lesion, the mucosal patterns are unclear, while visible microvessels appear to have abnormal courses and conspicuous dilation.

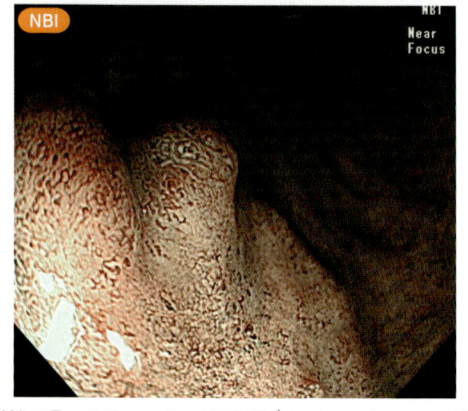

NBI Near Focus observation: HQ290 (structure enhancement A7). On the lesser curvature side of the lesion, the microvascular structure presents a fine network pattern that is characteristic of differentiated adenocarcinoma. The visibility of the lesion boundaries is better than in NBI normal (without magnifying) observation.

Endoscope/Light source : GIF-HQ290/EVIS LUCERA ELITE (Olympus) (normal observation, Near Focus), GIF-H260Z/EVIS LUCERA SPECTRUM (Olympus) (magnifying endoscope).
NBI setup : Structure enhancement A5/A7/A8, color mode 1

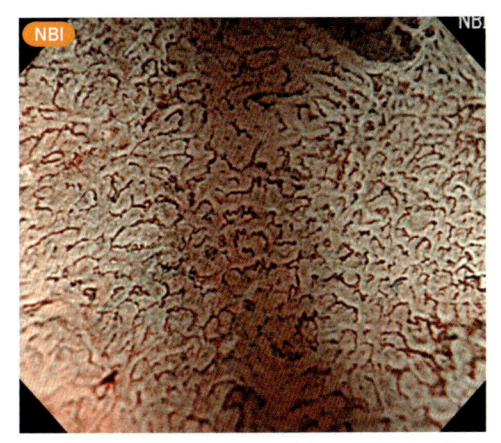

NBI magnifying observation of the proximal side of lesion, using the LUCERA GIF-H260Z.

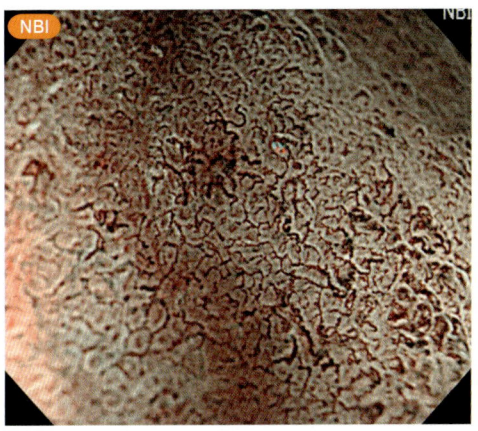

NBI magnifying observation of the lesser curvature side of lesion : As in NBI Near Focus observation, microvascular structures with fine network patterns can be recognized.

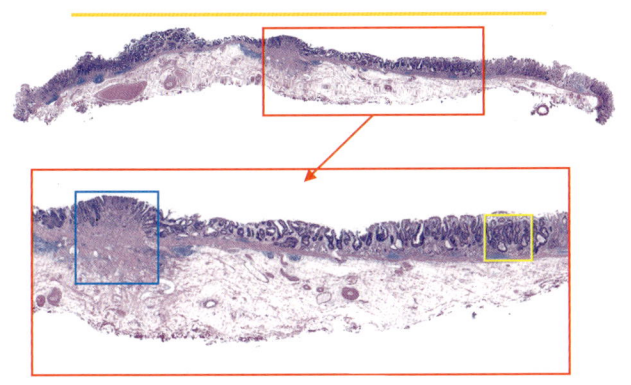

Magnified image of ESD specimen. Rupture of muscularis mucosae is recognized in the biopsy scar (blue frame). The depth of the tumor remains in the LPM.

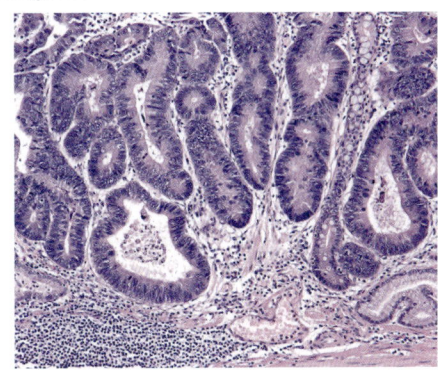

Findings inside the yellow frame in the magnified image : An image of well or moderately differentiated adenocarcinoma is observed. Pathological diagnosis : type 0-IIc, 24×22 mm, UL-IIs, pT1a (M), ly0, v0, pHM0, pVM0.

Comment

In this case, we used the LUCERA GIF-H260Z for the preoperative evaluation and the ELITE GIF-HQ290 for ESD marking, so we were able to compare the observation findings from both systems. The lesion presented typical findings of 0-IIc differentiated carcinoma regardless of which observation method was used. Images obtained in NBI observation using the ELITE system are brighter overall than the LUCERA system and suitable for observation of a wide field. In this case, abnormal microvascular structures such as the fine network patterns confirmed in the preoperative observation using the H260Z can be observed at a lower magnification so the lesion extent could be evaluated in less time.

▶**Observation tips** With the HQ290 system, the maximum magnification is not as high as on its predecessor, the H260Z, so better image quality can be obtained when observing a wide area from a relatively far view. To obtain a well-focused image, it is helpful to use the cap attachment as in a conventional procedure.

(Kamba, S., Sumiyama, K., Tajiri, H.)

Case 36 Diagnosis of histological type of early gastric carcinoma

Male in his 60s **Purpose** Detailed observation of gastric lesion
Location Greater curvature on the mid body **Macroscopic type** 0 - Ⅱc

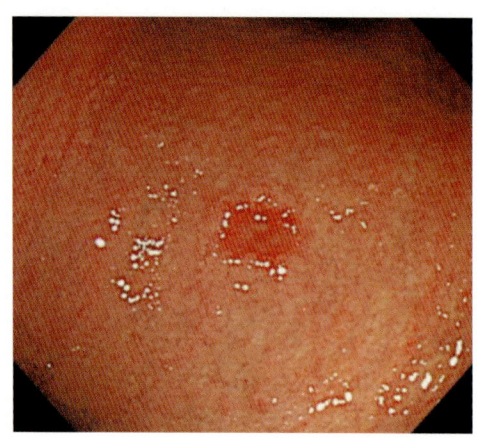

WLI normal observation (far view): An erythematous depressed lesion with a 15-mm diameter is recognized on the greater curvature of the middle body.

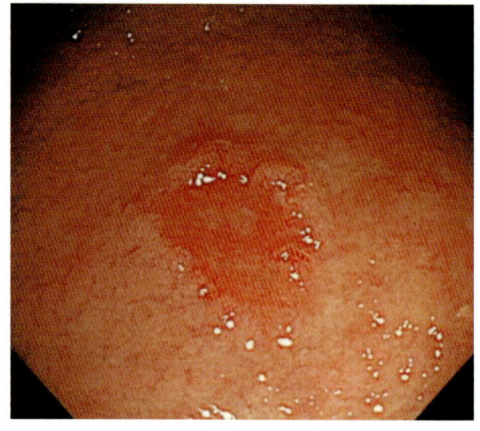

WLI normal observation (near view): The depression is accompanied with light elevations in the surroundings, where a mixed presence of erythematous and discolored areas is observed.

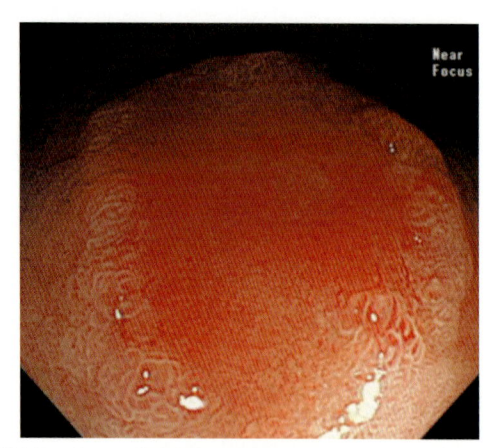

WLI Near Focus observation: On the depression on the center of the lesion, the marginal crypt epithelium has disappeared and irregular microvessels are observed, though less clearly.

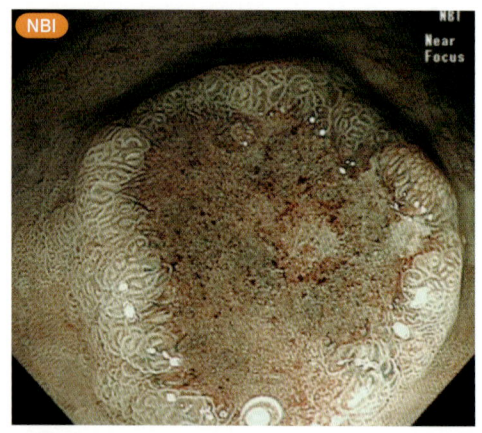

NBI Near Focus observation: Extremely dense mucosal microstructures and irregular microvessels are recognized in the area coincident to the depression's boundaries.

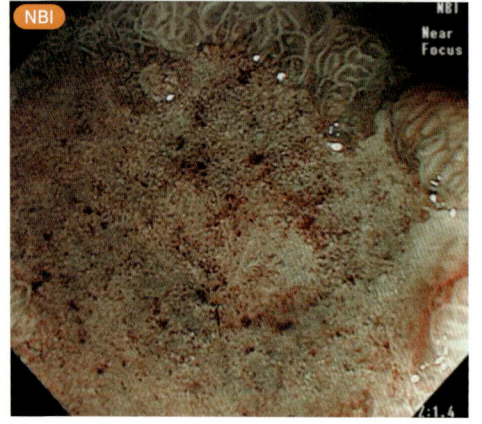

NBI Near Focus + 1.4× electronic zoom observation: Uneven, irregular mucosal microstructures are observed in the depression. Microvessels are dilated, tortuous, variable in diameters and uneven in shapes. The network pattern is destroyed and corkscrew patterns can be observed.

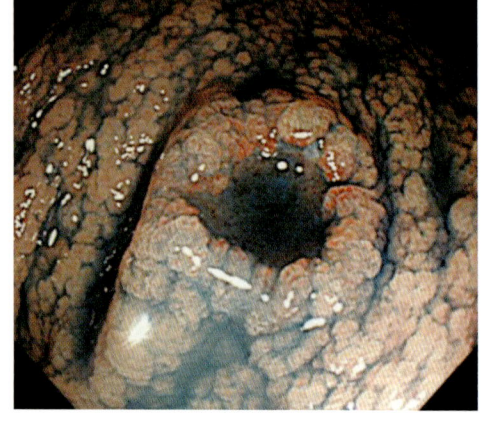

Indigo carmine-sprayed normal observation: Dye has accumulated on the depression surface, making the depressed area clearly recognizable.

Endoscope：GIF-HQ290（Olympus）　Light source：EVIS LUCERA ELITE（Olympus）
NBI setup：Structure enhancement B8, color mode 1

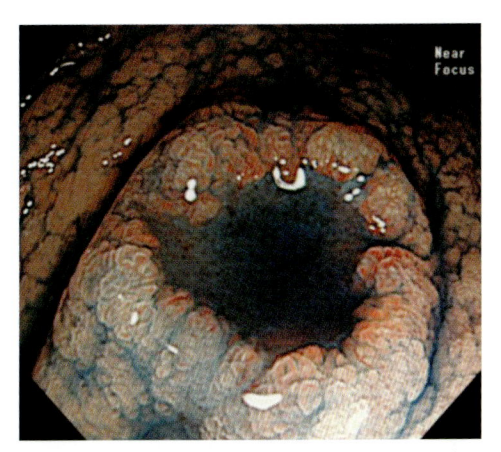

Indigo carmine-sprayed Near Focus observation： Normal marginal crypt epithelium remains in the elevated area around the depression so it is clear that the lesion is localized in the depressed surface.

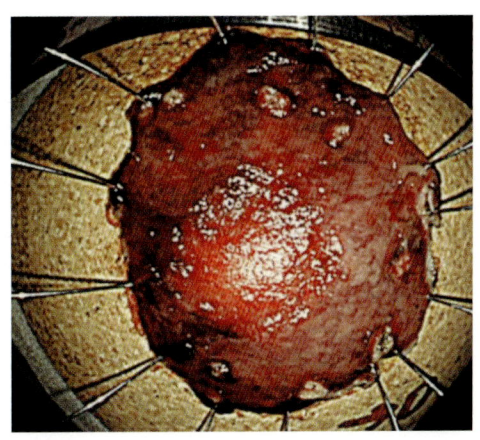

ESD resected specimen：On the 40×30 mm specimen, a 0-Ⅱc tumor with dimensions of 15×14 mm is recognized.

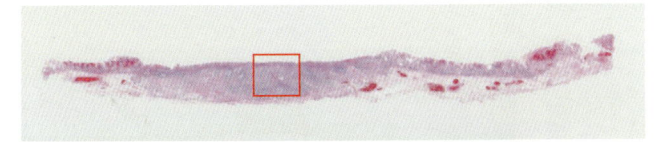

Image through a loupe.

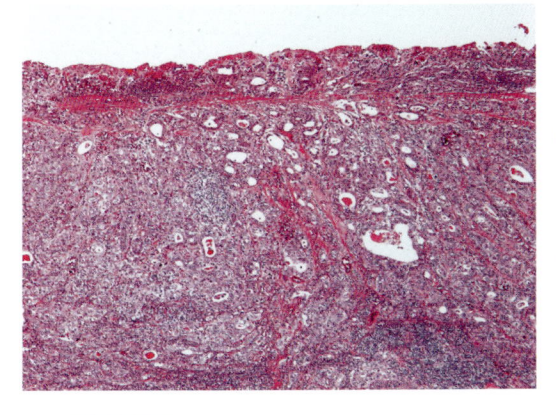

Microscopic pathology（HE, 40×）：The tumor has grown from a small tubular shape to a fused glandular structure, and small cluster invasion with unclear glandular cavity formation is observed in the invaded region. The tumor penetrates across the submucosal layer, and the deepest point reaches about 1 mm in the submucosal layer, where vascular invasion is also observed. Adenocarcinoma（tub2＞tub1, por2）, pT1b2（SM2）, ly1, v2.

Comment

Since a moderately differentiated carcinoma has a narrow gland duct orifice, it presents highly dense, fine mucosal microstructures, which are often unclear, when viewed with magnifying endoscopy. The microvascular structures have a deformed network pattern, and advanced irregularities in diameters and courses are observed. Approximately 80% of undifferentiated carcinomas present corkscrew patterns.

▶**Observation tips** Because the lesion in this case was located on the greater curvature of the middle gastric body, observation was susceptible to respiratory movement during magnifying endoscopy. To minimize this, we had the patient hold his breath. Also, in NBI Near Focus mode electronic zoom observation, when a zoom ratio of 2.0× was used, the image would be destabilized by cardiac motion. Consequently, in order to obtain clear images, we used a zoom ratio of 1.4×. This case is a typical example in which the histological type can be estimated from the observations of the mucosal microstructures and microvascular structures.

（Mochizuki, S., Fujishiro, M., Koike, K.）

Case 37 Diagnosis of histological type of early gastric carcinoma

Male in his 70s **Purpose** Detailed observation before endoscopic treatment of early gastric carcinoma
Location Posterior wall of middle body **Macroscopic type** 0-IIc

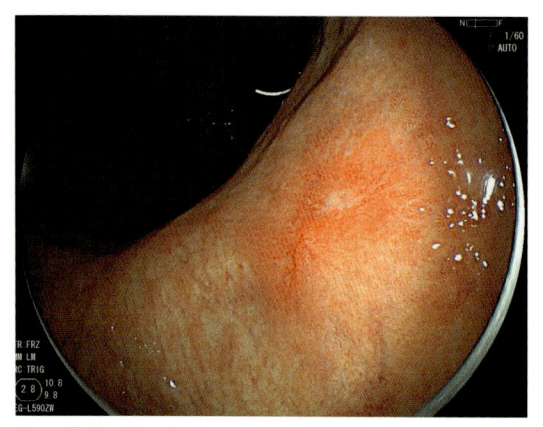

Normal white-light observation: An erythematous, depressed lesion in the atrophic mucosa on the posterior wall of the middle body. The erythematous area has an overall size of less than 20 mm. An extremely erythematous area exists inside and a depression to which white coat is attached is observed on the inner position. At this point, a differentiated carcinoma is suspected.

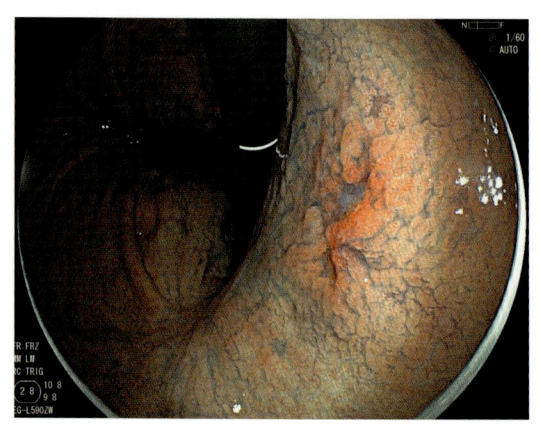

Normal chromoendoscopy: The depression surface is enhanced in the region corresponding to the highly erythematous area.

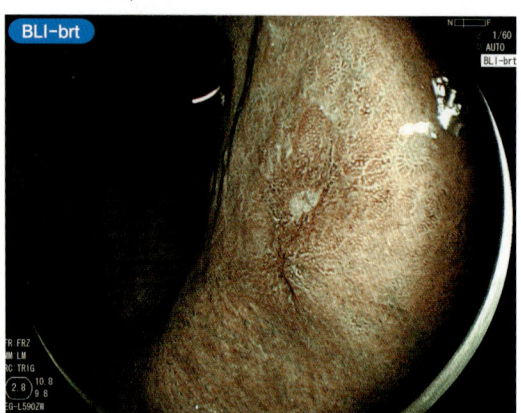

BLI-bright normal observation: The lesion is imaged as a brownish area and the difference in the surface patterns can be recognized even in the far view.

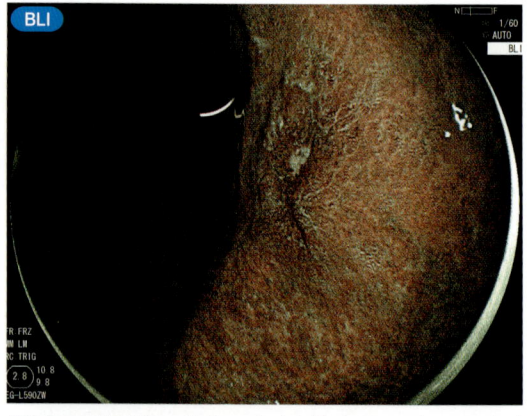

BLI observation: The entire image is dark. The lesion can be recognized as a dark brownish area but the details are unclear.

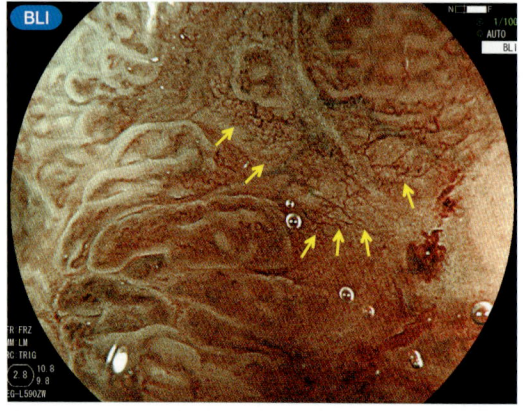

BLI magnifying observation: Anterior wall side of the depressed surface. No network is formed and vessels with irregular diameters and courses are observed (arrows). The surface microstructures are not recognized on the depressed surface.

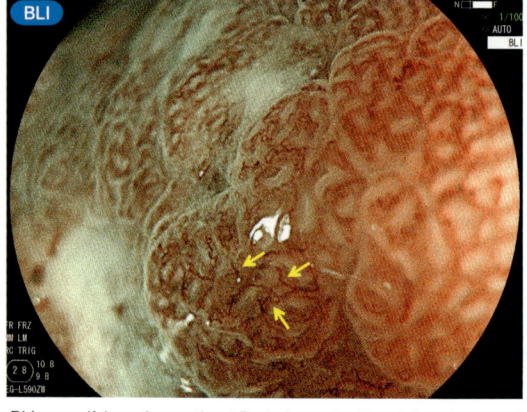

BLI magnifying observation: Posterior wall side of the depressed surface. Vessels with irregular diameters and courses that appear to be surrounding the crypt orifice (arrows) can be seen below the interfoveolar epithelium of the non-neoplastic fundic gland presenting linear surface microstructures.

Endoscope：EG-L590ZW（Fujifilm）　Light source：LASEREO（Fujifilm）
BLI setup：BLI―Structure enhancement A6, color enhancement C1；BLI-bright―Structure enhancement A5, color enhancement C1

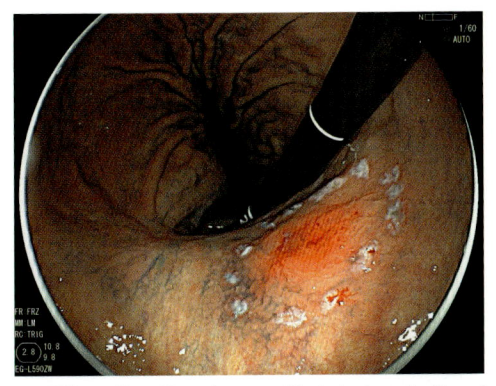

Pre-ESD marking：The region around the lesion is marked based on the BLI observation findings. The white coat on the depressed surface has fallen off after the magnifying observation so it is determined that there is no mucosal defect. The lesion is treated as a lesion without ulcerative change.

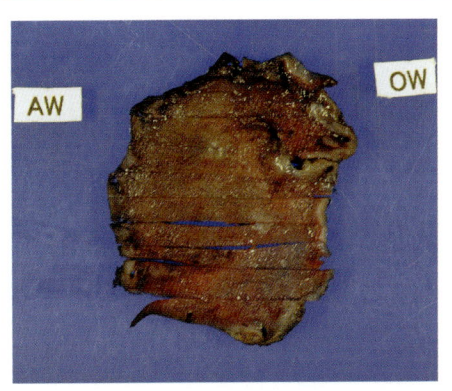

Macroscopic view of ESD-resected specimen：8×8 mm 0-Ⅱc lesion on the 40×30 mm ESD specimen. The lesion is observed in a position almost coincident to the depressed surface.

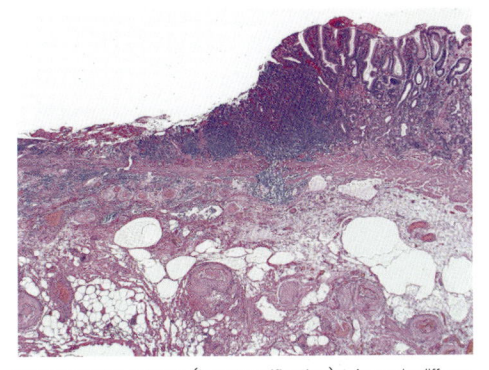

Pathological specimen（low magnification）：A poorly differentiated adenocarcinoma remaining in the mucosa is recognized in the position almost coincident to the depressed surface. The focus contains prominent lymphocytic interstitium and no finding suggesting ulcerative change such as fibrosis of the submucosal layer is recognized. Adenocarcinoma（por）, pT1a（M）, UL（－）, ly（－）, v（－）, pHM0, pVM0.

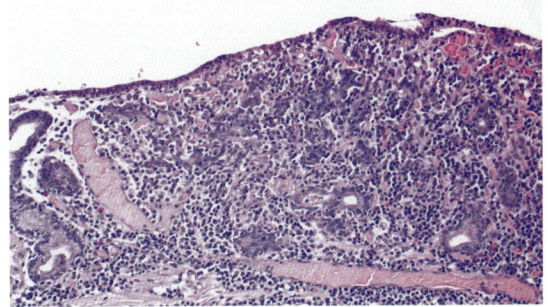

Pathological specimen（high magnification）：The lesion contains an area where a poorly differentiated carcinoma coated with non-neoplastic epithelium invades the middle layer of the mucosa.

Comment

This is a case of undifferentiated intramucosal carcinoma on the posterior wall of the gastric middle body. In normal observation, it is observed as an erythematous lesion in the atrophic mucosa and suspected to be a differentiated carcinoma. The irregular vessels in the depression that are observed in BLI magnifying observation are not the corkscrew-type vessels typical of undifferentiated gastric carcinoma, nor do they form a network that would suggest a ductal structure. However, their courses are disorderly, which is consistent with undifferentiated gastric carcinoma. As irregular vessels are also recognized below the epithelium of the surrounding mucosa presenting regularly arranged surface microstructures, the lesion is suspected to be a carcinoma invading below the non-neoplastic epithelium.

▶Observation tips　A highly erythematous lesion like this case tends to cause bleeding by contact in magnifying observation because of blood congestion. Therefore, such a lesion should be observed cautiously since bleeding will cause a deterioration in observation conditions. As bleeding occurs most easily inside the lesion, approach the lesion from the normal mucosa on the distal side of the lesion while increasing the magnification gradually, and observe the lesion in the counter clockwise direction from the posterior wall side to the proximal side and anterior side. Observe and evaluate as quickly and cautiously as possible. If too much time is take on this procedure, observation will become impossible due to bleeding.

(Takeuchi, Y., Uedo, N., Tomita, Y.)

Case 38 **Diagnosis of histological type of early gastric carcinoma**

Male in his 70s　*Purpose*　Detailed observation of gastric lesion　*Location*　Posterior wall of antrum
Macroscopic type　0-Ⅱa

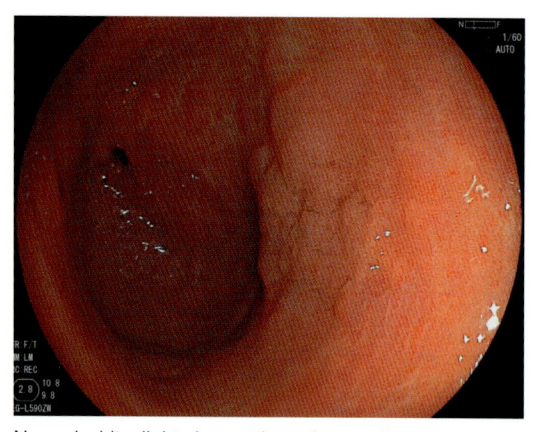

Normal white-light observation : A normally colored lesion of about 20 mm with slight height irregularities on the posterior wall of the antrum. The demarcation is unclear.

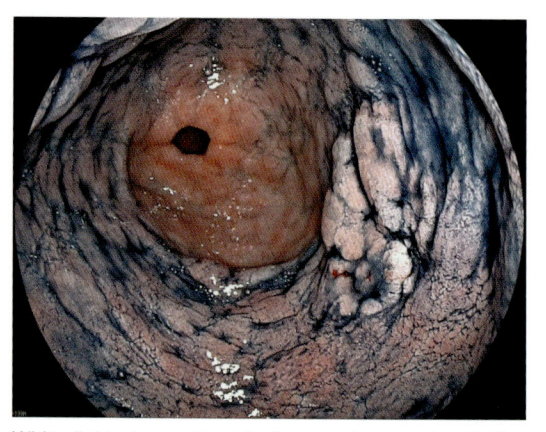

White-light observation : Indigo carmine spraying clarifies that the lesion is elevated. Indigo carmine has accumulated in a groove shape inside the tumor, helping to clarify the tumor's surface irregularities.

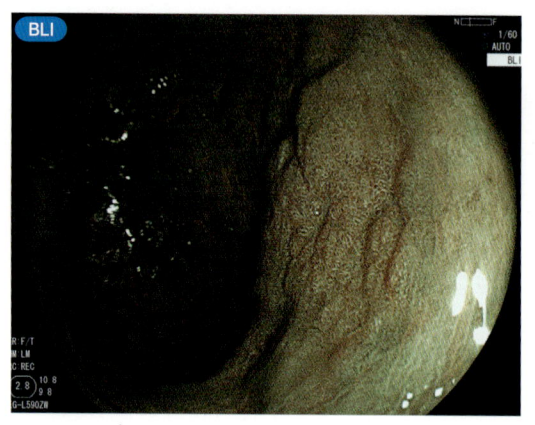

BLI mode (structure enhancement B7, color enhancement C3) non-magnifying observation : The lesion is recognized as a more brownish area than the surroundings and the demarcation between the neoplastic and non-neoplastic regions can be observed clearly.

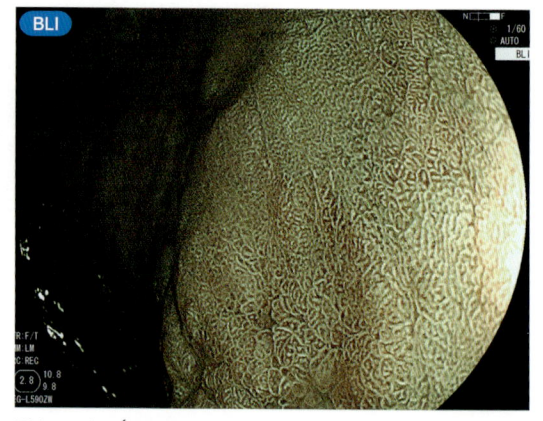

BLI mode (structure enhancement B7, color enhancement C3) low-magnification observation : Diagnosis of extent of the tumor on the posterior wall side. The surface structures of the tumor show that it has low architectural atypia even when compared with the ductal structures in the surrounding area. Slight orientation irregularities, size reduction and size irregularities can be recognized.

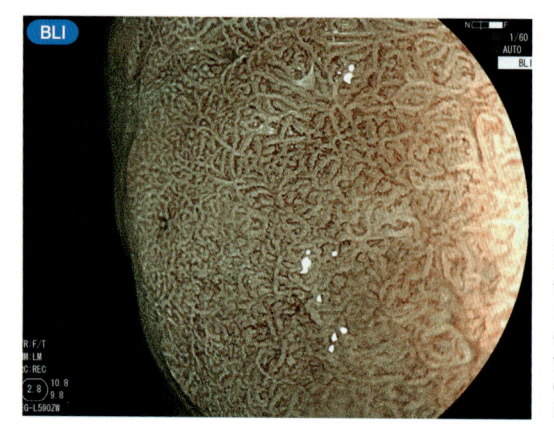

BLI mode (structure enhancement B7, color enhancement C2) medium-magnifying observation of the tumor margin on the greater curvature side : The micro structures are variable in size and orientation, and denser than those in the surrounding normal areas. The white margin structure reflecting the marginal crypt epithelium is maintained, but the overall structures are irregular. Irregular microvessels are also observed.

Endoscope : EG-L590ZW (Fujifilm)　Light source : LASEREO (Fujifilm)
BLI setup : Structure enhancement B7, color enhancement C3/C2

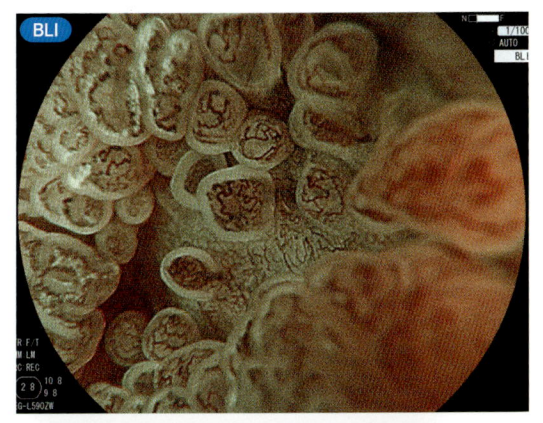

BLI mode (structure enhancement B7, color enhancement C2) high-magnification (full zoom) observation : Observation of the center of the lesion in water. The gland ducts are not fused and the surface microstructures are maintained, but size irregularities are noticeable and tortuous atypical vessels with irregular diameters are observed clearly in the interfoveolar area. A network of irregular microvessels can be observed in the depressed area.

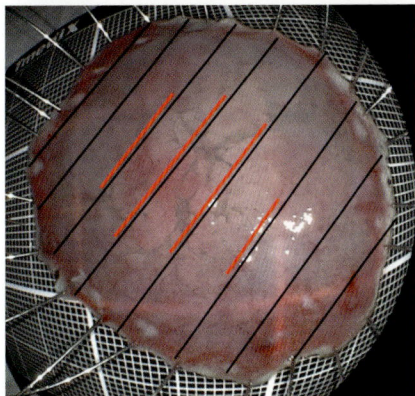

Resected specimen

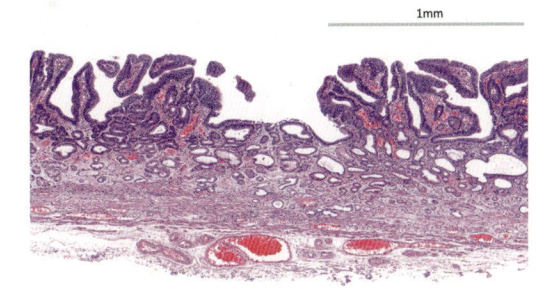

Pathological HE staining (center) : The tumor has grown in a tubular shape as if replacing the superficial layer, but the ductal structures are not dense. Gland ducts can be seen in the transverse direction on the surface layer of the groove-like area on the center. Considering the strong nuclear atypia, the tumor is diagnosed as a tub1 carcinoma. The groove-like area in the center seems to coincide with the area where the network of vessels was observed in the endoscopic observation.

Pathological HE staining (margin) : The tumor cells progress by replacing the superficial layer, while maintaining the ductal structures. Although there are areas in which differentiation from adenocarcinoma is difficult, the tumor is still in the category of low-grade atypia so the tumor is diagnosed as a well-differentiated adenocarcinoma. The gland ducts are densely proliferated, which coincides with the findings in the endoscopic observation of the margin.Final diagnosis : Early gastric carcinoma, tub1, pT1a (M), ly0, v0, pHM0, pVM0, UL (−).

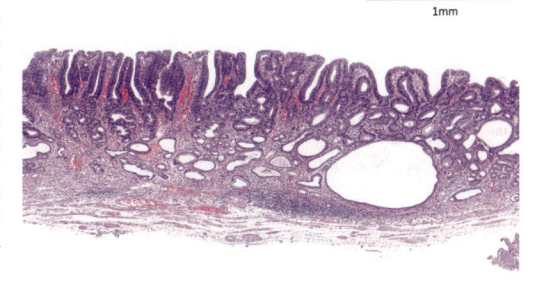

Comment

This is an example of a case where magnifying observation shows different-looking surface structures within a single tumor. Estimation of the pathological image from the surface microstructures observed with endoscopy is useful for estimating the histological type.

▶**Observation tips** When intestinal metaplasia is observed on the mucosa of surrounding tumor with BLI, the extent of the early gastric carcinoma can be diagnosed even with white light observation when light-blue crests are present, as in this case. As the gland ducts are dense and the crypt orifices are narrowed on the margin, there is some concern that the surface structures cannot be clearly visualized. With BLI, however, the surface structures can be observed clearly because the blue laser light contains the white light component. The microvessels in the depressed area can be seen clearly so the result is useful for the qualitative diagnosis.

(Miura, Y., Yamamoto, H.)

Case 39 Transnasal endoscopic observation of early gastric carcinoma

Male in his 80s Purpose Screening (follow-up) Location Greater curvature of gastric angulus
Macroscopic type Ca in adenoma (0-Ⅱa)

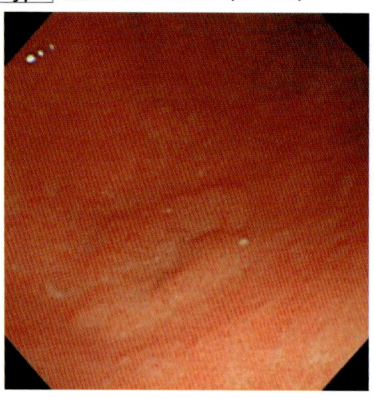

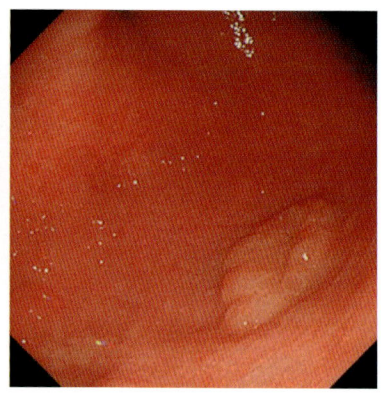

Normal WLI observations
Left：XP260NS—A 30 mm sized flat elevated lesion is observed on the greater curvature of the gastric angle. The center is slightly depressed, and uneven mucosa are also recognized.
Right：XP290N—A flat elevated lesion is recognized similarly. In overall, uneven mucosa and the demarcation with the surroundings can be observed clearer than the XP260NS.

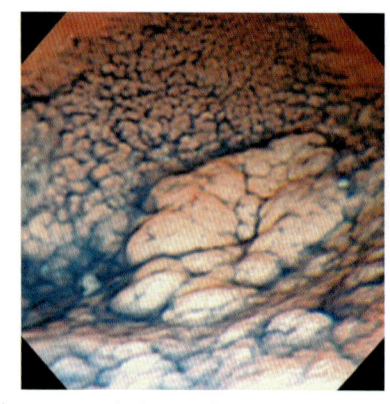

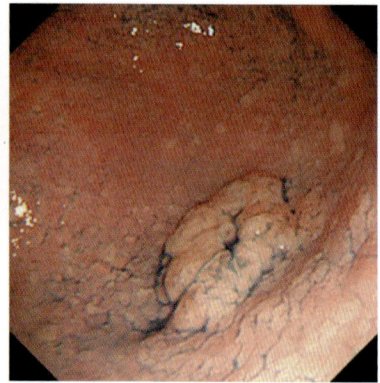

Indigo carmine-sprayed observation
Left：XP260NS—Image is clearer than WLI, and uneven mucosa with granule are noticeable.
Right：XP290N—Overall, the uneven mucosa looks slightly clearer than with the XP260NS, but no obvious difference is recognized.

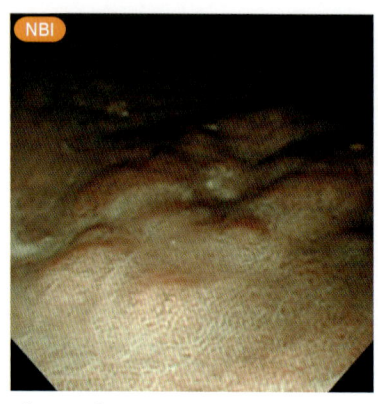

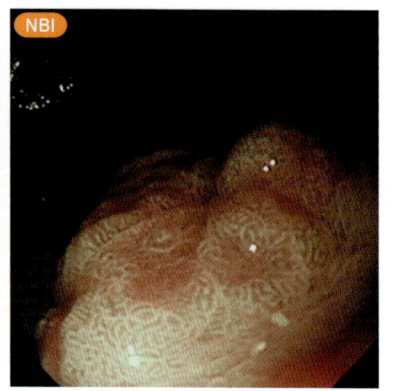

NBI close-up observation
Left：XP260NS—The close-up can enhance the uneven mucosa but the mucosal structures are only partially observable.
Right：XP290N—The close-up can observe the mucosal structures as well as uneven mucosa. Loss of mucosal microsurface pattern is recognized in a part of the lesion.

Endoscope : GIF-XP260NS & GIF-XP290N (Olympus)
Light source : EVIS LUCERA SPECTRUM (XP260NS), EVIS LUCERA ELITE (XP290N) (Olympus)
NBI setup : Structure enhancement A6, color mode 1 (EVIS LUCERA SPECTRUM [XP260NS])
Structure enhancement A6, color mode 1 (EVIS LUCERA ELITE [XP290N])

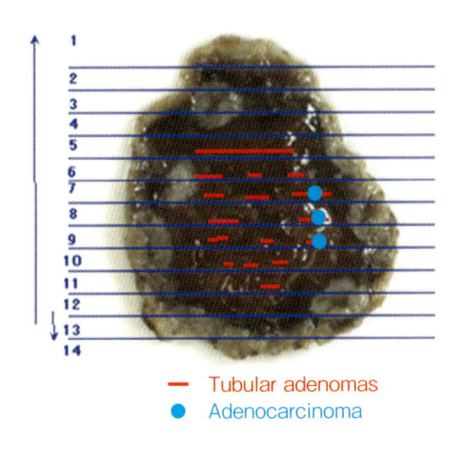

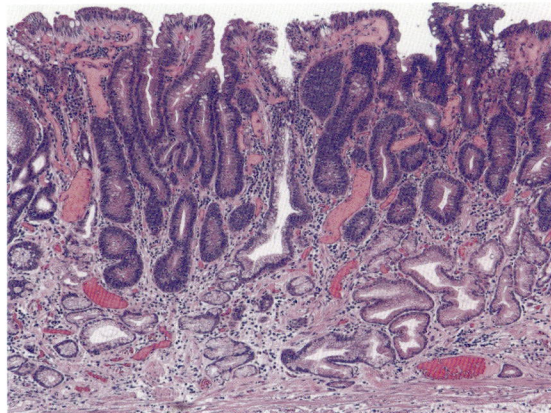

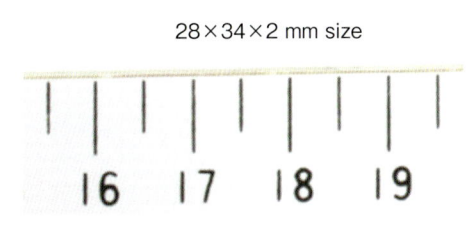

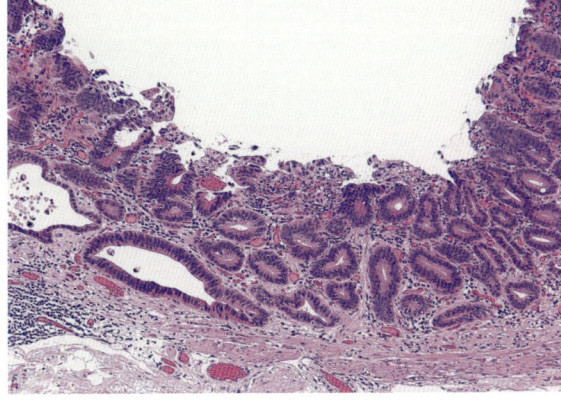

— Tubular adenomas
● Adenocarcinoma

28×34×2 mm size

Pathology
Left : Macroscopic view of a flat elevated lesion of 28×34 mm. Although mostly adenomatous, the adenocarcinoma components can be partially seen in the center of the depression.
Right : Microscopic view of the lesion. Upper : The adenomatous area in the lower part of mucosa contains non-neoplastic gland ducts. Low : The carcinomatous area occupies the whole mucosal layer where erosion has formed. Well differentiated tubular adenocarcinoma in adenoma (tub1, pM, ly0, v0, pHM0, pVM0)／

Comment
The main points that have been recommended for transnasal endoscopy procedure include sufficient stretching of the stomach, washout of mucus, close-up observation and, finally, indigo carmine staining. When the conventional slim transnasal endoscope (XP260NS) was used, the lesion was easily visible in indigo carmine-stained and close-up observation. However, when the XP260NS was used in NBI observation, the image was dark and adequate observation of the mucosal surface was difficult even in close-up observation. When the new XP290N was used, the image obtained in indigo-carmine staining was similar to that of the XP260NS. NBI super close-up observation, however, was much brighter and enabled visual recognition of the abnormal mucosal structures.

▶**Observation tips** The new XP290N slim transnasal endoscope uses a light source with higher brightness, allowing the use of objective optics that do not cause contrast to deteriorate in close-up observation. This has made it possible to manifest resolving power of the GIF-H260 class in super close-up (3 mm) (Kawai, T. et al. : Evolution of the ultra-thin endoscope. Dig. Endosc. 2013). As the mucosal structures can be observed in NBI super close-up observation, this endoscope is useful in endoscopic diagnosis (particularly qualitative diagnoses) of lesions.

(Kawai, T.)

Case 40 Early carcinoma in gastric remnant

Male in his 80s **Purpose** Suspicion of remnant gastric carcinoma
Location Posterior wall of anastomosis (after distal gastrectomy)

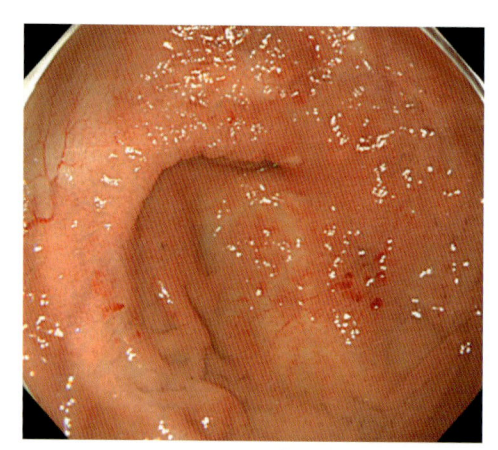

Normal WLI observation (far view): Remnant gastritis is noticeable after distal gastrectomy.

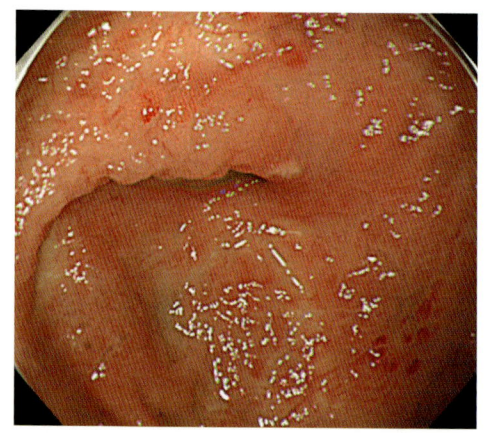

Normal WLI observation (near view): It is hard to recognize obvious lesions around the anastomosis.

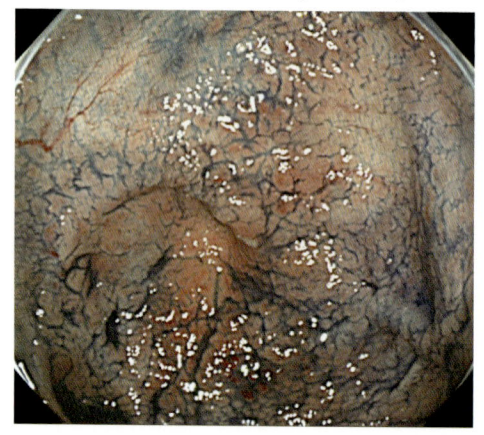

Normal chromoendoscopy (near view): Recognition of lesion is still hard after the indigo carmine spraying.

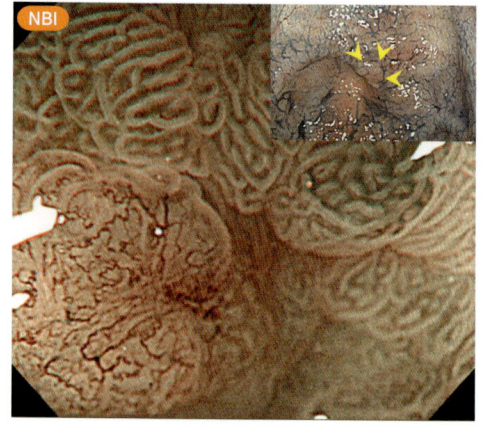

NBI observation (enlarged view of area indicated by arrows): A 5-mm sized mucosal area in which the ductal structures are unclear is recognized.

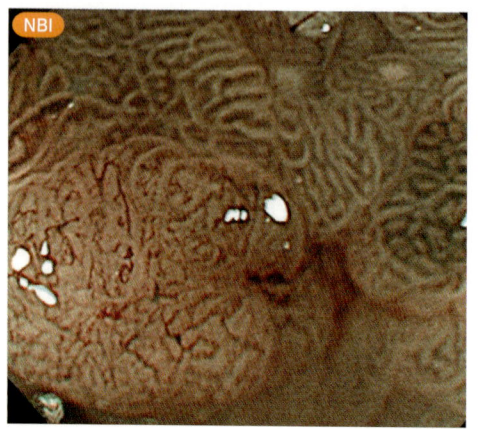

NBI observation: The demarcation line with the surrounding non-neoplastic mucosa is clear.

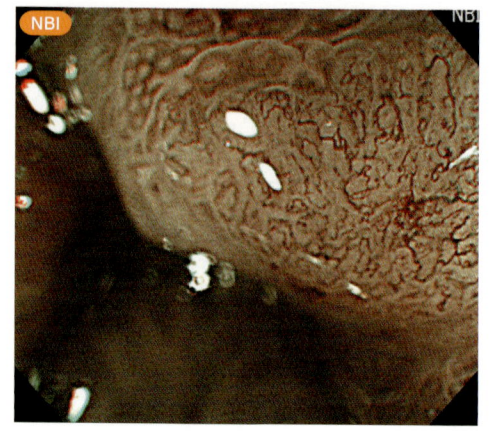

NBI observation: As abnormal vessels with noticeable dilation and tortuosity are observed, the lesion can be diagnosed as a carcinoma.

Endoscope：GIF-H260Z（Olympus）　Light source：EVIS LUCERA SPECTRUM（Olympus）
NBI setup：Structure enhancement B8, color mode 1（Normal observation—Structure enhancement A1； Chromoendoscopy—Structure enhancement A3）

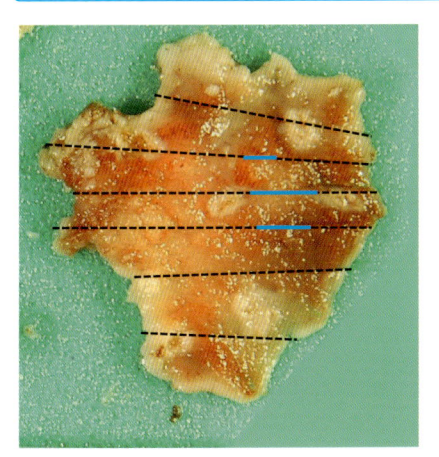

Mapping (specimen size 36×25 mm. lesion size 5×4 mm).

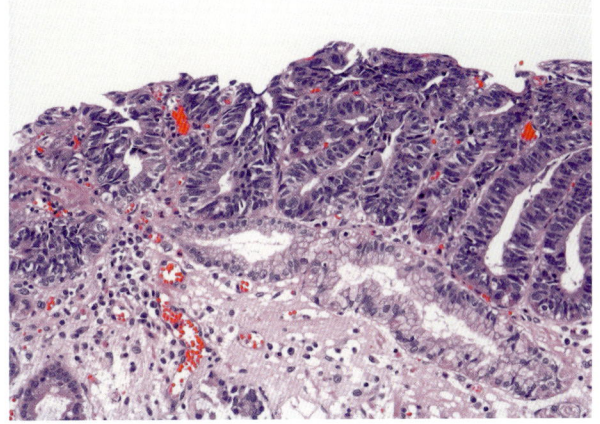

Pathological findings：Atypical columnar epithelium with enlarged nuclei has grown while forming irregular ductal structures. Early gastric carcinoma, 0-Ⅱa, tub1, T1a (M), 5×4 mm, UL (−), ly0, v0, HM (−), VM (−).

Comment

This is an example of early gastric carcinoma that cannot be recognized with WLI or chromoendoscopy, but can be recognized with NBI magnifying observation. The causes of the difficulty in the lesion recognition may include the presence of advanced remnant gastritis in the background and the small size of the lesion — just 5 mm.

▶Observation tips　NBI magnifying observation is useful for diagnosis of such a small carcinoma. Three main characteristics helped define this case as a carcinoma：①unclear ductal structures；②atypical vessels with noticeable dilation and tortuosity, and；③clear demarcation line from the non-neoplastic mucosa. Confirmation of these three characteristics can often be impossible with such small lesions. Special care is required to ensure differentiation from an inflammation.

(Sawai, H., Ono, H.)

Case 41 MALT lymphoma

Male in his 50s | Purpose | Abnormality found in health check
| Location | Gastric body and antrum | Macroscopic type | Superficial type (gastritis type)[1]

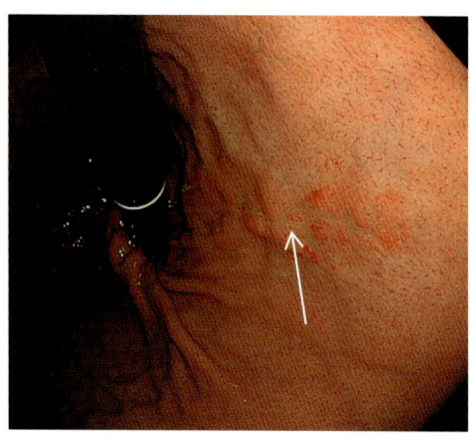

Normal WLI observation: An erythematous area with a discolored depression is visible in the lesser curvature of the upper gastric body.

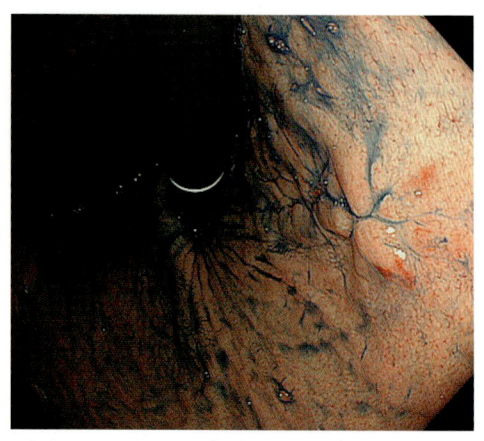

Normal chromoendoscopy (indigo carmine): The depression is more clearly visible by indigo carmine. The surrounding elevated area has a smooth surface.

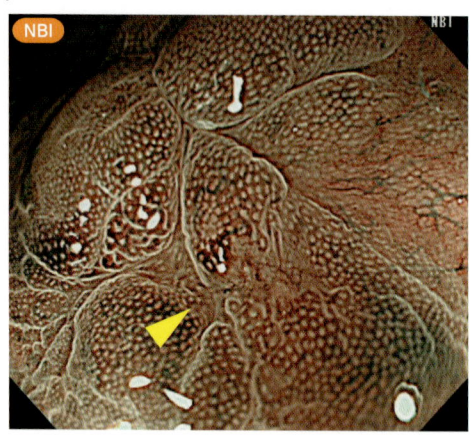

NBI low-magnification observation (area indicated by white arrow): Glossy mucosal superficial layer. The depressed area lacks the pit-like appearance and presents irregular microvessels. This finding suggests the presence of MALT lymphoma. The surrounding elevated area presents a regular pit-like appearance. This finding indicates that the surrounding area is uninvolved.

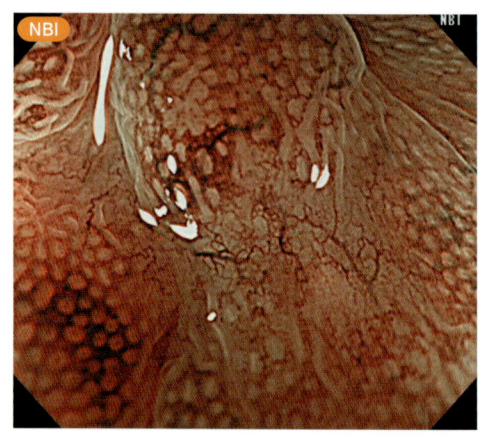

NBI high-magnification observation (area indicated by yellow arrowhead): Irregular microvessels are formed in the lesion. The irregular vessels have tortuosity without caliber change.

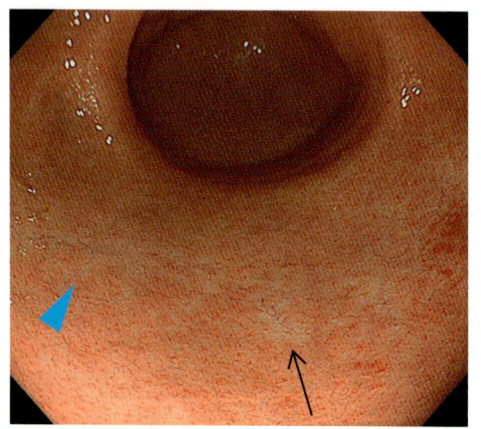

Normal WLI observation: Slightly irregular surface is observed in the greater curvature of the antrum. This lesion also shows color changes including a mixture of erythematous and discolored areas.

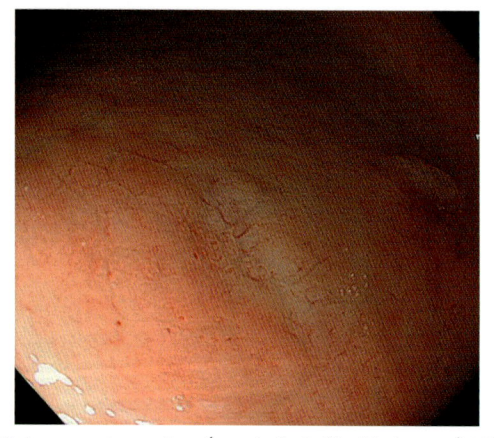

WLI close-up observation (area indicated by black arrow): The close-up view shows relatively large vessels in the discolored depressed area.

140

Endoscope : GIF-H260Z (Olympus)　Light source : EVIS LUCERA ELITE (Olympus)
NBI setup : Structure enhancement A8, color mode 1

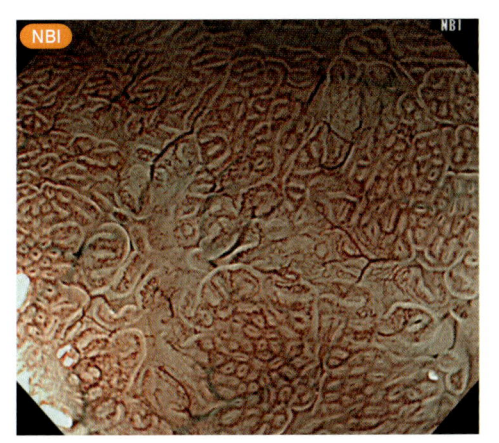

NBI magnifying observation (area indicated by blue arrowhead) : The lesions often show a discolored depression instead of a pit-like appearance. Branching vessels are observed, but changes in caliber and proliferation are not noticeable. Uninvolved surrounding regions show a regular pit-like appearance.

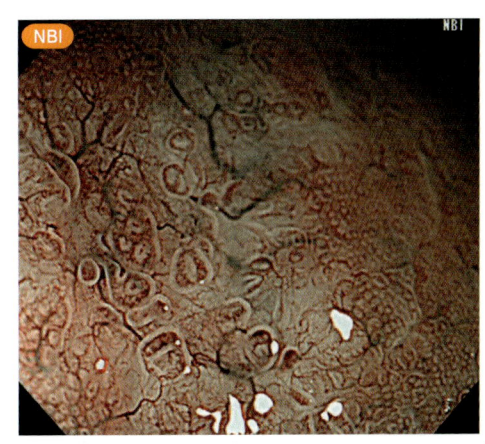

NBI magnifying observation (area indicated by black arrow) : Some regions with pit-like appearance varied in size, and some of them were also swollen or unclear (due to destroyed structures). The microvessels in regions with swollen pit-like appearance are branched continuously from the large vessels in the depressed area.

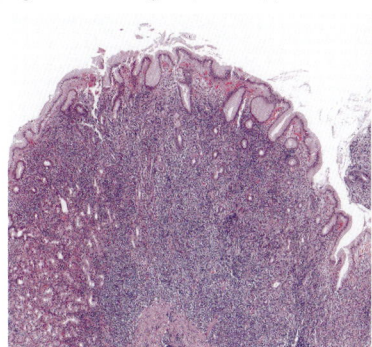

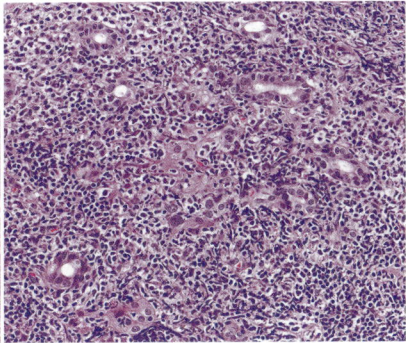

Left : Histological findings sampled from the area by blue arrowhead (H-E stain, ×100) : Small lymphocytes infiltrate the LPM.
Right : Histological findings (H-E stain, ×400) : A lymphoepithelial lesion (LEL) is revealed as infiltration of small lymphocytes among glandular epithelial cells in the LPM.

Comment

In normal WLI endoscopy, gastric MALT lymphoma present in several different ways : as a gastritis-like change, diffusion, ulcer or submucosal tumor. Differential points from gastric carcinoma include poorly demarcated boundaries, surface gloss, multicentricity, cobblestone mucosa and the presence of lymphoid follicle-like structures[2].

▶**Observation tips**　MALT lymphoma cells are often localized in proximity to muscularis mucosae. Therefore it is difficult to detect the presence of MALT lymphoma from minute changes of superficial mucosa. Indigocarmine is effective to evaluate the irregularity of the surface such as depressions and erosions. In NBI magnifying observation, these cases show "tree-like appearance" because the abnormal vessels resemble branches from the trunk of a tree[3]. These vessels show tortuosity but no caliber changes and disruption like gastric cancer cases[4].
Changes of glandular epithelial cells appear as swelling, size variation, lack of pit-like appearance. Whitish lymphoid follicle-like structures are sometimes observed. NBI magnifying observation is effective for targeted biopsy of such minute changes.

Reference
1) Nakamura, S. et al. : Journal of Japanese Society of Gastroenterology 2001 ; 98 : 624-635
2) Isomoto, H. et al. : Endoscopy 2008 ; 40 : 225-228
3) Nonaka, K. et al. : J Gastroenterol. Hepatol. 2009 ; 24 : 1697
4) Ono, S. et al. : Gastrointest. Endosc. 2008 ; 68 : 624-631

(Matsushima, K., Isomoto, H., Onita, K., Shikuwa, S.)

Case 42 MALT lymphoma

Female in her 60s **Purpose** Detailed observation of gastric lesion
Location Greater curvature of lower part of body **Macroscopic type** Superficial type (discolored)

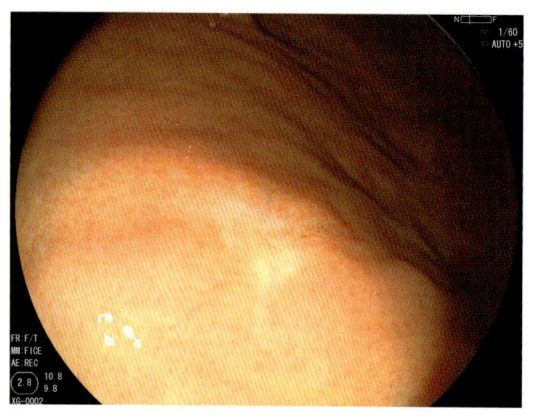

Conventional white-light image: A discolored small area about 10 mm in size surrounded by non-atrophic gastric mucosa is visible in the greater curvature of the lower third of the stomach.

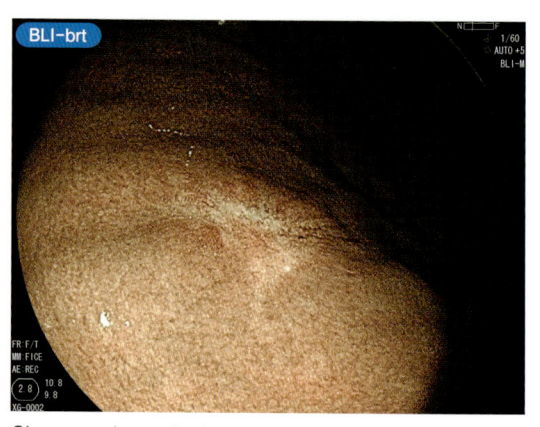

Chromoendoscopic image with BLI-bright mode: The non-atrophic mucosa has a uniform brownish color tone, while the lesion appears whitish.

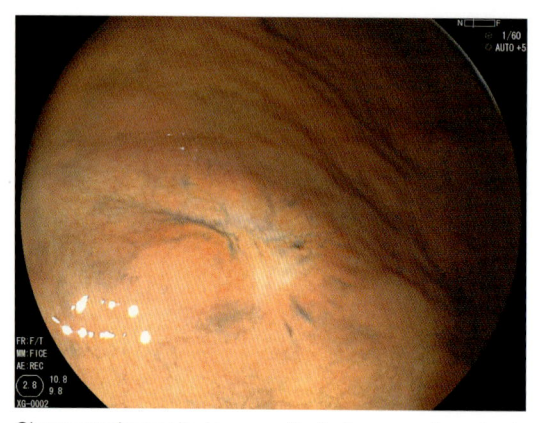

Chromoendoscopic image with indigo carmine dye: Demarcation of the lesion is not clear.

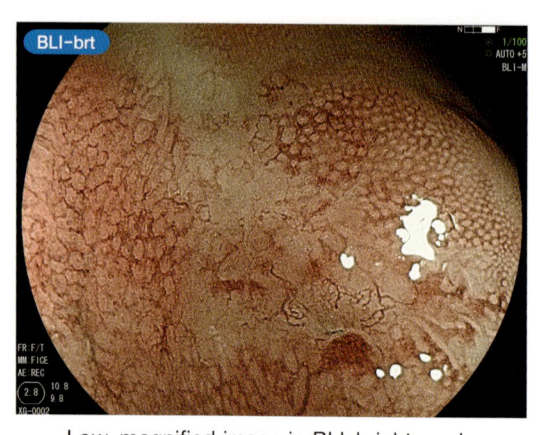

Low-magnified image in BLI-bright mode

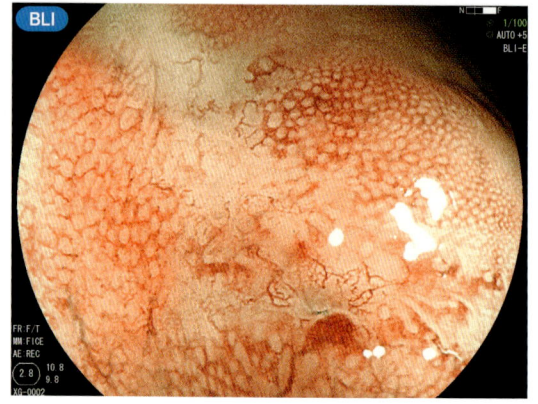

Low-magnified image in BLI mode: Although the regular microstructures in the surrounding area are visible, the microstructures in the lymphoma lesion have almost completely disappeared and irregular microvessels can be seen. The demarcation line is unclear.

Endoscope : Prototype (EG-L590ZW equivalent) (Fujifilm)　Light source : LASEREO (Fujifilm)
BLI setup : Structure enhancement A6, color enhancement C1.

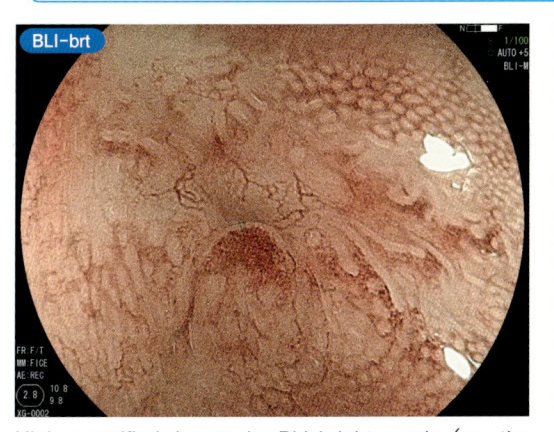

High-magnified image in BLI-bright mode (on the posterior wall side of lesion) :

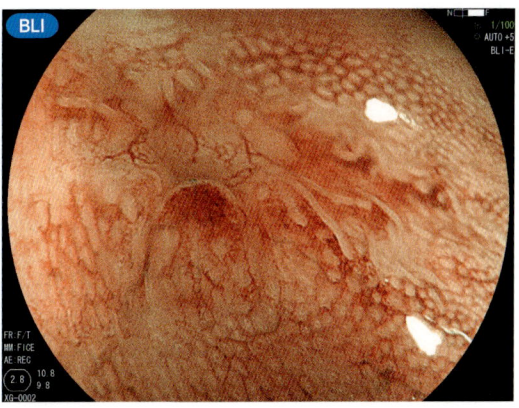

High-magnified image in BLI mode (on the posterior wall side of lesion) : The intervening parts are elongated and the gastric pits have been destroyed. The subepithelial capillary network (SECN) is also stretched and congested.

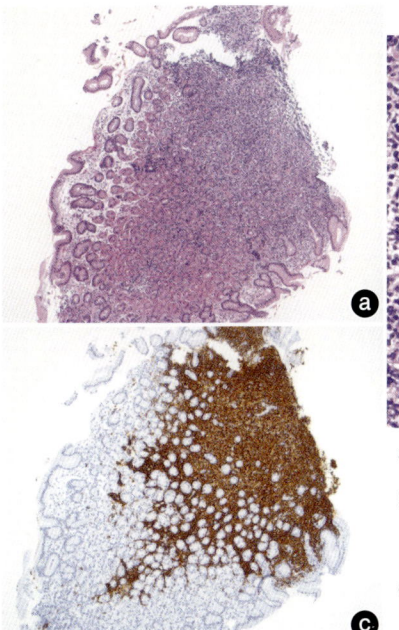

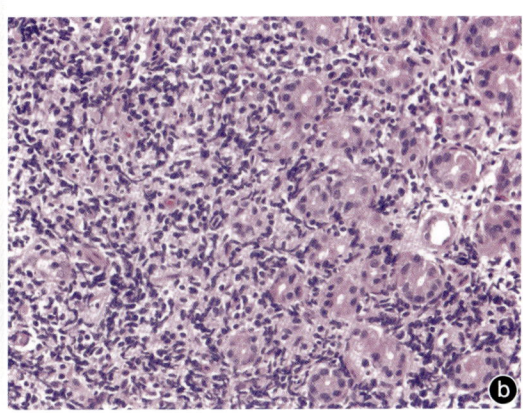

a : Histological image (hematoxylin-eosin, original magnification : 10×).
b : Histological image (hematoxylin-eosin, original magnification : 40×). Dense proliferation of small lymphoid cells with lymphoepithelial lesion is seen. The histological diagnosis is Wotherspoon grade 5.
c : Histological image (CD20, original magnification : 10×) : The lymphoma cells are CD3-negative and CD20-strongly positive.

Comment

This is a case of an API2-MALT-1 fusion-positive gastric MALT (mucosa-associated lymphoid tissue) lymphoma developed in the *H. pylori*-negative patient. Although the MALT lymphoma is a non-epithelial tumor, we can see the changes in the microsurface pattern induced by the invasion of lymphoma cells using magnifying endoscopy.

▶ **Observation tips** It has been reported that destruction of the normal gastric pits and appearance of abnormal vessels are typical in magnified endoscopic images of MALT lymphoma. These images reflect the histological findings of displacement and destruction of gastric glands by infiltration of lymphoma cells[1,2]. After treatment, the gastric pits and subepithelial capillary network (SECN) reappeared, while the abnormal vessels disappeared. We recommend magnifying endoscopy for target biopsies and evaluations after treatment.

Reference　1) Ono, S. et al. : Gastrointest Endosc 2008 ; 68 : 624-631
　　　　　　　2) Ono, S. et al. : J Gastroenterol Hepatol 2011 ; 26 : 1133-1138

(Ono, S.)

Case 43 Duodenal adenoma

Male aged 72   **Purpose** Preoperative examination of duodenal lesion
Location Inferior wall of duodenal bulb   **Macroscopic type** 0-Ⅱa

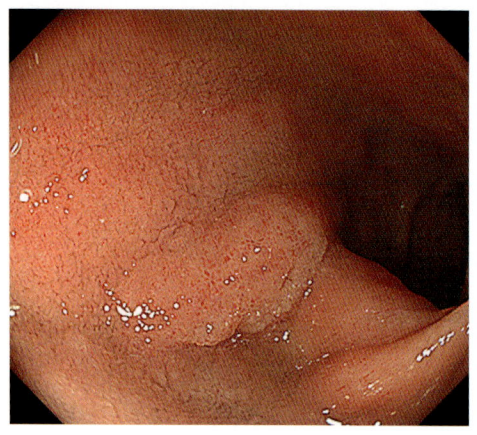

White light observation: Elevated lesion with a size of 10 mm and low height. Dot-shaped reddish area is observed in the lesion. The demarcation on the left side of the lesion is not clear.

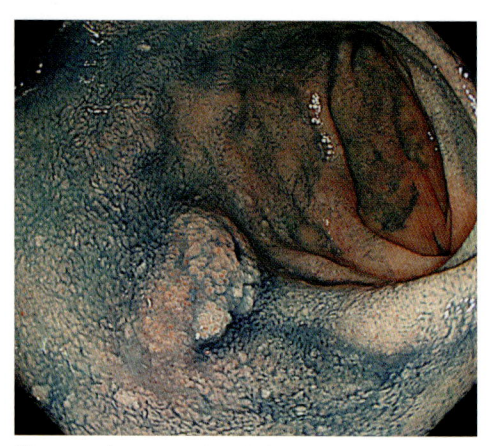

Chromoendoscopy using indigo carmine: The lesion demarcation is seen relatively clearly.

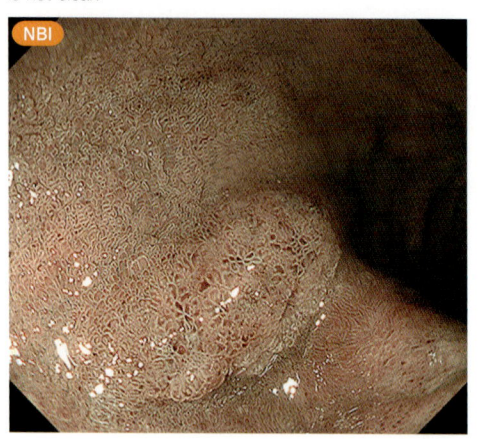

NBI non-magnifying observation: Like chromoendoscopy, NBI endoscopy can show the lesion demarcation relatively clearly.

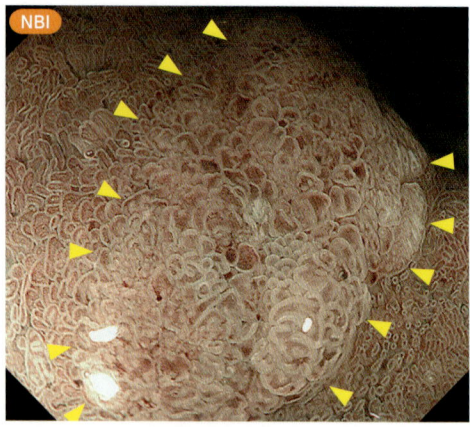

NBI magnifying observation: The demarcation from the surrounding normal mucosa is imaged clearly (arrowheads). The lesion contains large villous architecture with irregular sizes and shapes.

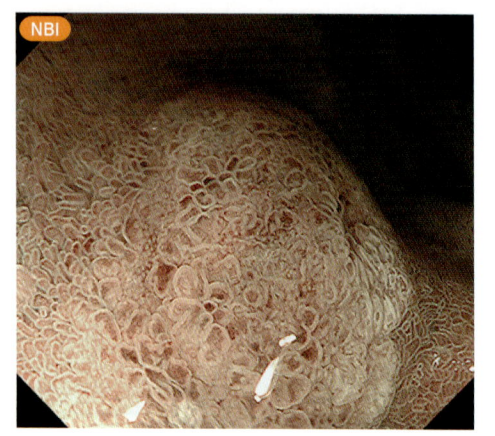

NBI magnifying observation of center of lesion: There is no sign of any unclear mucosal patterns or abnormal vascular proliferation.

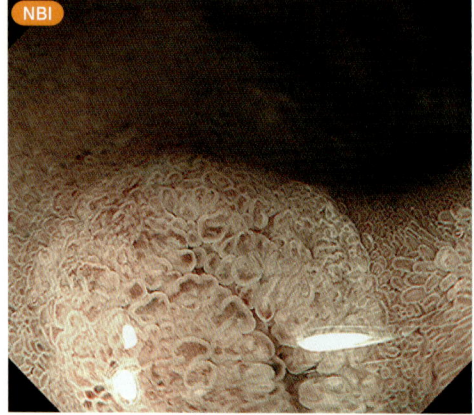

NBI magnifying observation of distal side of lesion: Thanks to NBI's increased brightness, the entire lesion is clear and bright even under magnifying observation.

Endoscope：GIF-H260Z（Olympus）　Light source：EVIS LUCERA ELITE（Olympus）
NBI setup：Structure enhancement B7, color mode 1

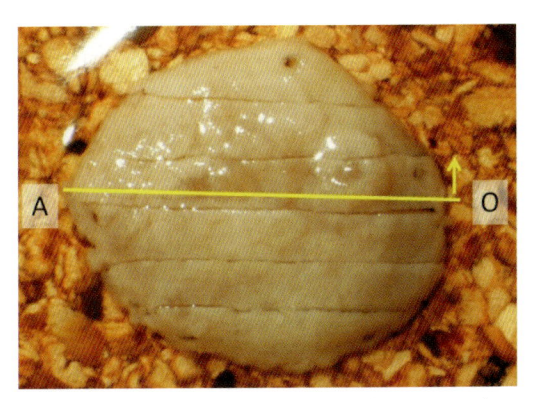

Macroscopic pathology：After en bloc resection with EMR using the snare method, the lesion is sliced as shown in the photo.

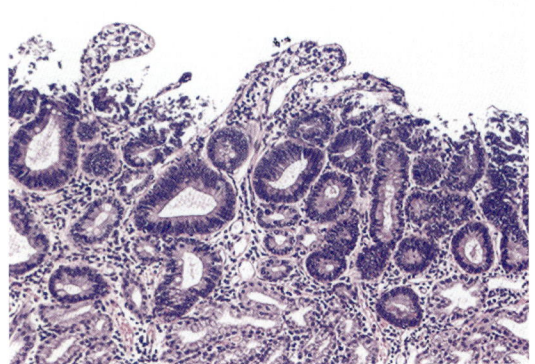

Microscopic pathology：Histologically, tumor cells with enlarged oval nuclei proliferate by forming gland ducts. The neoplastic ducts are of a relatively uniform size and the nuclei are arranged on the base side, so the lesion is diagnosed as a tubular adenoma with high-grade atypia.

Comment

This is a 10 mm elevated lesion found in the duodenum. Even under indigo carmine chromoendoscopy, the demarcation was hard to distinguish; however, under NBI magnifying observation, it was clearly and circumferentially visible. Since the lesion was located on the bulb, differentiation from non-neoplastic lesions such as ectopic gastric mucosa or non-epithelial tumors such as carcinoids was required. NBI magnifying observation showed that this case had the characteristics of an epithelial neoplastic lesion, including the presence of a localized lesion with clear demarcation and villous architecture with irregular sizes and shapes.

▶**Observation tips** Even when the lesion is relatively hard to distinguish from the surrounding area in terms of color tone and demarcation, accurate qualitative and extent diagnoses are possible with NBI magnifying observation. This can be achieved by identifying the differences between the surrounding normal villi and the lesion's villous architecture at half-zoom magification and then increasing the magnification and observing the mucosal patterns and microvascular structures in detail.

(Dobashi, A., Goda, K., Tajiri, H.)

Case 44 Duodenal adenoma

Male in his 40s   **Purpose** Detailed examination of duodenal lesion
Location Descending part of the duodenum   **Macroscopic type** 0 - IIc

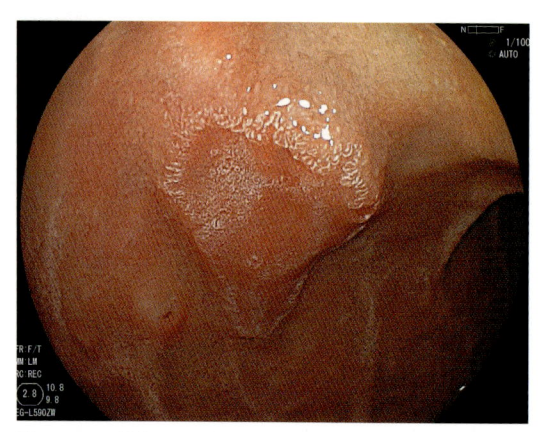

Non-magnifying white-light observation : A 25-mm depressed reddened lesion with a partially whitened area in the descending part of the duodenum.

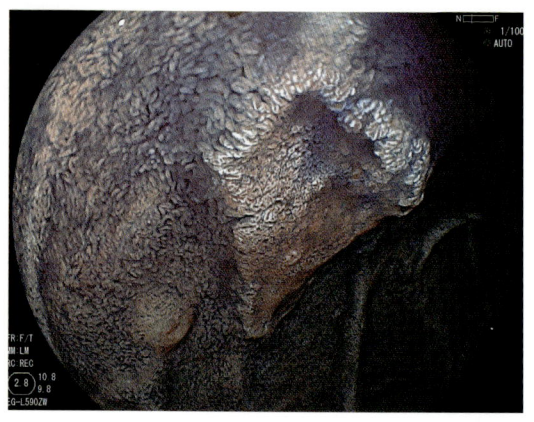

Non-magnifying chromoendoscopy : Indigo carmine-sprayed observation clarifies the demarcation between the lesion and surrounding area.

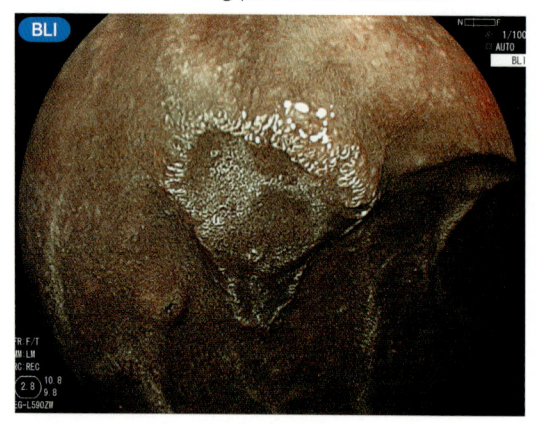

BLI non-magnifying observation : The lesion is more clearly visible.

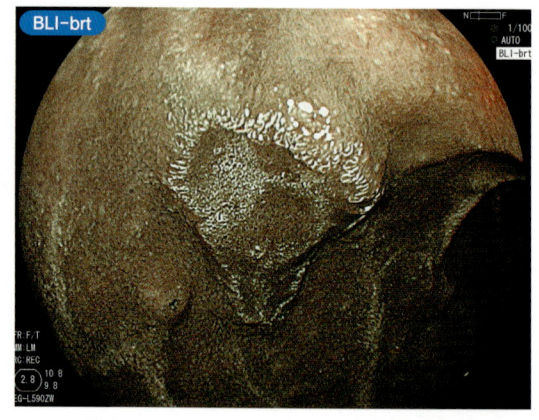

BLI-bright non-magnifying observation.

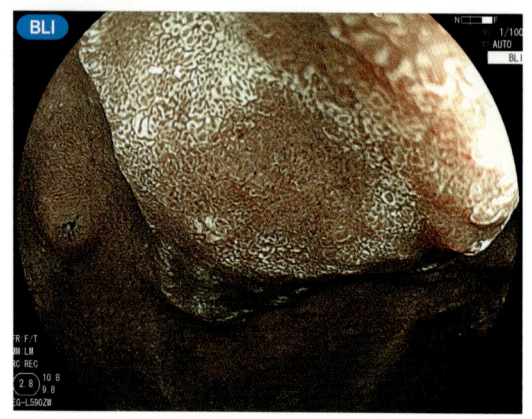

BLI low-magnification observation : The microsurface structure in the lesion can be seen. WOS is present in some regions. At this magnification, however, it is impossible to evaluate the microvascular architecture and microsurface structure.

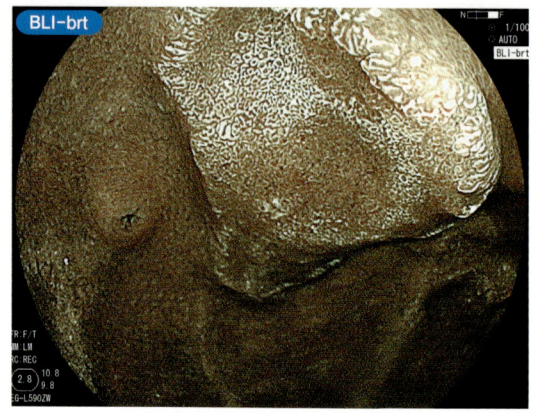

BLI-bright low-magnification observation.

146

Endoscope：EG-L590ZW（Fujifilm） Light source：LASEREO（Fujifilm）
BLI setup：BLI—Structure enhancement B8, color enhancement C1；BLI-bright—Structure enhancement B8, color enhancement C1

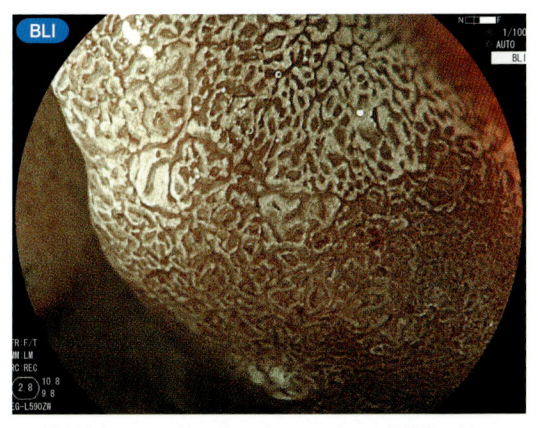

BLI high-magnification observation：WOS with a reticular pattern can be seen. The microvascular architecture in this lesion is not visualized.

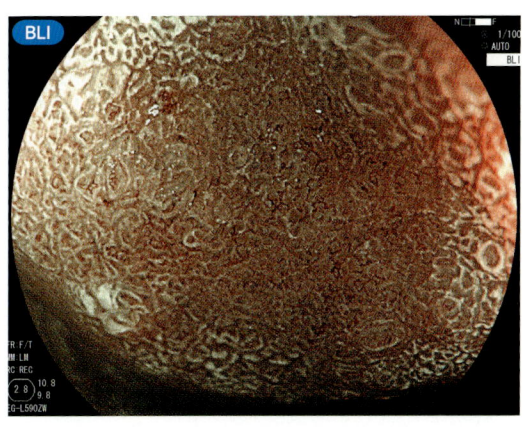

BLI high-magnification observation：The microsurface structure and microvascular architecture can be seen. The microsurface structure and microvascular architecture are regular.

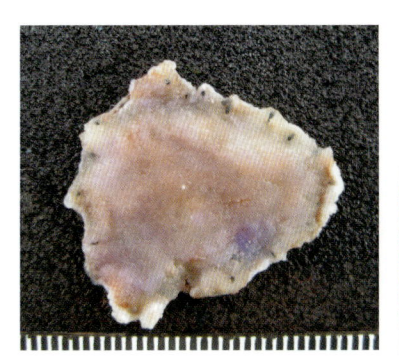

ESD-resected specimen：The specimen is 30×20 mm with a 25×18 mm Ⅱc lesion.

Loupe image

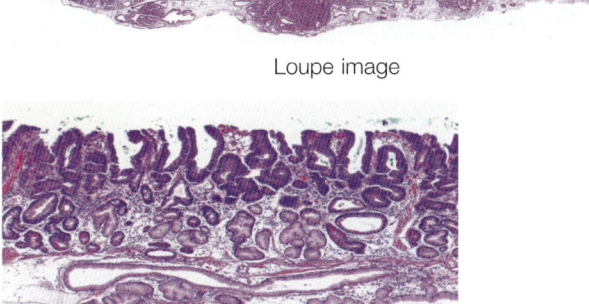

Low-magnification image：Tubular adenoma of the duodenum, severe atypia, HM0, VM0.

Comment

Duodenal adenoma is often accompanied by WOS covering all or part of the lesion. The color ranges from whitish to light reddish depending on the state of distribution. While BLI observation shows the WOS more clearly and facilitates recognition of the microsurface structure, it also makes observation of microvascular architecture more difficult. In this case, the microsurface structure, for which the WOS is used as an alternative optical sign, was observed to have a reticular pattern. As the microsurface structure and the microvascular architecture were regular, this lesion was judged to be an adenoma. In this case, the BLI mode was more suitable than the BLI-bright mode as it provided higher contrast under magnification, enabling more detailed magnifying observation.

▶**Observation tips** The findings in BLI magnifying observation are evaluated based on the microsurface structure and microvascular architecture. When both are observable as in this case, diagnosis can be based on both of them. When the microvascular architecture is obscured due to the WOS, the adenoma can be diagnosed based on observation of the microsurface structure.

(Yoshida, S.)

Case 45 Duodenal carcinoma

Male in his 60s　**Purpose**　Preoperative examination of duodenal lesion
Location　Descending part of the duodenum　**Macroscopic type**　0-Ⅱa

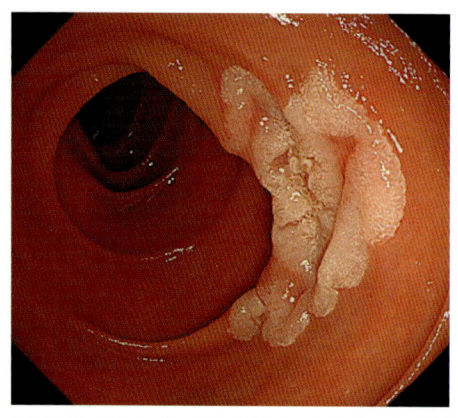

WLI far-view observation：A whitish elevated lesion about 30 mm in size. The margin is irregular like pseudopodia and accompanied by surface irregularities. Poor distensibility of the wall is found.

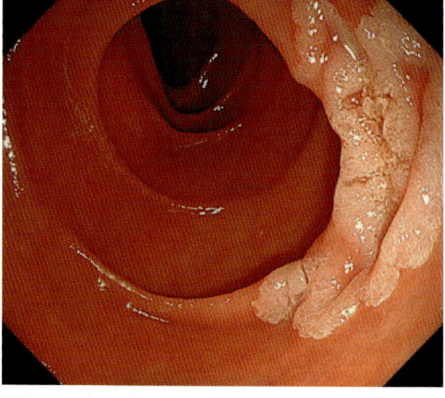

WLI near-view observation：As the entire lesion presents a milk-white color tone, we call it a milk-white mucosa（MWM）, entire type. Reddish depressions are also found in some places.

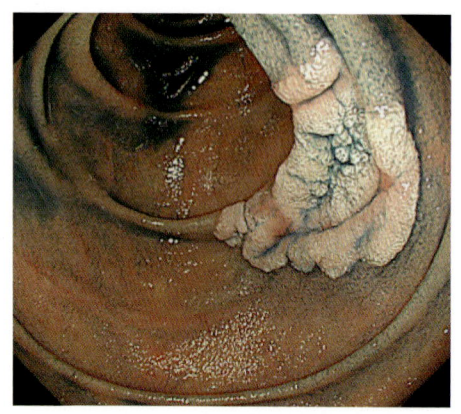

Indigo carmine chromoendoscopy：The lesion demarcation and height irregularities can be observed more clearly.

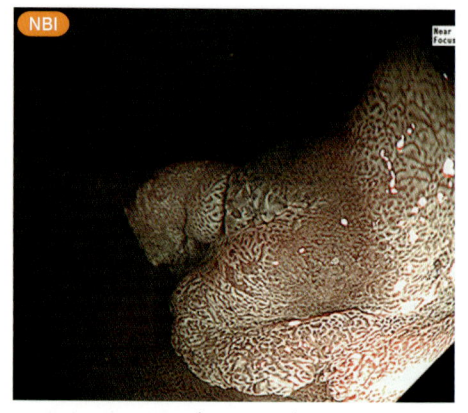

NBI magnifying observation（Near Focus）：The reddish depression （MWM-negative area） on the left margin of the lesion ranges from very small to disappeared.

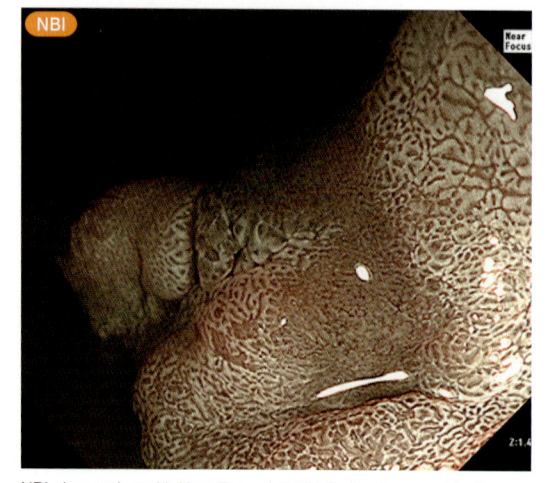

NBI observation with Near Focus＋1.4×electronic zoom：In the area where the mucosal pattern is very small or hard to recognized, microvessels with network patterns are observed, suggesting the presence of a lesion somewhere between a high-grade adenoma and an adenocarcinoma.

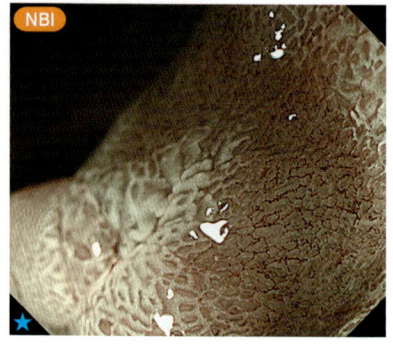

NBI high-magnification observation with the H260Z：The network pattern is more clearly visualized. However, the new system's HQ290 can capture anomalies in the mucosal patterns and vascular structures with a level of quality just as good as the conventional magnifying endoscope.

148

Endoscope : GIF-HQ290 (GIF-H260Z with image marked ★) (Olympus)
Light source : EVIS LUCERA ELITE (Olympus)　NBI setup : Structure enhancement A7, color mode 1

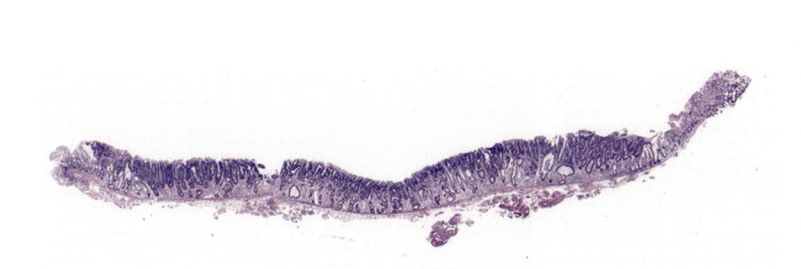

Magnified image (HE) : After en bloc resection of the lesion with ESD, the reddish depression shown in the NBI image is cut and subjected to histological examination.

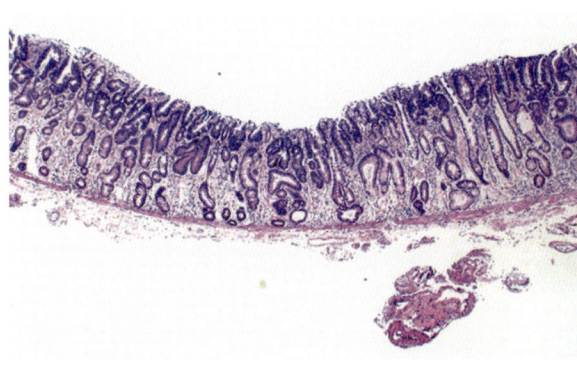

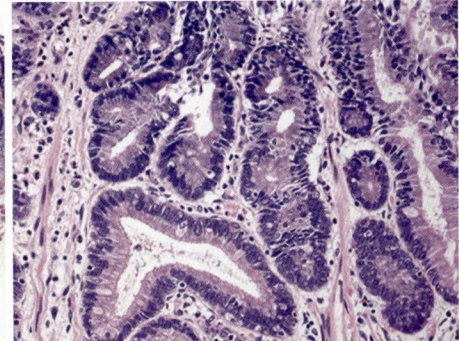

Left : Pathology (HE, low magnification). **Right** : Pathology, (HE, high magnification).
Histologically, most of the lesion is adenoma. However, in the position coincident to the reddish depression, branching and abnormal courses of gland ducts as well as appearance of nucleoli, enlargement of nuclei and disturbance of polarity are observed. As a result, the lesion is diagnosed as a well-differentiated adenocarcinoma. Final diagnosis : well differentiated adenocarcinoma in adenoma. Type 0 - Ⅱa, pM, ly0, v0, pHMX, pVM0.

Comment

This is a relatively large-sized elevated lesion in the duodenum. WLI observation is sufficient to assess it as an adenomatous lesion. In NBI magnifying observation of the reddish depression, small mucosal patterns on the proximal side can be seen, as well as network patterns, strongly suggesting the presence of a well-differentiated adenocarcinoma.

▶**Observation tips** This lesion is basically whitish with reddish depression in some areas. The HQ290 endoscope with Dual Focus capability is easy to manipulate thanks to its button-controlled magnification method, and magnification operation is easy, as well, thanks to the extended depth of focus. This enables quick observation of a few reddish areas and, in the Near Focus mode, detection of those areas where the mucosal patterns are small or unclear. When the electronic zoom is used, it is possible to find the abnormal vessels that present network patterns, which is useful for identification of adenocarcinoma inside the adenoma.

(Dobashi, A., Goda, K., Tajiri, H.)

Case 46 Duodenal carcinoma

Female in her 50s **Purpose** Detailed examination of duodenal lesion
Location Inferior wall of duodenal bulb **Macroscopic type** 0-Ⅱa+Ⅱc

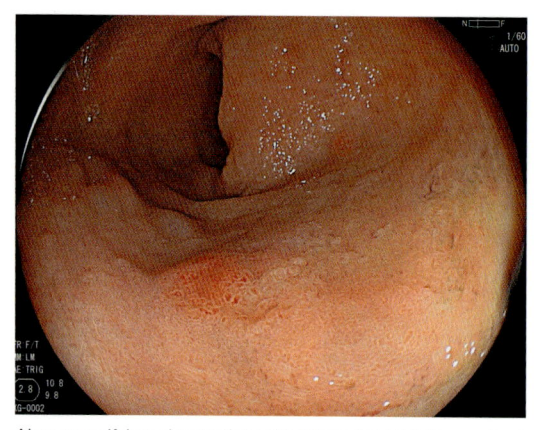

Non-magnifying observation with White-light : A 6 mm-sized elevated lesion accompanied by erythematous areas and irregular depressions on the inferior wall of the duodenal bulb.

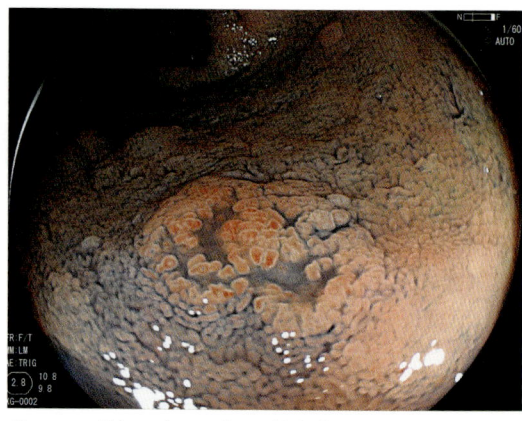

Non-magnifying observation with Indigo carmine-sprayed : The mucosal patterns on the elevation are larger than the villous architecture on the background duodenal mucosa. In some parts, these patterns present the erythematous color tone.

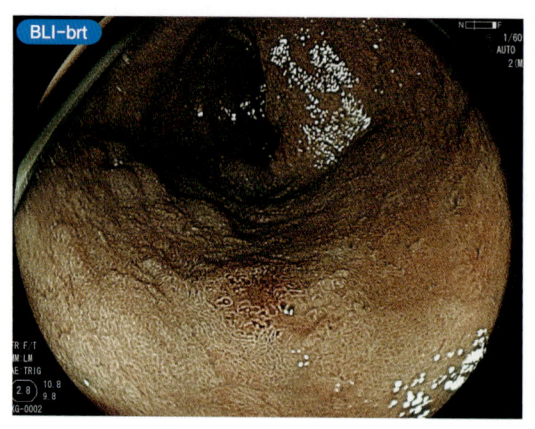

Low-magnifying observation with BLI-bright mode : The entire lesion can be imaged from a relatively far view. Enlarged mucosal patterns and irregular depression surfaces are observed.

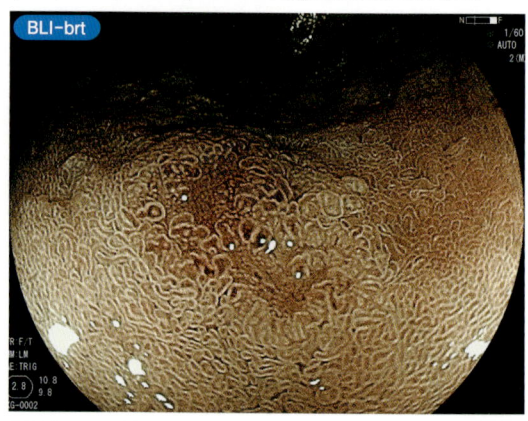

Middle-magnifying observation with BLI-bright mode : Even without indigo carmine spraying, the villous architecture of the surrounding duodenal mucosa is clearly visible. In addition, the enlarged granular mucosal patterns of the lesion and the fine mucosal patterns of the depressed area are visible.

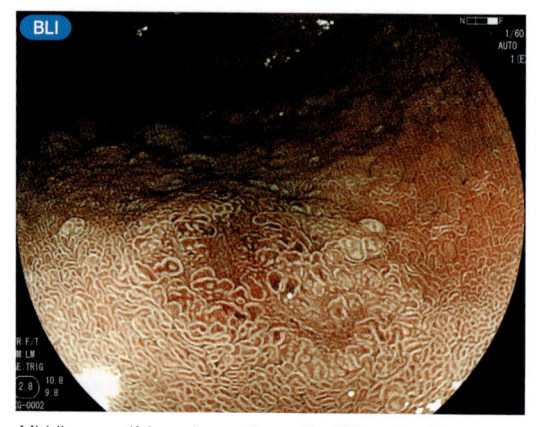

Middle-magnifying observation with BLI mode : The overall image is more reddish than the BLI-bright mode image. The mucosal patterns are visible with an enhanced sense of the differences in height.

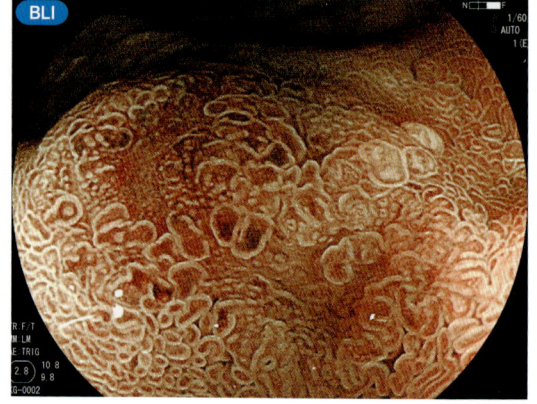

High-magnifying observation with BLI mode : The depressed area on the distal side presents relatively uniform fine mucosal patterns.

Endoscope：Prototype（EG-L590ZW equivalent）（Fujifilm）　　Light source：LASEREO（Fujifilm）
BLI setup：BLI—Structure enhancement B6, color enhancement C1；BLI-bright—Structure enhancement B8, color enhancement C1

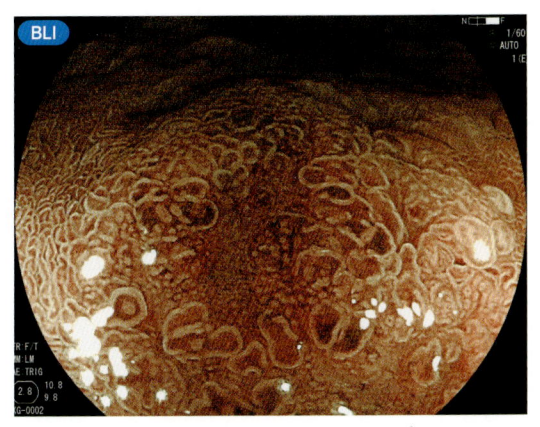

High-magnifying observation with BLI mode（distal side of lesion）：On the distal side of the lesion, depressed areas with fine pit patterns can be seen in uneven mucosal patterns containing loop-shaped vessels.

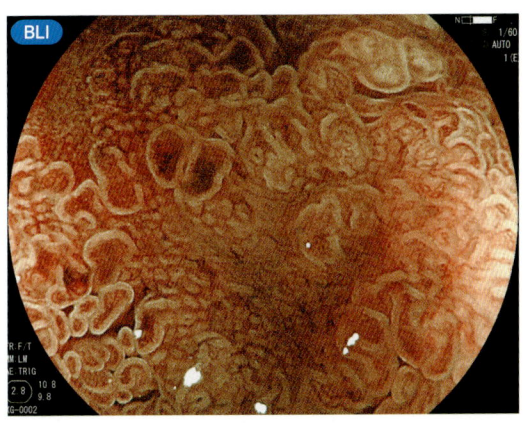

High-magnifying observation with BLI mode（proximal side of lesion）：On the proximal side of the lesion, the mucosal patterns of some depressed areas are unclear and irregular vascular patterns are observed.

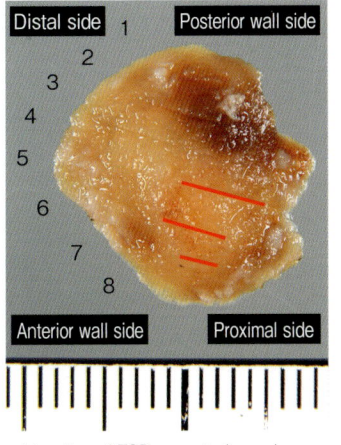

Mapping of ESD-resected specimen

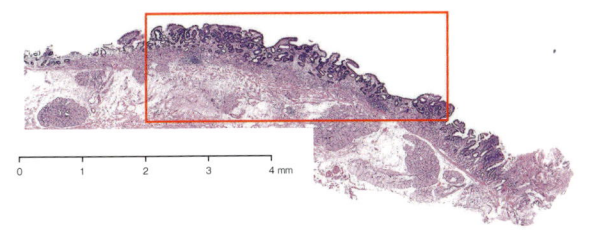

Loupe images of sections in the resected specimen：Adenocarcinoma tubulare, very well differentiated, tub1, Type 0-Ⅱa+Ⅱc, 6×5 mm, depth m, ly（−）, v（−）, pHM0, pVM0.（inside red rectangle）

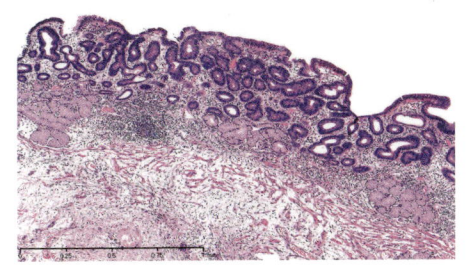

Low-magnification image：Densely proliferated neoplastic ductal glands can be seen. Although their degree of atypia is not high, certain gland ducts present relatively irregular branching and tumor cells are occasionally exposed on the surface layer, so the lesion is diagnosed as a very well-differentiated carcinoma.

Comment

Magnifying observation in the BLI-bright or BLI mode can image the ductal structures clearly without the help of indigo carmine spraying. The gland duct patterns in the elevated area are larger than those on the normal duodenal mucosa in the surrounding area, and the diameters and shapes are irregular. In BLI high-magnification observation, the irregular mucosal patterns and the internal loop-shaped vessels are both enhanced. In the depressed region, relatively uniform micromucosal patterns are mixed with areas where the mucosal structures are unclear, and irregular vascular patterns are observed. Based on the BLI observation findings, the lesion is diagnosed as a very well-differentiated duodenal carcinoma（intramucosal cancer）.

▶Observation tips　In BLI magnifying observation, factors leading to a suspicion of malignancy include enlargement of the surface mucosal patterns, proliferation of loop-shaped vessels, unclear mucosal patterns in the depressed area and the appearance of irregular microvessels. Since the lumen in the duodenum is relatively narrow, BLI observation is suitable because of the ease of obtaining surface layer information and of enhancing height irregularities.

（Yagi, N.）

Case 47 Duodenal carcinoma

Male in his 40s **Purpose** Detailed examination of duodenal lesion
Location Descending part of the duodenum **Macroscopic type** Flat elevation (0-Ⅱa type)

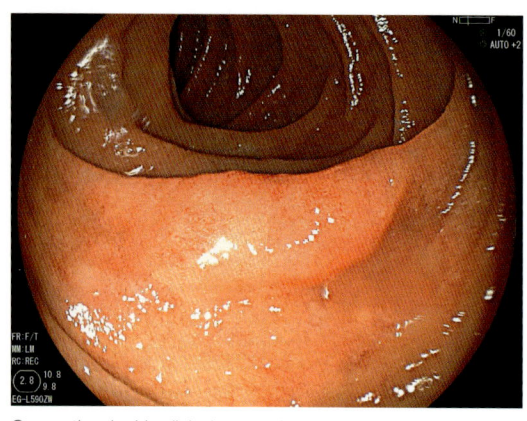

Conventional white-light image: A flat elevated lesion about 15 mm in diameter in the descending part of the duodenum. The color is almost the same as the background mucosa.

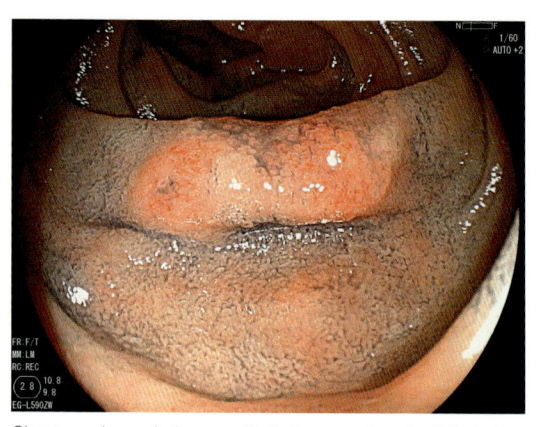

Chromoendoscopic image with indigo carmine dye: A shallow depression on the lesion appears.

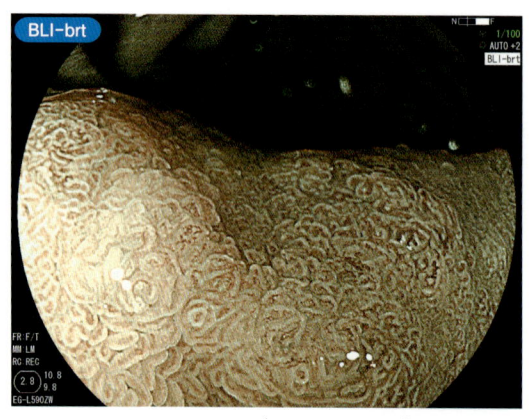

BLI-bright mode (low magnification)

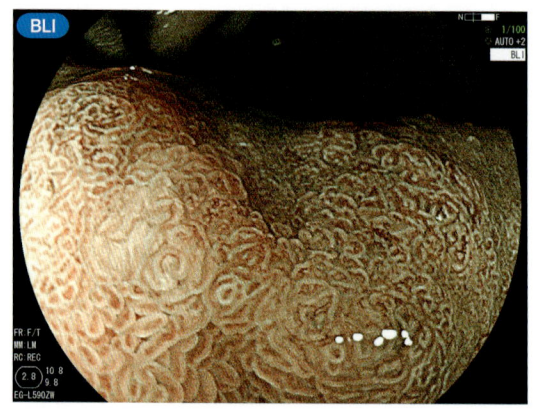

BLI mode (low magnification): Tubular or ridge-shaped microstructures can be seen. The demarcation between the tumor and the background is unclear.

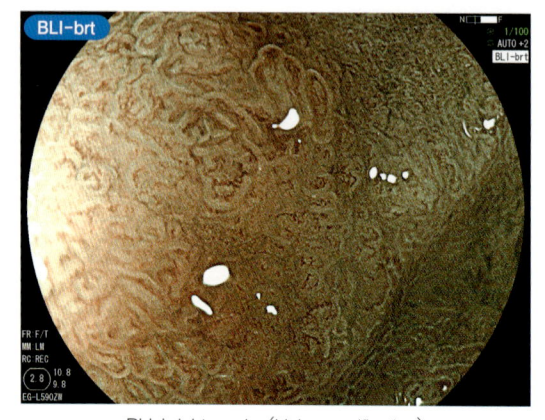

BLI-bright mode (high magnification)

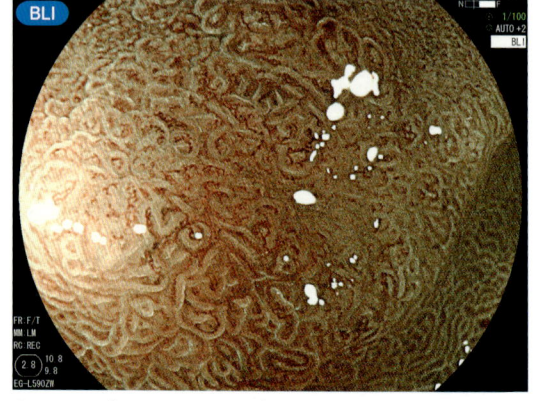

BLI mode (high magnification): On the proximal side of the lesion, severe irregularities in the microstructures can be seen. In addition, there is no sign of any marginal villous epitheliums and the microstructures have disappeared. Microvessels with irregular diameters run in irregular patterns and no WOS (white opaque substance) can be seen.

Endoscope：EG-L590ZW（Fujifilm）　　Light source：LASEREO（Fujifilm）
BLI setup：Structure enhancement A6, color enhancement C1

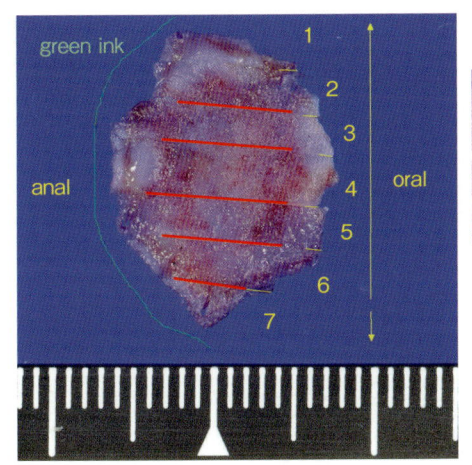

Macroscopic image of resected specimen: A Ⅱa lesion in size 17 mm×15 mm, Tubular adenocarcinoma (tub1), pM, ly (−), v (−), pHM (−), pVM (−).

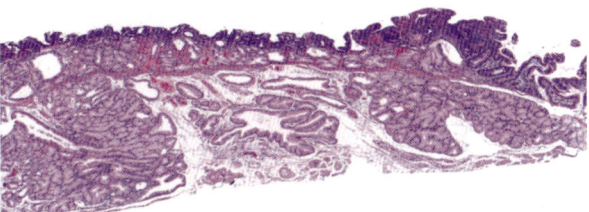

Histological image (hematoxylin-eosin)：Histological image of slice No. 3 is shown. The cells with enlarged nuclei form irregular glandular ducts. On the distal side, polarity is maintained for the most part, but atypical glandular ducts which have dropped can also be seen.

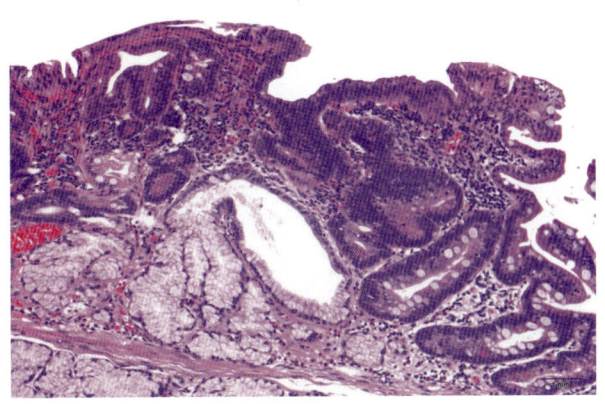

Histological image (hematoxylin-eosin)：High-magnification histological image of the proximal side of slice No. 3 is shown. It is the same region shown in the two images at the bottom of the page on the left. Glandular ducts with severe architectural atypia and enlarged nuclei can be seen.

Comment

Duodenal tumors are relatively rare and endoscopic diagnosis has not been established. This case is one where differentiation between the duodenal adenoma and duodenal carcinoma is histologically difficult. In conventional white-light imaging, the lesion appeared relatively smooth, but magnified images showed irregular microstructures.

▶Observation tips Adenomas with severe atypia and intramucosal carcinomas show unclear microstructures and microvessels with an irregular network pattern in magnified endoscopic images[1]. Whitening of the mucosa (which is equivalent to the presence of WOS) is often observed with duodenal adenoma ; however, when the atypism of the adenoma advances, the whitening of the mucosa remains only on the margin[2]. Because whitening of the mucosa was not observed and the microstructures had partially disappeared in this case, the lesion was suspected to be an adenoma with severe atypia or intramucosal carcinoma.

Reference 1) Yoshimura, N. et al.：Hepatogastroenterology 2010；57：462-467
2) Yoshimura, N. et al.：Gastroenterol Endosc 2007；49（Suppl. 1）：840

(Ono, S.)

Featured Article

Pathological correlative approach to magnified images

In the past, the pathological diagnosis was the "final diagnosis" and there is no doubt that pathology has proven critical in supporting diagnoses of many gastrointestinal diseases. Now, however, endoscopy has at last entered the micro world. The resolution of magnifying endoscopes is now at the micrometric level, and the measurement scales used by endoscopists and pathologists are already identical. The time when things were visible only through the pathological eye is over. Now things are visible with both endoscopy and pathology.

Nevertheless, people are slow to change and when they speak of the endoscopy-pathology correlation (hereinafter referred to as the "correlation"), they often want to check if the observation made by endoscopy is correct. Two decades ago, this might have been appropriate ; today that is no longer the case. Because so much more information is available, the correlation cannot be permitted to remain a simple matter of double-checking the results.

Pathologists do work hard. They must deal with a vast amount of standards, guidelines and classification methods. However, it is very difficult to follow everything including issues that do not appear in the standards. Aside from GI-friendly pathologists, that is, pathologists with a special interest in the GI tract, ordinary pathologists would find it difficult to go beyond what is written in the standards. But for this correlation to be of true value, it is essential to go beyond the standards.

A correlation should never be ended by simply reading words such as "WDTA*, invasion pT1a (M)" written in the pathological report. Is this "WDTA" a WDTA lesion with a low degree of atypia that proliferates by replacing the mucosal superficial layer or one with a high degree of atypia that infiltrates the LPM but advances by crawling through the intermediate layer without exposing itself to the superficial layer? Their magnified images are completely different.

Figure shows images obtained with a case with the pathological diagnosis of WDTA (provided by the courtesy of Dr. Junichi Kodaira at Keiyukai Sapporo Hospital ; the areas enclosed by the yellow dotted lines [e] are the neoplastic ducts). In this case, the endoscopist who was concerned about the unclear demarcation line (DL) marked out the area himself and sliced the ESD specimen in order to inform the pathologist that these would definitely be the regions of interest. When the specimen was observed microscopically, it was found that the tumor was indeed a WDTA tumor. The surface layer was found to be coated with non-neoplastic epithelium, while the tumor was determined to be progressing horizontally in the LPM (LPM invasion). These findings are logical for explaining why the DL is unclear. This conclusion would be impossible to reach by reading only the standard information provided in the pathological report.

Detailed degree of differentiation, morphology of tumor nest, mode of invasion and development, status of muscularis mucosae, courses/distribution/diameter of vessels, distributions of lymphoid follicles and ectopic ducts, conditions of background mucosa and so on—the real interest in the correlation lies in what is not written in the pathological report, and goes beyond simple double-checking.

*Well differentiated tubular adenocarcinoma (tub 1)

(Ichihara, S.)

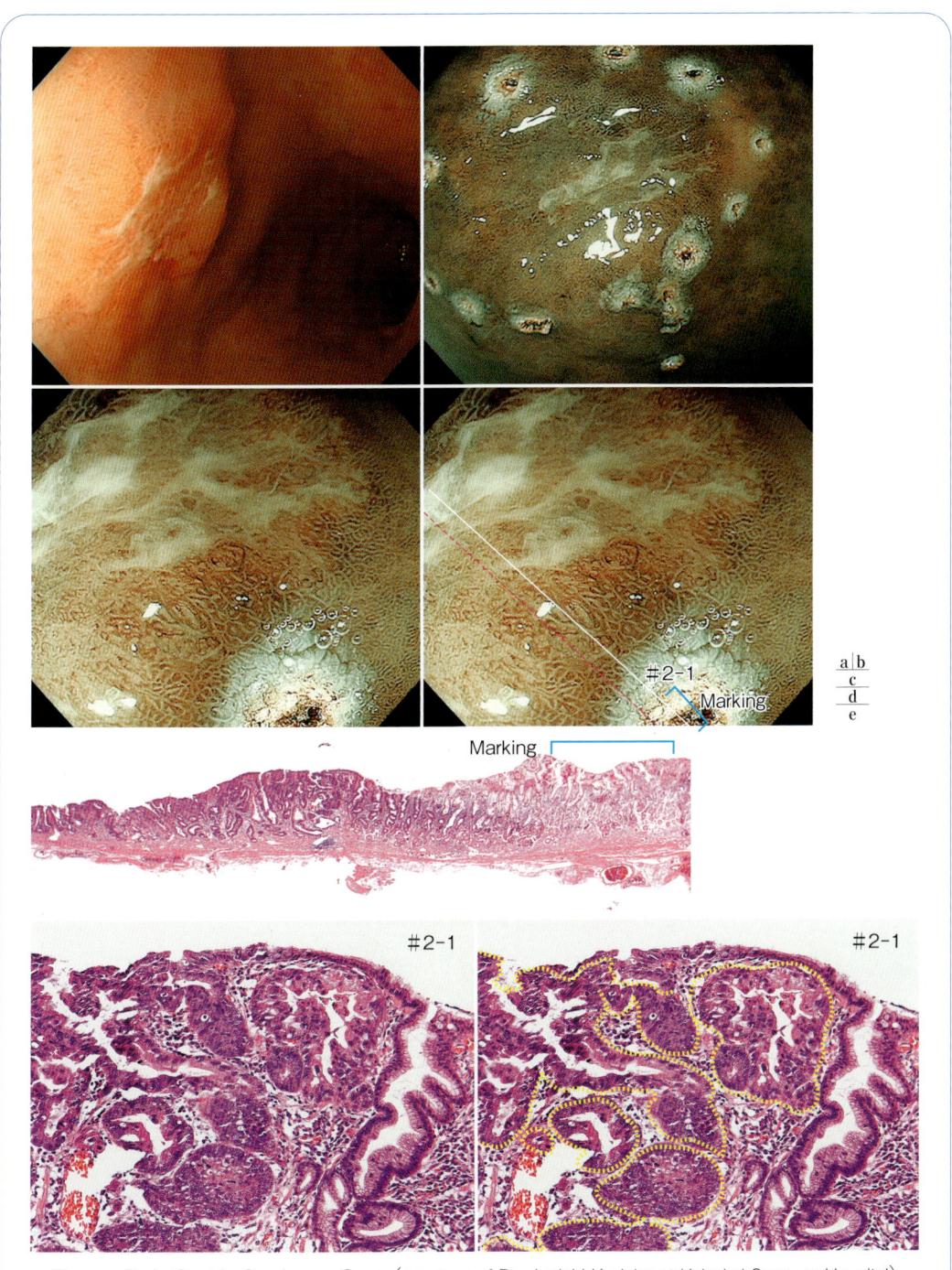

Figure Early Gastric Carcinoma Case (courtesy of Dr. Junichi Kodaira at Keiyukai Sapporo Hospital)
a : Endoscopic image b : Marking
c : The demarcation line is unclear. Presentation of the region of interest by the endoscopist for the pathologist. The photo on the right shows the slice line position.
d : Magnified image (left-right inverted according to the endoscope)
e : The surface layer is coated with non-neoplastic epithelium, while the tumor progresses inside the LPM (LPM invasion). The areas enclosed by the yellow dotted lines are the neoplastic ducts.

Colon and Rectum

See page 4 for explanation of abbreviations.

Colon and Rectum

General Theory : How to Observe These Regions with NBI or BLI

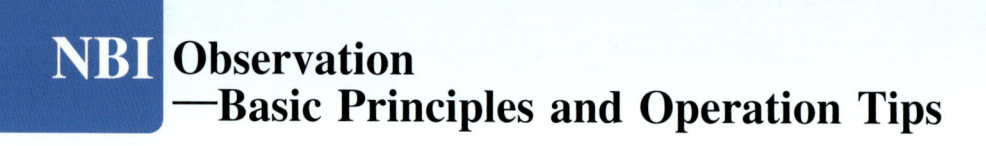

NBI Observation
—Basic Principles and Operation Tips

I. Principles of qualitative lesion diagnosis with NBI

As the microvessels on the superficial layer of normal mucosa and hyperplastic lesion are very small and sparse, it is difficult to recognize them with NBI's current wavelength settings. In neoplastic lesions, on the other hand, microvessels in the superficial layer can be seen because they are enhanced in brown. Furthermore, in the case of carcinoma, irregularities in vascular diameter, disorderly vascular courses and disrupted distribution are observed following the invasion and proliferation of carcinoma cells, infiltration of inflammatory cells and interstitial reactions. NBI's image enhancement function makes it possible to recognize pit-like structures (surface patterns, **Fig. 1**) without using a dye[1].

The characteristics noted above make it possible to diagnose colorectal lesions—including differentiation between neoplasm and non-neoplasm, differentiation between adenoma and carcinoma, and invasion depth of early carcinoma—by using NBI observation[1] to analyze the visibility of microvessels, variation in vascular diameter and distribution, and irregularities in surface patterns.

II. Basic findings of NBI magnifying observation of colon tumors

1. Vascular pattern[1]

With colorectal tumors, an increase in the degree of histological atypia typically leads to increased vascularization, as well as to increased diameter and density of microvessels. As previously mentioned, it is usually difficult to visualize microvessels in the normal mucosa and hyperplastic lesions with NBI observation at the current wavelength settings because diameter of superficial microvessels is very small and sparse. With neoplastic lesions, on the other hand, diameter of microvessels is larger and more densely concentrated, so they are easier to see when enhanced with a brownish color tone.

In NBI magnifying observation of adenomatous lesions, the superficial microvessels on the mucosae between pits are enhanced using a brownish color tone, making them stand out against the surrounding area and allowing them to be clearly recognized as a capillary network. With a carcinoma, differences in vascular diameters, disorderly vascular courses, and uneven distribution are observed following the invasion and proliferation of carcinoma cells, the infiltration of inflammatory cells, and interstitial reactions. This means that differentiating a neoplastic from a non-neoplastic colorectal lesion and an adenoma from a carcinoma is possible by analyzing the findings from NBI magnifying observation such as microvessel visibility and the uniformity/irregularity of vascular diameter and distribution. Even so, there are still cases in which it can be difficult to make a qualitative analysis of tumors from the

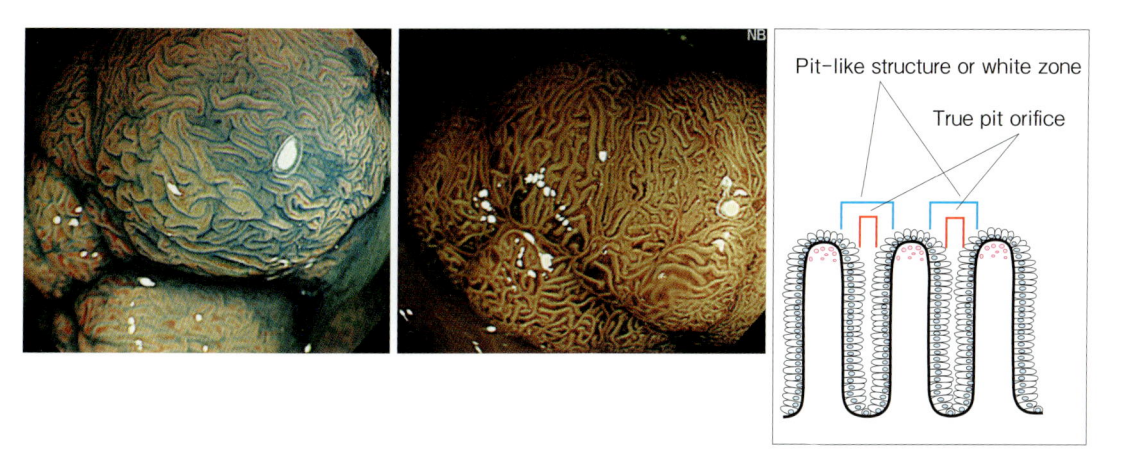

Fig. 1 Real Status of Surface Pattern (pit-like structure or white zone) (CF-H260AZI)
The structure shown above and referred to as the pit-like structure or the white zone has both a crypt opening (CO) and a marginal crypt epithelium (MCE) (Yao, K. et al.). Since colorectal lesions have many slight elevations, as well as tangled, tortuous gland ducts, NBI light is rarely able to enter the pits perpendicularly. As a result, very little illumination reaches the inside of pits, making them too dark to properly observe ; instead, the structure combining the CO and MCE which appears white is observed as if it were a pit. Therefore, the pit-like structure observed with NBI looks thicker than the true pit orifices in which indigo carmine dye is accumulated. In the region where the light enters the inside of pits perpendicularly, light is not scattered inside the true pit orifices so the inner cavity of each pit looks black.

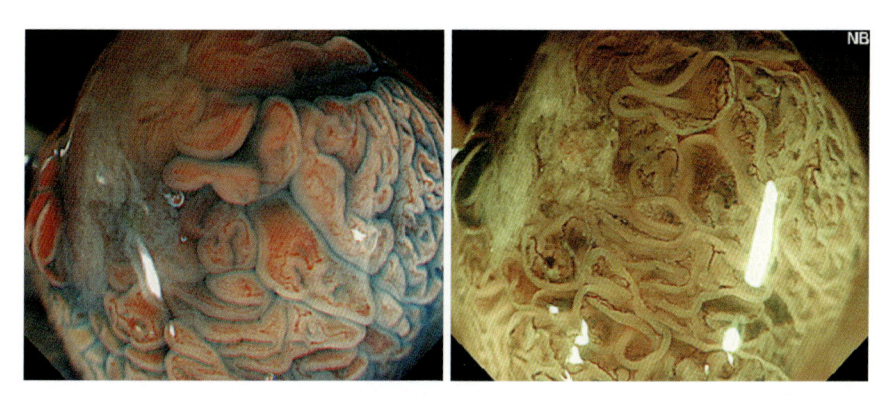

Fig. 2 Tubulovillous Adenoma and NBI Magnifying Observation Findings (CF-H260AZI)
The vascular pattern in this case is clearly irregular as indicated by the disorderly courses and uneven distribution. However, a surface pattern with a regular tubulovillous structure can be observed, so it is likely that an accurate histological diagnosis is possible.

vascular pattern found in NBI magnifying observation (**Figs. 2-4**). Therefore, it is important to perform a comprehensive evaluation based on the surface pattern described below.

2. Surface pattern[1)]

In NBI magnifying observation of an adenomatous lesion, the surface microvessels on the mucosae between pits are shown in brown and can be recognized as a capillary network. The pit-like structures that do not include vessels appear as white zones. When NBI structure enhancement function is used under these circumstances, the pit-like structures can be diagnosed indirectly (**Fig. 1**). In the case of a carcinoma,

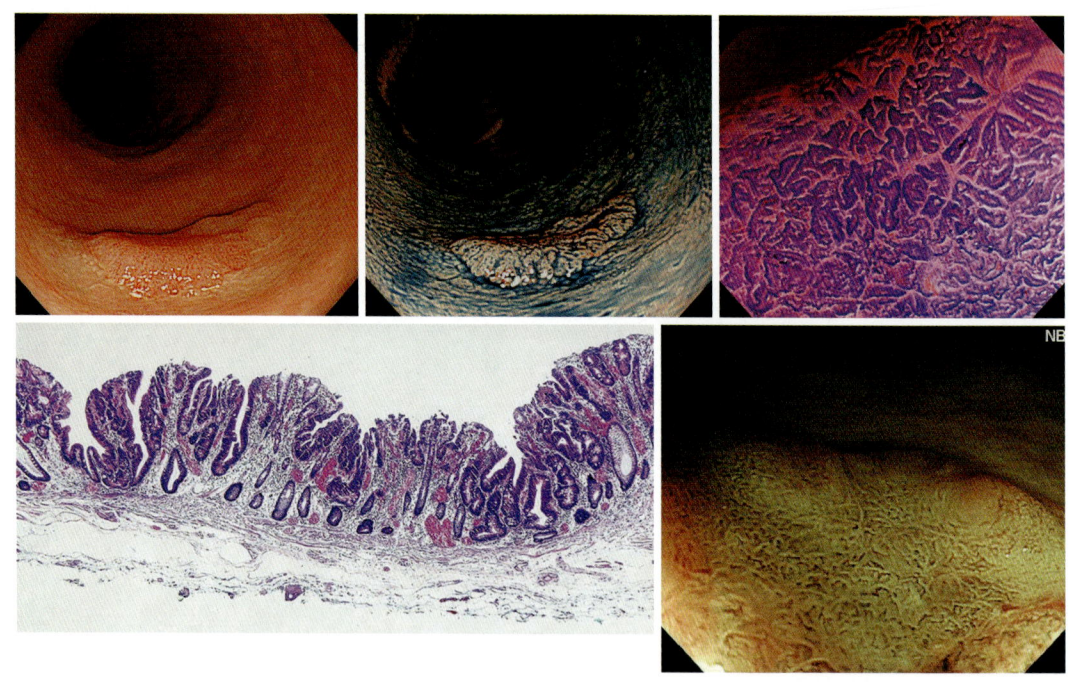

Fig. 3 Superficial Carcinoma with Low-Grade Atypia and NBI Magnifying Observation Findings (CF-H260AZI)
   In this case, the vascular pattern should be diagnosed as highly irregular due to the disorderly courses, uneven distribution and the presence of avascular areas. However, the surface pattern is not as irregular, so an accurate histological diagnosis is possible. Since a regular surface pattern is visible even in the avascular areas, deep invasion is unlikely.

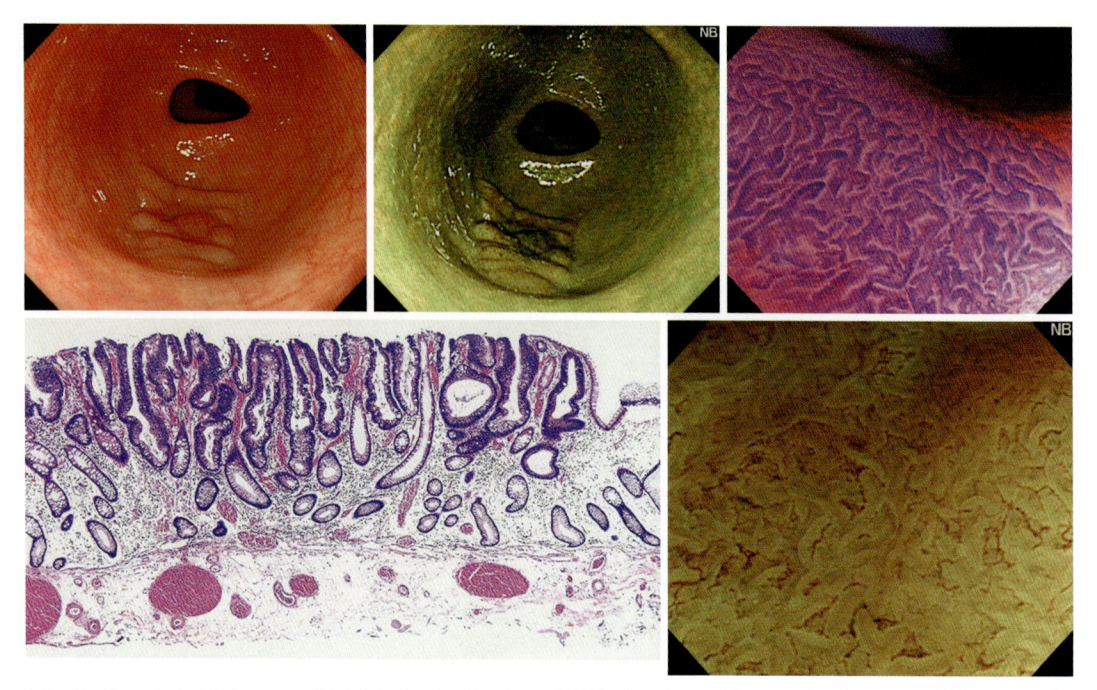

Fig. 4 Superficial Adenoma with High-Grade Atypia and NBI Magnifying Observation Findings (CF-H260AZI)
   In this case, the vascular pattern should be diagnosed as clearly irregular due to the disorderly courses, irregular margin and uneven distribution. However, the surface pattern is relatively regular, so an accurate histological diagnosis is possible. Since a regular surface pattern is observed even in the avascular areas, deep invasion is unlikely.

variation in vessel diameter, disorderly vascular courses, uneven distribution, and destruction of the pit-like structures and interfoveolar mucosae are observed following the invasion and proliferation of carcinoma cells, infiltration of inflammatory cells, and desmoplastic reactions.

While diagnostics based exclusively on the microvascular architecture has been established for the squamous epithelium regions of the laryngopharynx and esophagus that do not have a glandular structure, evaluation of the surface patterns is as very important as the evaluation of the microvascular architecture using magnifying observation for diagnosis of tumors in the columnar epithelium regions on Barrett's esophagus, the stomach, and intestine, etc.

III. Knack and pitfall of NBI magnifying observation

1. Findings in NBI magnifying observation in relation to macroscopic type and development pattern[2),3)]

    Fig. 5 shows the differences in vascular pattern between macroscopic types of adenoma. NBI magnifying observation of an elevated colorectal adenoma shows a regular surface pattern, and, with most elevated adenomas, a qualitative diagnosis is possible based on the surface pattern. In NBI magnifying observation of a flat-depressed colorectal adenoma, on the other hand, the surface pattern is not always clear, but a regular vascular pattern can be seen. In general, however, the vascular

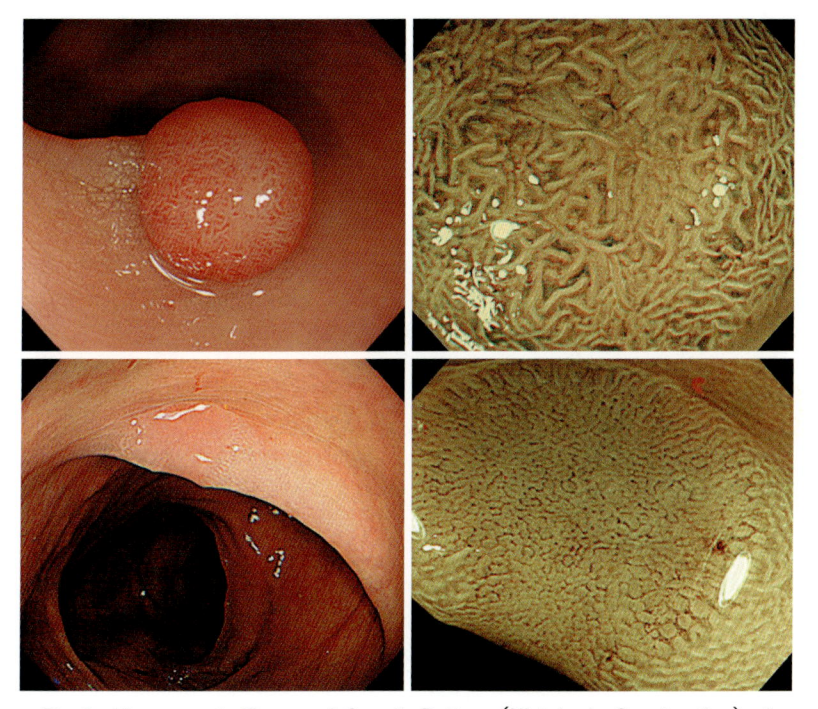

Fig. 5 Macroscopic Type and Growth Pattern (Histologic Construction) of Tumor and NBI Magnifying Observation Findings (CF-H260AZI)

The images in the upper row show an elevated adenoma in which the glandular structure is entangled in a complicated way to form the elevation. As a result, the surface pattern is more useful for a qualitative diagnosis than the vascular pattern. The images in the lower row show a flat adenoma. In this case, the surface pattern is unclear but the vascular pattern is regular enough for a qualitative diagnosis. As these images show, the vascular pattern or surface pattern can be difficult to recognize depending on the properties and condition of each lesion. What is important is to select or combine them as appropriate.

and surface patterns of flat tumors (including the flat-depressed tumor and LST-NG), vary widely, frequently making it difficult to make a qualitative diagnosis based on the findings from NBI magnifying observation alone. When evaluation of the findings from NBI magnifying observation of a flat tumor (including the flat-depressed tumor and LST-NG) is difficult, conventional pit pattern diagnosis using a dye supported by magnifying observation is critical for accurate diagnosis. By having a good understanding of where NBI magnifying observation is effective and where it is not, you will be able to select the technique—NBI magnifying observation or pit pattern diagnosis—most appropriate to the conditions of the case.

2. System setting for NBI magnifying observation

To evaluate the surface pattern, it is important to set the structure enhancement to A8 and the color mode to 3. With this setup, the surface pattern can be diagnosed with properly focused magnifying observation.

Proper focus is as important in magnifying observation is as it is in pit pattern diagnosis. However, compared to early esophageal and gastric carcinomas, many colorectal lesions show elevated appearance and height irregularities, making it difficult to get the entire image in focus at the same time. It is therefore recommended to record an accurately focused image from each part of the lesion. Meanwhile, the rough vascular pattern can be observed if they are in a deep color. When proceeding to NBI magnifying observation, make sure to take conscious effort to focus the surface pattern accurately.

IV. Classifications of NBI magnifying observation findings adopted in Japanese institutions

In Japan at this time, several classifications exist for NBI magnifying observation findings. The representative classifications are described below.

1. Sano Classification (Fig. 6)[4),5)]

The Sano Classification evaluates the microvascular architecture alone. In this classification, the capillary pattern (CP) is defined as the meshed capillary arrangement surrounding a pit. Based on its visibility, size variation, tortuosity and disruption, a CP is classified as type I, II, IIIA or IIIB. CP type I is a pattern of normal, hyperplastic polyps that precludes visual identification of microvessels. CP type II is a pattern of adenoma in which microvessels of similar size appear to be surrounding a pit. CP type IIIA is observed in carcinomas. CP type IIIB is observed in deep submucosal (SM) invasive carcinomas.

2. Hiroshima Classification (Fig. 7)[6)]

The Hiroshima Classification comprehensively evaluates both the pit-like structures (surface pattern) and microvascular architecture. The surface pattern is given the priority in diagnosis. In this classification, type A includes normal or discolored lesions with invisible microvessels. Type B includes lesions observed indirectly by their clear and regular pit-like structures or lesions observed with regular vascular pattern. Type C includes lesions lacking a specific structure or with irregular surface pattern ; this type is subclassified into C1-C3. Type C3 includes lesions with an unclear surface pattern, with avascular areas (AVAs), and interspersed with irregular microvessels or fractured microvessels. Although an irregular surface pattern is observed in types C1 and C2, they differ in the degree of heterogeneity of vascular diameter and distribution.

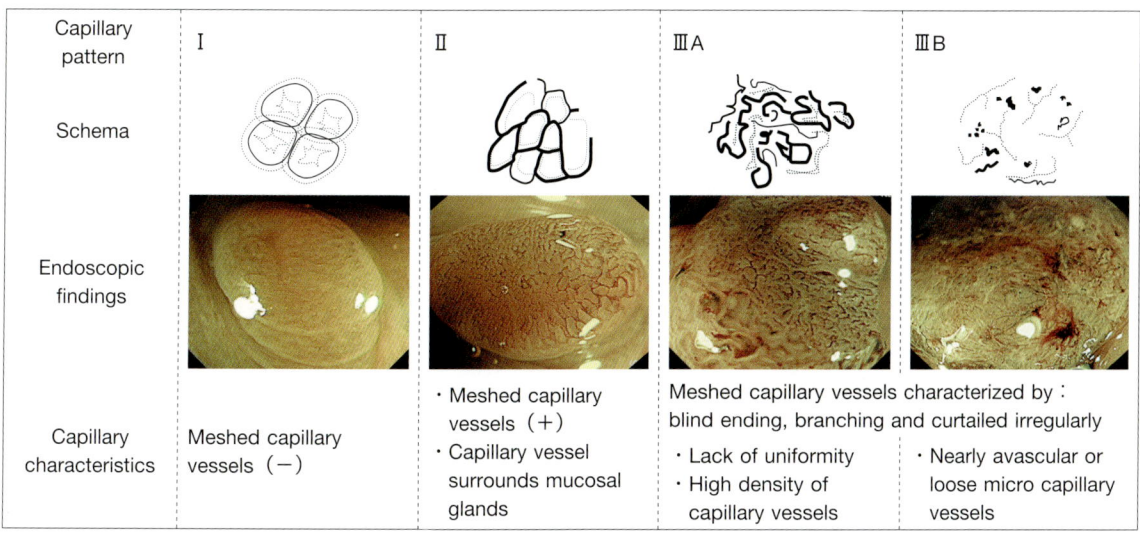

Capillary pattern	I	II	IIIA	IIIB
Schema				
Endoscopic findings				
Capillary characteristics	Meshed capillary vessels (−)	・Meshed capillary vessels (＋) ・Capillary vessel surrounds mucosal glands	Meshed capillary vessels characterized by : blind ending, branching and curtailed irregularly ・Lack of uniformity ・High density of capillary vessels	Meshed capillary vessels characterized by : blind ending, branching and curtailed irregularly ・Nearly avascular or loose micro capillary vessels

Fig. 6　Sano Classification

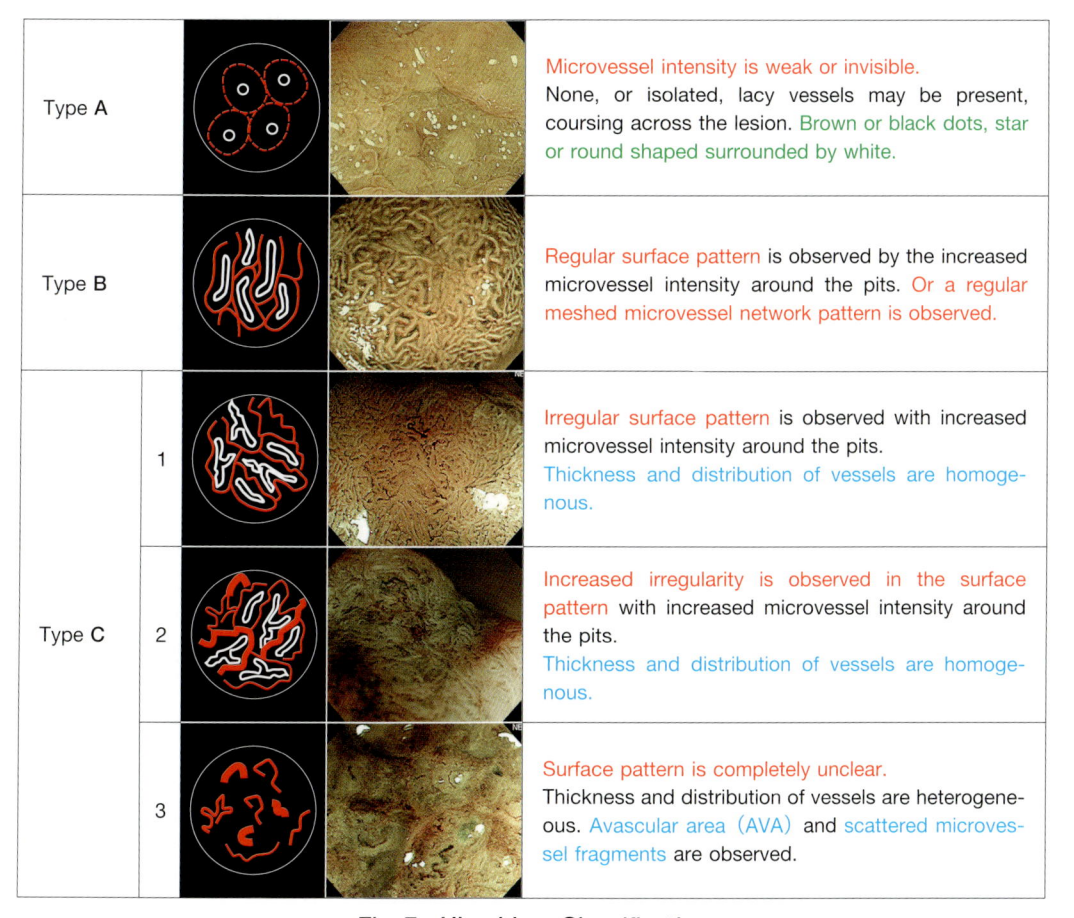

Type A				Microvessel intensity is weak or invisible. None, or isolated, lacy vessels may be present, coursing across the lesion. Brown or black dots, star or round shaped surrounded by white.
Type B				Regular surface pattern is observed by the increased microvessel intensity around the pits. Or a regular meshed microvessel network pattern is observed.
Type C	1			Irregular surface pattern is observed with increased microvessel intensity around the pits. Thickness and distribution of vessels are homogenous.
	2			Increased irregularity is observed in the surface pattern with increased microvessel intensity around the pits. Thickness and distribution of vessels are homogenous.
	3			Surface pattern is completely unclear. Thickness and distribution of vessels are heterogeneous. Avascular area (AVA) and scattered microvessel fragments are observed.

Fig. 7　Hiroshima Classification

normal pattern   faint pattern   network pattern

dense pattern   irregular pattern   sparse pattern

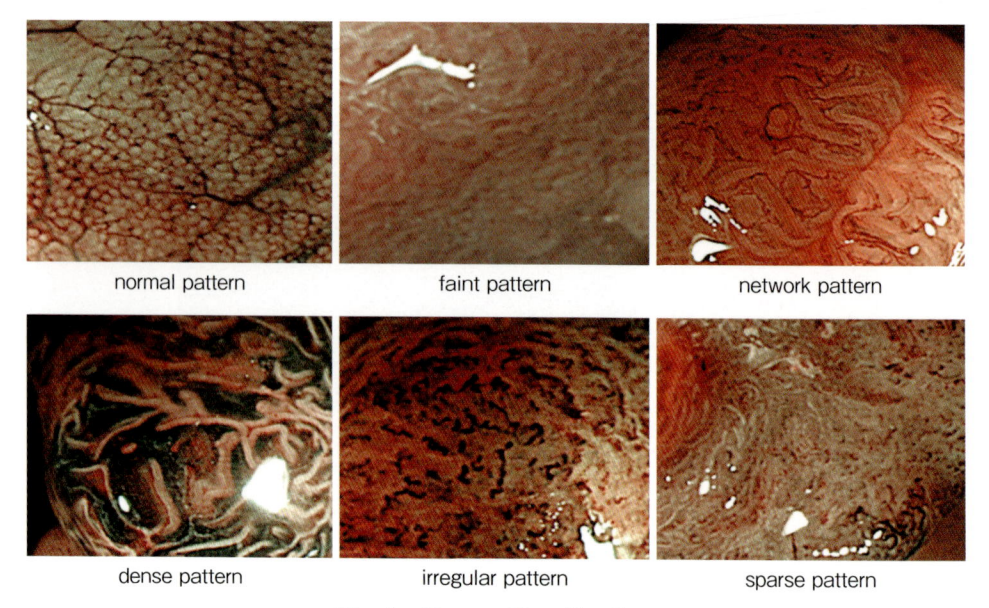

Fig. 8   Showa Classification

3. Showa Classification (Fig. 8)[7]

The Showa Classification evaluates pit-like structures and microvascular architecture, and expresses their characteristics morphologically. This classification differs from the category-based classification systems described above. In lesions with a faint pattern, the microvessels surrounding the pit are more difficult to identify visually, as can be seen in hyperplastic polyps, for example. In tubular or tubulovillous adenomas with a network pattern, microvessels of a similar size form an elliptical network among the pits. In tubular adenomas with a dense pattern, the microvessels are thick and dense and the epithelium looks thickly congested. In a deep SM invasive carcinoma with an irregular pattern, the microvessels show size variation, high tortuosity, disruption-inducing continuity and little deterioration. In deep SM invasive carcinoma with a sparse pattern, fewer microvessels than normal are seen in the recess.

V. NICE Classification[1),8)-10)]

At the international level, the NICE (NBI International Colorectal Endoscopic Classification, **Table 1**) classification system has established simple, yet effective standards for classification using close-up observation with a high-resolution endoscope. This classification system features three categories—Types 1, 2 and 3—based on three characteristics: ①color, ②vessels and ③surface pattern. Type 1 is an index for hyperplastic lesions, while Type 2 is an index for adenoma or mucosal/SM shallow invasive carcinoma, and Type 3 is an index for SM deep invasive carcinoma. The biggest advantage of this system is that it enables any endoscopist in the world to diagnose a hyperplastic lesion that does not need treatment or a deep SM invasive carcinoma that requires surgery. In Europe and North America where the "Resect and Discard Trial" is common practice, the ability to differentiate tumors from non-tumors at the minute lesion level is considered of critical importance, making the NICE Classification invaluable.

Table 2 shows the relationship between the NICE Classification and the Sano, Hiroshima and Showa Classifications. The table shows the approximate relationship although some details might be different, and the information in Types 1 and 3 of the

Table 1　NICE Classification*

	Type 1	Type 2	Type 3
Color	Same or lighter than background	Browner relative to background (verify color arises from vessels)	Brown to dark brown relative to background ; sometimes patchy whiter areas.
Vessels	None, or isolated lacy vessels present, coursing across the lesion	Brown vessels surrounding white structures**	Has area (s) of disrupted or missing vessels
Surface pattern	Dark or white spots of uniform size, or homogeneous absence of pattern	Oval, tubular or branched white structures** surrounded by brown vessels	Amorphous or absent surface pattern
Most likely pathology	Hyperplastic	Adenoma***	Deep submucosal invasive cancer

*Can be applied using colonoscopes with or without optical (zoom) magnification
**These structures (regular or irregular) may represent the pits and the epithelium of the crypt opening.
***Type 2 consists of Vienna classification types 3, 4 and superficial 5 (all adenomas with either low or high grade dysplasia, or with superficial submucosal carcinoma). The presence of high grade dysplasia or superficial submucosal carcinoma may be suggested by an irregular vessel or surface pattern, and is often associated with atypical morphology (e. g., depressed area).

Table 2　Relationship between NICE Classification and Sano/Hiroshima/Showa Classifications

	Type 1	Type 2	Type 3
Color	Same or lighter than background	Browner relative to background (verify color arises from vessels)	Brown to dark brown relative to background ; sometimes patchy whiter areas.
Vascular pattern	None, or isolated lacy vessels present, coursing across the lesion	Brown vessels surrounding white structures**	Has area (s) of disrupted or missing vessels
Surface pattern	Dark or white spots of uniform size, or homogeneous absence of pattern	Oval, tubular or branched white structures** surrounded by brown vessels	Amorphous or absent surface pattern
Sano Classification	Type I	Types II-IIIA	Type IIIB
Hiroshima Classification	Type A	Types B-C2	Type C3
Showa Classification	Faint pattern	Network pattern　Irregular pattern　Dense pattern	Sparse pattern

CF-H260AZI
(LUCERA)

CF-HQ290L/I
(LUCERA
ELITE)

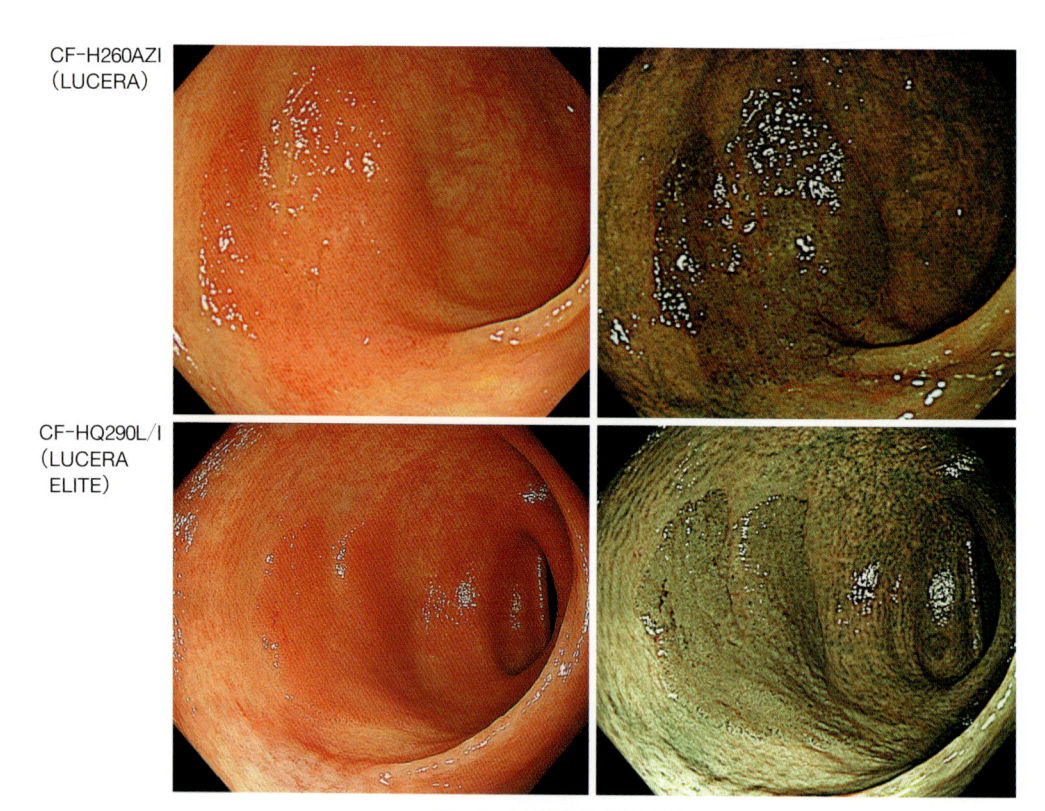

Fig. 9 LUCERA ELITE System
This figure shows normal endoscopic images of the same lesion, using the LUCERA CF-H260AZI for the upper-row images and the LUCERA ELITE CF-HQ290L/I for the lower-row images. The comparison shows that the CF-HQ290L/I is obviously brighter, higher in resolution and clearer than the CF-H260AZI. Although the positioning of the lesion in the frame is different because the field of view of the CF-HQ290L/I is 30 degrees larger (170°) than that of the CF-H260AZI, the wider field of view does not produce images that look like fisheye-lens images.

NICE Classification is almost identical to other classifications. However, some Japanese magnifying endoscopists find a more general category like Type 2 of the NICE Classification to be inadequate for their needs because it does not enable differentiation between adenoma and carcinoma, nor does it facilitate meticulous qualitative diagnosis. Seen in this light, the shortest route to unifying the classification of findings in NBI magnifying observation may be to establish subcategories for NICE Classification Type 2 based on detailed examination of the findings in NBI magnifying observation. At present, a team convened by the Japanese Ministry of Health, Labour and Welfare is conducting a multicenter study, which covers the significance of each category of findings in NBI magnifying observation. The outcome of this project is widely anticipated, and, while arguments about the results would no doubt be endless, there can be little argument that it would at least be necessary to discuss the addition of the findings proper to serrated lesions as a subtype of NICE Classification Type 1, including the SSA/P (sessile serrated adenoma/polyp), which is currently receiving a great deal of attention.

VI. New NBI endoscopic diagnosis using the LUCERA ELITE System

So far, we have discussed some of the basics of NBI observation and outlined the existing classifications. This book contains images taken with the new LUCERA ELITE system as seen in **Fig. 9**, for example. We hope that the readers of this book will also see and appreciate NBI diagnosis images obtained using a new light source.

References
1) Tanaka, S., Sano, Y. : Aim to unify the narrow band imaging (NBI) magnifying classification for colon tumors : current status in Japan from a summary of the consensus symposium in the 79th annual meeting of the Japan Gastroenterological Endoscopy Society. Dig Endosc 2011 ; 23 : S131-S139
2) Oba, S., Tanaka, S, Oka, S. et al. : Characterization of colorectal tumors using narrow-band imaging magnification : combined diagnosis with both pit pattern and microvessel features. Scand J Gastroenterol 2010 ; 45 : 1084-1092
3) Takata, S., Tanaka, S., Hayashi, N. et al. : Characteristic magnifying narrow-band imaging features of colorectal tumors in each growth type. Int J Colorectal Dis 2012 ; 28 : 459-468
4) Machida, H., Sano, Y., Hamamoto, Y. et al. : Narrow-band imaging in the diagnosis of colorectal mucosal lesions : a pilot study. Endoscopy 2004 ; 36 : 1094-1098
5) Ikematsu, H., Matsuda, T., Emura, F. et al. : Efficacy of capillary pattern type ⅢA/ⅢB by magnifying narrow band imaging for estimating depth of invasion of early colorectal neoplasms. BMC Gastroenterol 2010 ; 10 : 33
6) Kanao, H., Tanaka, S., Oka, S. et al. : Narrow-band imaging magnification predicts the histology and invasion depth of colorectal tumors. Gastrointest Endosc 2009 ; 69 : 631-636
7) Wada, Y., Kudo, SE., Kashida, H. et al. : Diagnosis of colorectal lesions with the magnifying narrow-band imaging system. Gastrointest Endosc 2009 ; 70 : 522-531
8) Oba, S., Tanaka, S., Sano, Y. et al. : Current status of narrow-band imaging magnifying colonoscopy for colorectal neoplasia in Japan. Digestion 2011 ; 83 : 167-172
9) Hewett, DG., Kaltenbach, T., Sano, Y. et al. : Validation of a simple classification system for endoscopic diagnosis of small colorectal polyps using narrow-band imaging. Gastroenterology 2012 ; 143 : 599-607
10) Hayashi, N., Tanaka, S., Hewett, DG. et al. : Validation of the Narrow Band Imaging (NBI) International Colorectal Endoscopic (NICE) Classification for prediction of colorectal lesions with deep submucosal invasive carcinoma. Gastrointest Endosc 2013 ; 78 : 625-632

(Tanaka, S.)

Colon and Rectum

General Theory : How to Observe These Regions with NBI or BLI

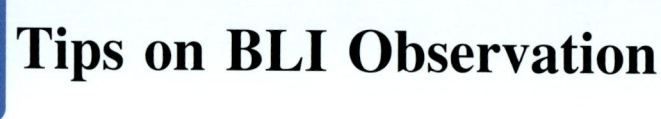

Tips on BLI Observation

I. Appropriate use of BLI modes in colorectal tumor observation

In Blue Laser Imaging (BLI) observation of a colorectal tumor using the LASEREO (Fujifilm) laser light source-based endoscope, it is important to select the optimum mode from the BLI and BLI-bright modes[1)-3)]. The brightness of the BLI-bright mode is useful in observation of the distant view (**Fig. 1**). Although contrast is not quite as good as in the BLI mode, the brightness of the BLI-bright mode enables visualization of the vascular courses of benign lesions and the surrounding mucosa. In observation of the whole tumor from a closer distance, the BLI mode shows the tumor margins more clearly than the BLI-bright mode despite its lower brightness (**Fig. 2**). In addition, the FICE (Flexible spectral Imaging Color Enhancement) mode available with Fujifilm's laser endoscopes enhances image clarity and can be expected to remain useful in future examinations.

In magnifying observation, there is not much difference between the BLI and BLI-bright modes, although the BLI mode is generally more suitable for observing superficial vessels and structures because it offers enhanced contrast of microvessels (**Fig. 3**). In cases where the field of view is dark, the BLI-bright mode may be able to provide a better view than the BLI mode. Simply select the mode best suited to the individual conditions of each case. Contrast can also be enhanced in both modes by the applying structure enhancement. However, use of this mode should be considered carefully as it renders a rougher image.

II. NBI Classification in BLI magnifying observation

The Hiroshima Classification, one of the current NBI (Narrow Band Imaging) classifications, has been reported as applicable to BLI magnifying observation of a colorectal neoplasm by the multicenter study of the Fukuoka University Chikushi Hospital and the Kyoto Prefectural University of Medicine[4)]. Further study is currently underway to determine the applicability of the Sano Classification. Parts of these studies are presented in the remainder of this section.

The target lesions are 104 neoplastic lesions, including 62 adenoma, 34 intramucosal and shallowly invaded submucosal carcinomas and 8 deeply invaded submucosal carcinomas. Each lesion is observed using BLI and NBI magnifying observation and diagnosed based on the Sano and Hiroshima Classifications in order to examine the accurate diagnosis rates of the histopathological diagnoses and the concordance rates of NBI and BLI.

The results do not present significant differences because the accurate diagnosis rates of the Sano Classification in magnifying observation were 73. 1% (76/104) with BLI and 76% (79/104) with NBI, while those of the Hiroshima Classification were

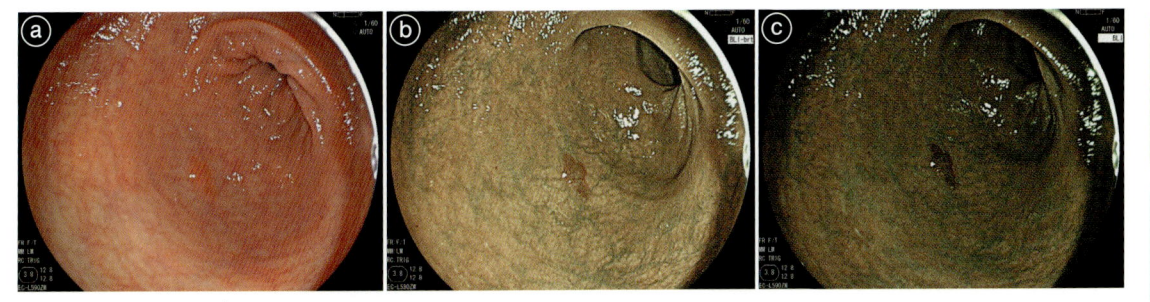

Fig. 1 Intramucosal Carcinoma in Rectum Ra
a : Distant view with white-light imaging.
b : BLI-bright distant view. High tumor visibility and bright overall field.
c : BLI distant view : High tumor visibility but relatively low brightness.

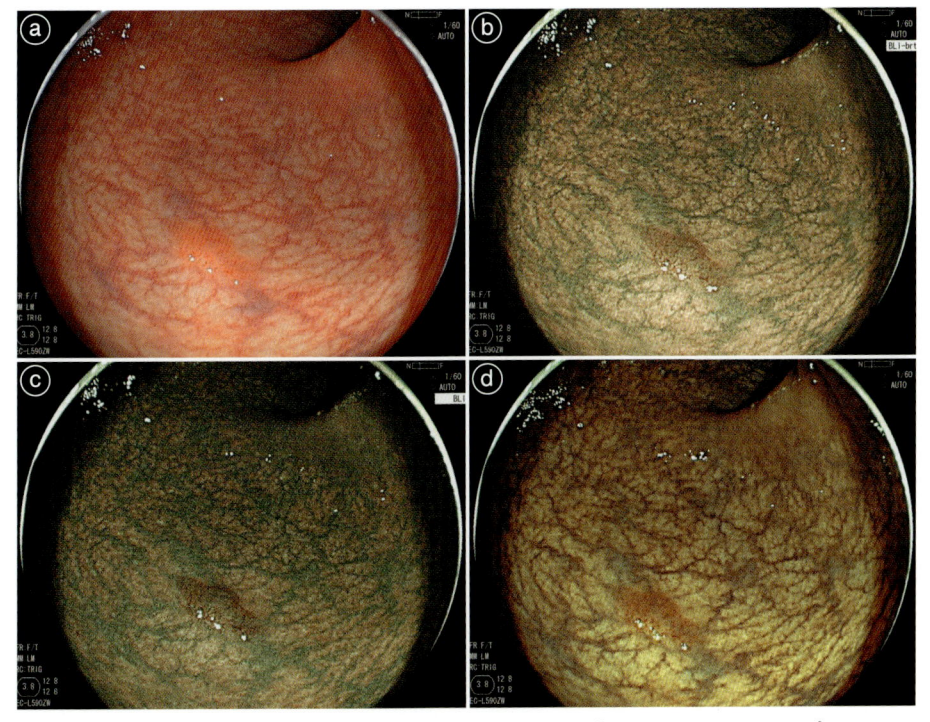

Fig. 2 Intramucosal Carcinoma in Rectum Ra (same tumor as Fig. 1)
a : Endoscopic image with white light.
b : BLI-bright image : The field of the tumor is bright, but the contrast of the tumor margin is low.
c : BLI image : The contrast of the tumor margin is good.
d : FICE image : The tumor visibility is good.

74.0% (77/104) with BLI and 77.9% (81/104) with NBI. Additionally, the concordance rate between BLI and NBI were 81.7% in the Sano Classification, and 74.0% in the Hiroshima Classification. When the reproducibility of diagnoses was examined by two endoscopists (Y., N. and H., T.), the results were very satisfactory : The intraobserver variability of the Hiroshima Classification of the BLI results, is k=0.893 (Y., N.) and 0.851 (H., T) while that of the Sano Classification is k=0.834 (Y., N.) and

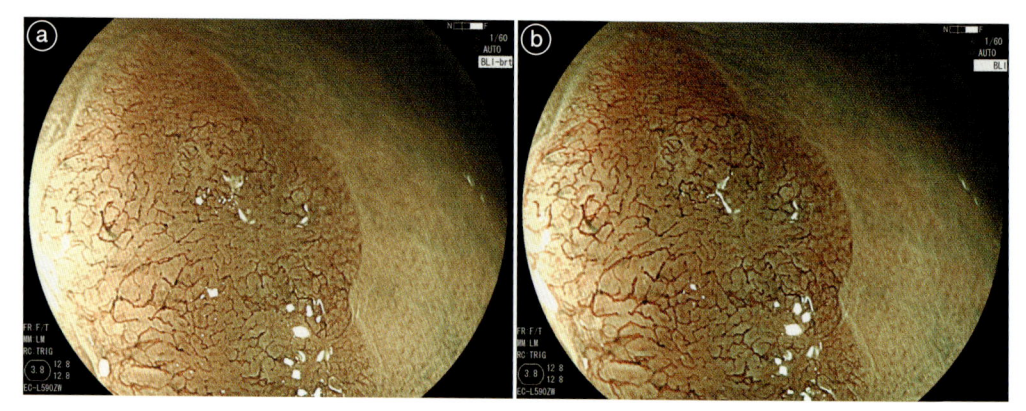

Fig. 3 Difference between BLI and BLI-bright Modes in Magnifying Observation (same tumor as Fig. 1)
a : BLI-bright image.
b : BLI image : The contrast of the microvessels is greater than in the BLI-bright mode image. As the surface pattern has type Vi pits and the vascular pattern presents tortuosity, the lesion is diagnosed as Type C1 of the Hiroshima Classification.

Table BLI Magnifying Diagnosis Capability of Colorectal Tumors (n=314)

	Number	HP	Ad	M	sSM	dSM
Type A	39	39				
Type B	159	2	142	14		1
Type C1	92		26	56	8	2
Type C2	13			9	2	2
Type C3	11			1	1	9

HP : hyperplastic polyp, Ad : adenoma, M : intramucosal cancer, sSM : shallowly invaded submucosal cancer, dSM : deeply invaded submucosal cancer

Accuracy rate
(39+142+64+11+9)/314=265/314=84.4%

0.926 (H., T.). The inter-observer variability of the Hiroshima Classification is k=0.863 and that of the Sano Classification is k=0.872.

In addition, our university observed 314 cases of neoplastic and non-neoplastic colorectal lesions and achieved favorable results, with an overall accurate diagnosis rate of 84.4%, an accurate neoplastic/non-neoplastic diagnosis rate of 99.4%, and an accurate deeply invaded SM carcinoma diagnosis rate of 94.3%[5] (**Table**). The results suggest that NBI classification enables satisfactory diagnoses of BLI images. In BLI observation, we first observe the surface pattern and use the vascular pattern observations as an auxiliary means of diagnosis[6]. The types identified with the classification are shown below together with their BLI images[3] (**Fig. 4**).

Type A has a circular or oval surface pattern. The vascular pattern in the superficial layer is almost unrecognizable, but regarded as the index of a hyperplastic polyp.

Type B requires careful diagnosis because it has either a papillary pattern or tubular pattern, and the vascular pattern for each is quite different. Differentiation is possible based on the surface pattern[2].

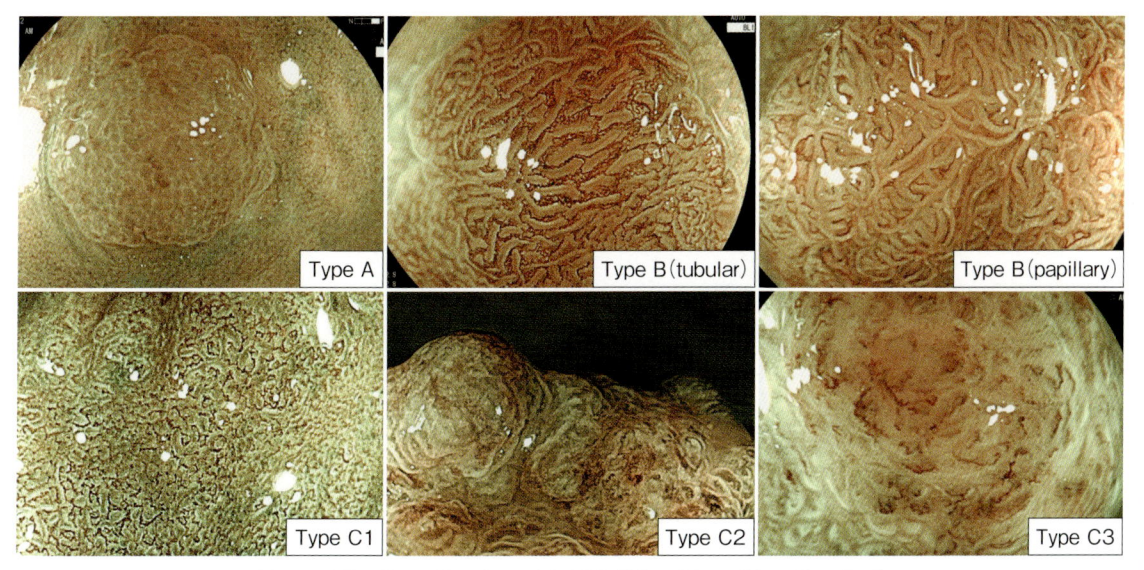

Fig. 4 NBI Classification with BLI (Hiroshima Classification)
Type A is a hyperplastic polyp, Type B an adenoma, Type C1 between an adenoma and a shallowly invaded submucosal carcinoma, Type C2 between an intramucosal and deeply invaded submucosal carcinomas, and Type C3 a deeply invaded submucosal carcinoma.

Namely, the papillary pattern presents a type Ⅳ pit-like structure with a flat, smooth margin, while its vascular pattern presents irregular sizes and tortuosity and does not form a network. The tubular pattern, on the other hand, presents a type ⅢL surface pattern or ⅢS pit-like structures, while its vascular pattern forms a uniform network resembling hexagons with no size irregularities. Type B is mainly regarded as the index for adenoma.

Type C1 does not have a surface pattern with type ⅢL or Ⅳ pit-like structures but shows irregular structures equivalent to what are called the type VI pits. The vascular pattern shows irregular vessels accompanied with tortuosity and irregular sizes (about 1.5 times the normal size). With Type C2, an uneven vascular pattern and a surface pattern with unclear margin are observed in addition to the irregularities observed with Type C1. According to our study, Type C1 is a lesion somewhere between an adenoma and a shallowly invaded submucosal carcinoma, and Type C2 is the index for a lesion between the intramucosal and shallowly invaded submucosal carcinoma (**Table**). Since all of the patterns partially include a deeply invaded SM carcinoma, it is desirable that additional detailed examinations using other means are included in actual clinical practice, such as pit pattern diagnosis using crystal violet chromoendoscopy and EUS. With Type C3, the surface pattern shows that the type VN pit-like structures have disappeared and the vascular pattern includes avascular areas and disruption or interruption of noticeable dilated vessels. Type C3 almost coincides with the deeply invaded submucosal carcinoma.

Ⅲ. Tips on BLI magnifying observation

Compared to NBI, BLI magnifying observation images the surface pattern in a relatively whitish color tone. The magnification ratio of the optical zoom is up to 135×, but it is preferable to use a slightly lower magnification than the maximum, when diagnosing colorectal tumors (**Fig. 5**). The magnification ratio can be adjusted by referring to the gauge on the top right of the screen. The optical magnification is

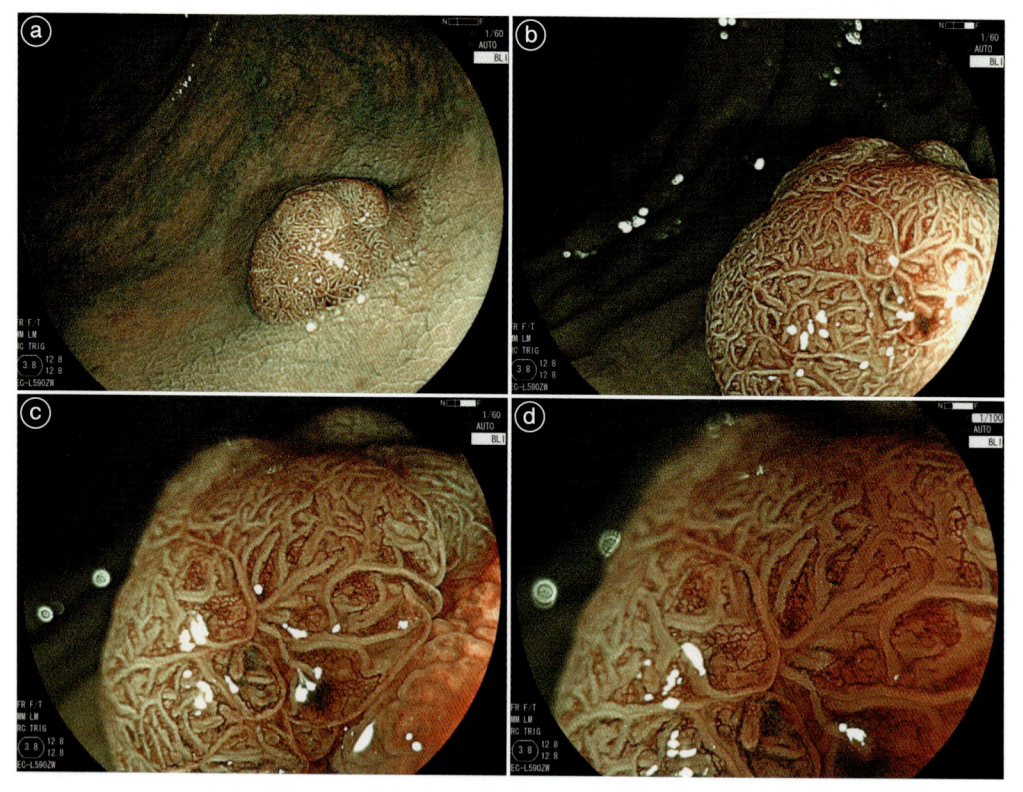

Fig. 5
a : I sp 10 mm in the rectum (Rb) (Later EMR led to the pathological diagnosis that the lesion is an adenoma.)
b : 50-60× observation in the 3rd step of magnification gauge.
c : 80-90× observation in the 5th step of magnification gauge : The surface pattern presents type Ⅳ pit-like structures and the vascular pattern presents tortuosity and dilation. The lesion is diagnosed as the papillary pattern of Hiroshima Classification Type B.
d : 120-135× observation in the 7th step of magnification gauge.

available in seven steps, at 50-60× in the 3rd step, 80-90× in the 5th step and 120-135× in the 7th step. In actual clinical practice, the 5th step is most useful even in high-precision qualitative diagnosis of colorectal tumors because of the ease of focusing and use. Higher magnifications are also available, but the resulting images are grainy and coarse, so they are usually intended for research purposes only and are rarely used in actual clinical practice.

Conclusion

In the above, the authors describe the details of colorectal tumor observation using BLI. The LASEREO laser endoscope has two narrow-band imaging modes (BLI and BLI-bright modes) so that satisfactory qualitative diagnosis is possible by selecting the optimum mode according to the distance from the lesion and the magnification ratio.

References

1) Yoshida, N., Yagi, N., Yanagisawa, A. et al. : Image-enhanced endoscopy for diagnosis of colorectal tumors in view of endoscopic treatment. World J Gastrointest Endosc 2012 ; 4 : 545-555

2) Yoshida, N., Yagi, N., Inada, Y. et al. : Therapeutic and Diagnostic Approaches in Colonoscopy. Amornyotin S (ed) : Endoscopy of GI Tract. 2013, In Tech—Open Access Company. Available from URL : http://www.intechopen.com/books/endoscopy-of-gi-tract/therapeutic-and-diagnostic-approaches-in-colonoscopy.
3) Yoshida, N., Yagi, N., Inada, Y. et al. : Significance and positioning of NBI/BLI in the algorithm of diagnosis/treatment of colorectal lesions : This is how we think—usefulness of Blue Laser Imaging in colorectal polyp diagnosis (in Japanese [title translated]). Intestine 2013 ; 17 : 277-280
4) Yoshida, N., Hisabe, T., Inada, Y. et al. : The ability of a novel blue laser imaging system for the diagnosis of invasion depth of colorectal neoplasms. J Gastroenterol (in press)
5) Yoshida, N., Yagi, N., Inada, Y. et al. : Ability of a novel blue laser imaging system for the diagnosis of colorectal polyps. Dig Endosc 2014 ; 26 : 250-258
6) Kanao, H., Tanaka, S., Oka, S. et al. : Narrow-band imaging magnification predicts the histology and invasion depth of colorectal tumors. Gastrointest Endosc 2009 ; 69 : 631-636

(Yoshida, N., Naito, Y., Ito, Y.)

Case 48 Hyperplastic polyp

Female aged 65 | **Purpose** Follow-up after colon polypectomy
Location Sigmoid colon | **Macroscopic type** 0-IIa

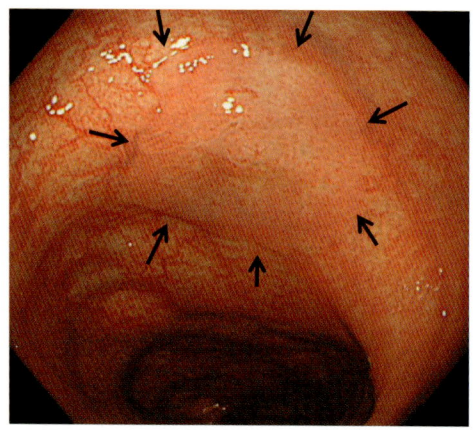

WLI observation : A slightly elevated lesion with a diameter of about 20 mm and whitish color tone is recognized in the sigmoid colon (arrows).

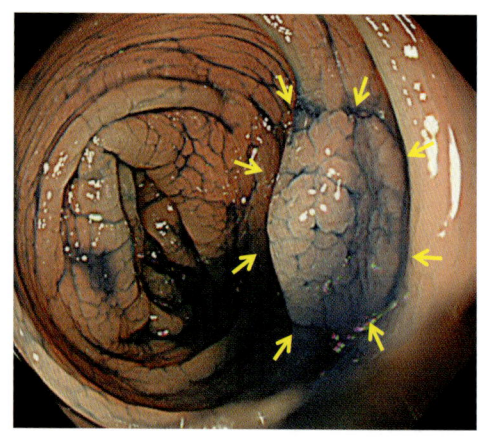

Indigo carmine chromo endoscopy : The granular changes on the surface layer and the tumor margin (arrows) are observed clearly.

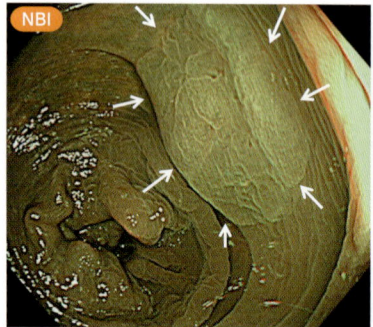

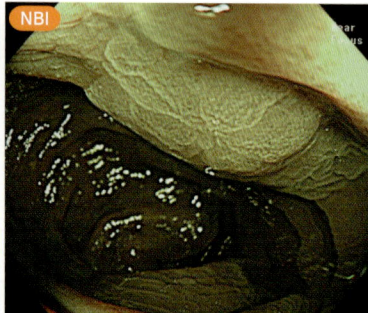

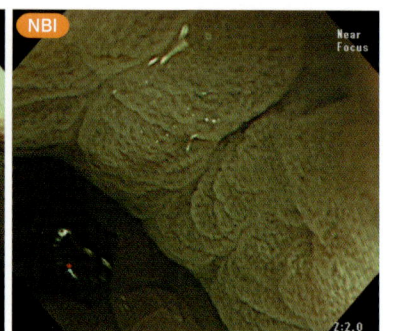

NBI normal observation shows the border of tumor clearly. The surface properties present height irregularities [Left ; arrows]. NBI magnifying observation shows that the vessels surrounding the pits are not dilated. [Middle : Low magnification (optical zoom, Near Focus 45×). Right : High magnification (optical zoom, Near Focus 45×, electronic zoom 2×)] In addition, the presence of dilated vessels as specified with the SSA/P in the deep of mucosal layer is not observed.

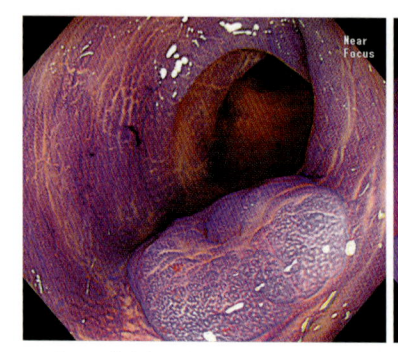

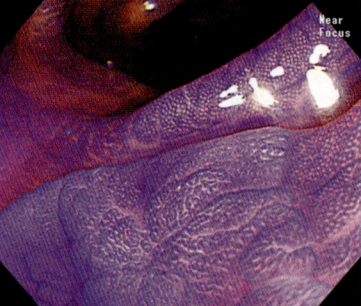

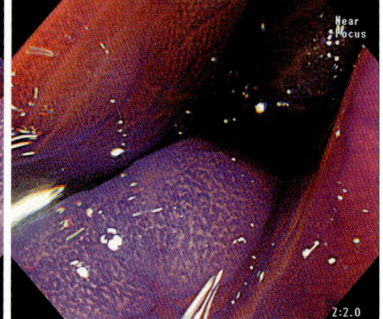

Crystal violet chromo endoscopy : As watched in WLI observation, the lesion is slightly elevated and the mucosal surface layer presents granular changes [Left, optical zoom 45×]. Using the electronic zoom shows that the ductal outlets are mainly asteroid shaped pits (type II pits), confirming that the lesion is a hyperplastic lesion. [Middle : Low magnification (optical zoom Near Focus 45×, electronic zoom 1.4×). Right : High magnification (optical zoom Near Focus 45×, electronic zoom 2×)]. Obviously neoplastic tumor's pits are not recognized.

Endoscope : CF-HQ290I (Olympus).　　Light source : EVIS LUCERA ELITE (Olympus)
NBI setup : Structure enhancement A8, color mode 3

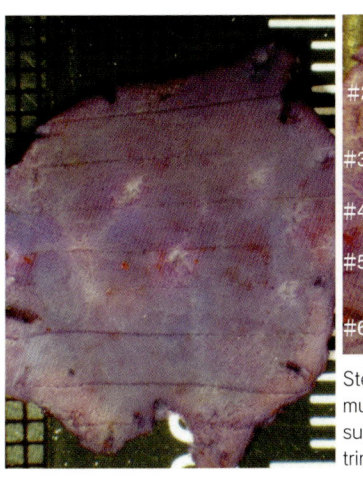

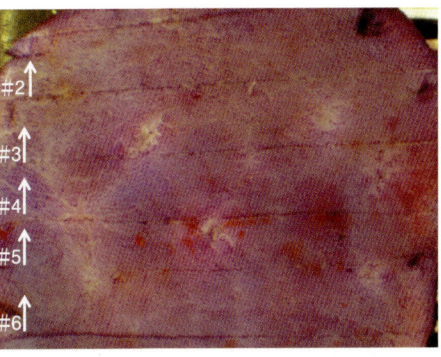

Stereoscopic observation (specimen fixed after EMR, left) : A few whitish mucosal depressions that seem to be inverted are recognized on the surface layer of the lesion. The specimen in question is sectioned and trimmed up (right). Sections #2-6 are shown below.

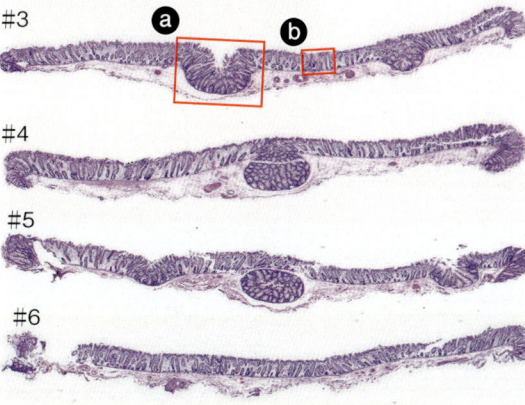

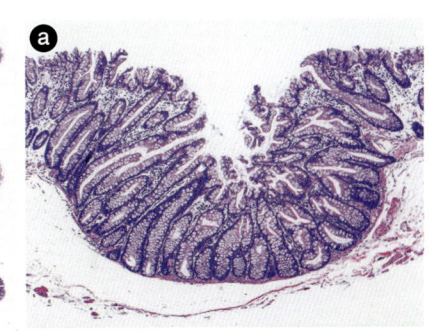

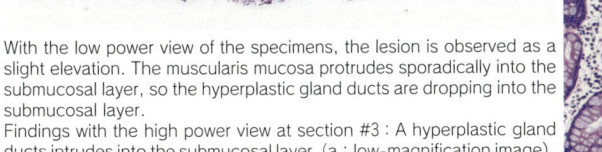

With the low power view of the specimens, the lesion is observed as a slight elevation. The muscularis mucosa protrudes sporadically into the submucosal layer, so the hyperplastic gland ducts are dropping into the submucosal layer.
Findings with the high power view at section #3 : A hyperplastic gland ducts intrudes into the submucosal layer (a : low-magnification image). The nuclear atypicality is poor, and the surface differentiation is maintained (b : high-magnification image). Based on the above, the lesion is diagnosed as a 35×25 mm, flat type hyperplastic polyp.

Comment

A hyperplastic polyp (HP) is a whitish polyp with a size of about 5 mm that grows in large numbers in the region from the rectum to the sigmoid colon. It is defined as a non-tumorous lesion, therefore, endoscopic treatment is not indicated and it is generally left untreated. Nevertheless, some HP lesions have sizes over 10 mm sized like the present case. If such a lesion is detected on the right side colon, the differentiation from sessile serrated adenoma/polyp (SSA/P) is required. If it is produced on the right side colon, cautious preoperative examinations become necessary considering the complication with traditional serrated adenoma (TSA). Therefore, this case is subjected to endoscopic resection.

▶**Observation tips** Unlike SSA/P, the lavage of attached mucus using hot water is easy with the HP. It is seen as a whitish nodular elevation in normal observation, while observed to have type Ⅱ pits in magnifying observation. There is no noticeable enlarged pits or dilated vessels surrounding with the pits, like those found with SSA/P. There is little sign of the dilated vessels transversing at the deep mucosal layer that are diagnosed typical with SSA/P.

(Saito, S., Ikegami, M., Tajiri, H.)

Case 49 SSA/P (sessile serrated adenoma/polyp)

Male aged 52 *Purpose* Detailed examination after positive fecal occult blood test
Location Cecum *Macroscopic type* 0-Ⅱa

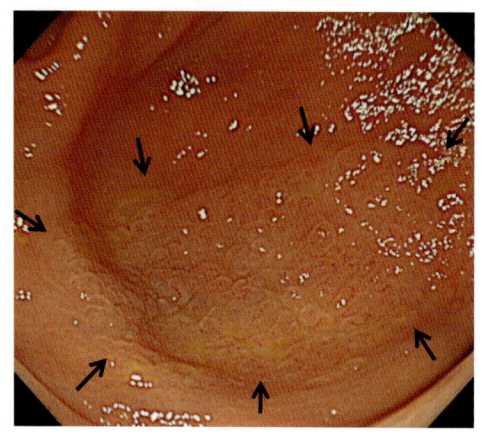

WLI observation: A slightly elevated lesion with a size of about 30 mm diameter and normal color tone is observed in the cecum. It is partially coated by yellowish mucus.

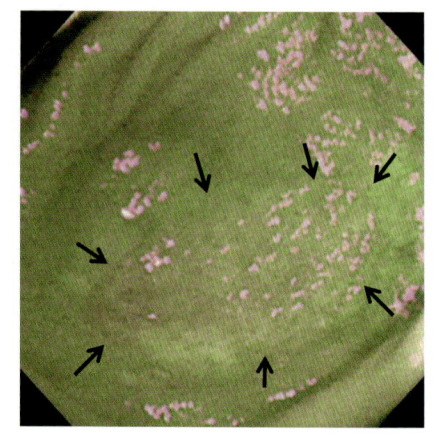

AFI observation: The color of the lesion is observed with the same dark greenish tone as the normal mucosa, the margin is shown slightly changed to magenta color.

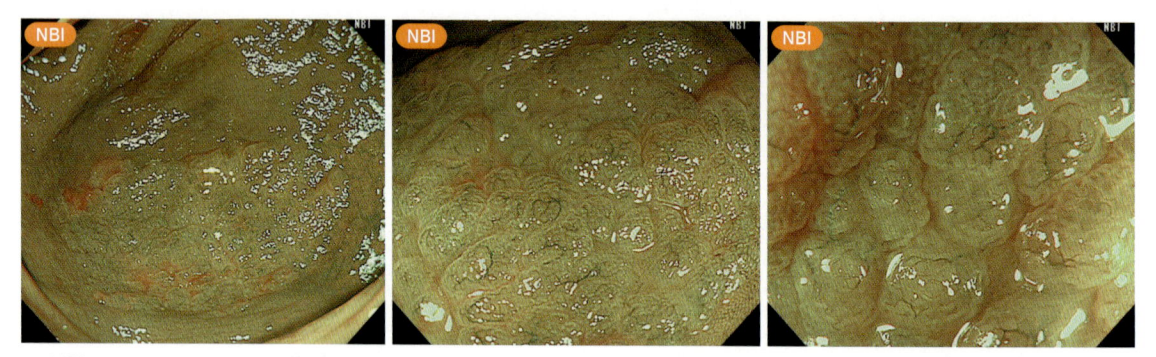

NBI normal observation: The borders are observed clearly, and the adhered mucus showing to reddish changed color on the surface of tumor (left).
NBI magnifying observation: The vessels surrounding the pit of glands are not dilated, but dilated vessels can be partially observed in the deep mucosal layer. Nevertheless, the surface pattern is possible to observe (middle: low magnification, right: high magnification).

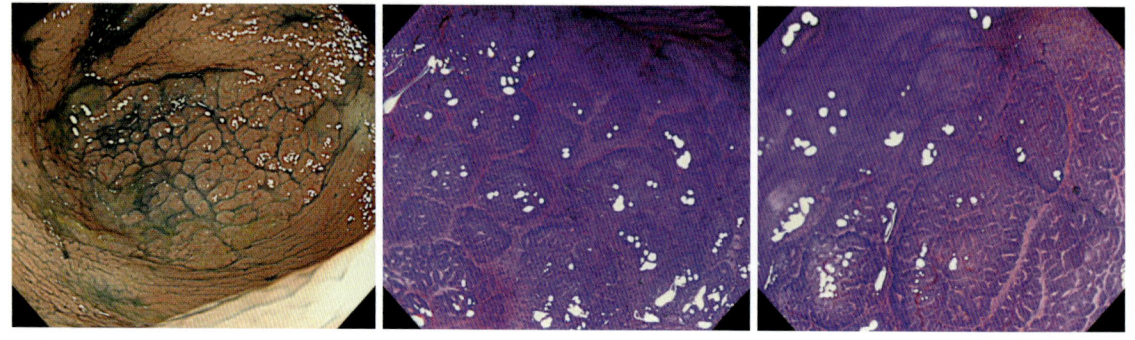

Indigocarmine, chromoendoscopy: The granular change of the surface layer is imaged clearly (left). In contrast, the crystal violet chromoendoscopy confirms that the lesion is a hyperplastic lesion mainly composed with asteroid shaped pits (type Ⅱ pits) (middle: low magnification, right: high magnification).

Endoscope：CF-FH260AZI（Olympus）　　Light source：EVIS LUCERA ELITE（Olympus）
NBI setup：Structure enhancement A8, color mode 3

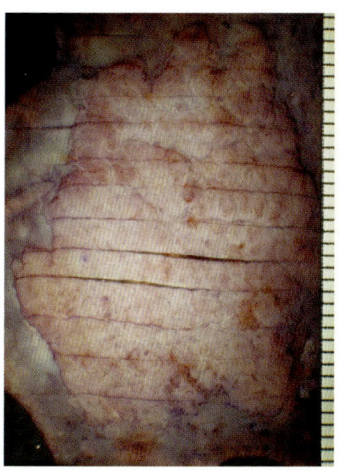

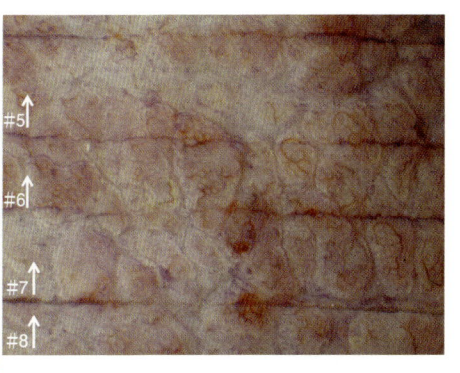

Stereoscopic image（specimen fixed after ESD, left）：The specimen is sectioned and trimmed（right, high power view）.

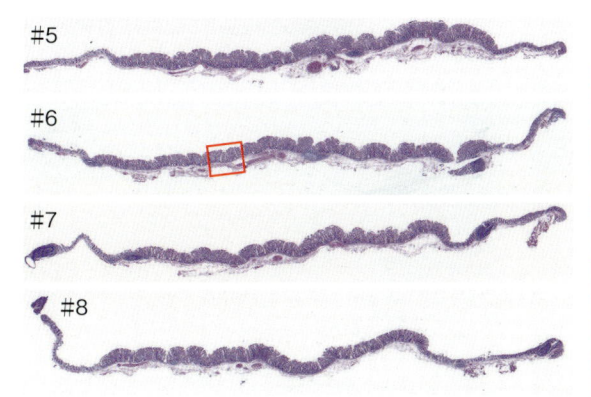

Magnified image：The lesion is observed as a slight elevation accompanied with growth of serrated duct glands.

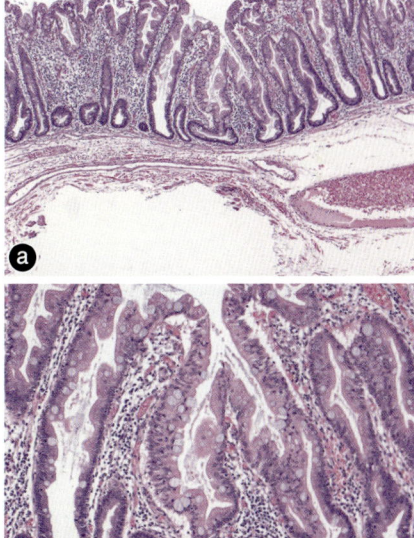

High power view：The gland ducts are dilated near the bottom of glands, and inverted T and L-shaped (like boots shaped) deformations are recognized（a：low power view）. The differentiation from bottom to surface is maintained and nuclear atypia is rarely found（b）. Based on the above, the lesion is diagnosed as a 0-Ⅱa, 35×25 mm sessile serrated adenoma/polyp (SSA/P), pHM0, pVM0.

Comment

Since one of the histopathological features of SSA/P is the structural atypia at the bottom of gland, differentiation from a large hyperplastic polyp is difficult to differentiate with superficial observation using by endoscope. However, there is also a possibility of indirect recognition of serrated gland ducts by observing gland ducts that have been dilated by the accumulation of a large amount of mucus pooling. In addition, the tortuous dilated vessels that seem to branch in the deep mucosal layer, as seen in the NBI magnifying observation image, is another feature characterizing as SSA/P.

▶ **Observation tips** A thick covering with the mucus is often observed with SSA/P, and a coating of reddish mucus is sometimes found together with the pit of glands as a black dots pattern in NBI observation. The mucus coating is therefore regarded as one of the characteristic features of SSA/P. This case was subjected to ESD for en bloc resection because the color turned slightly magenta in AFI observation, the lesion was large and there was undeniable infiltration of cancerous gland ducts from the bottom into the submucosal layer.

(Ide, D., Saito, S., Ikegami, M.)

Case 50 SSA/P (sessile serrated adenoma/polyp)

Male aged 69 **Purpose** Colonoscopy for periodic follow-up after EMR of early colon carcinoma
Location Ascending colon **Macroscopic type** 0-Is

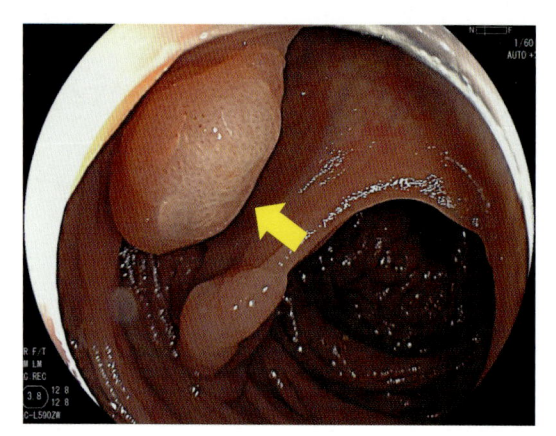

Normal white-light observation: A whitish flat elevated lesion with a diameter of 23 mm and coated with mucus is discerned (arrow).

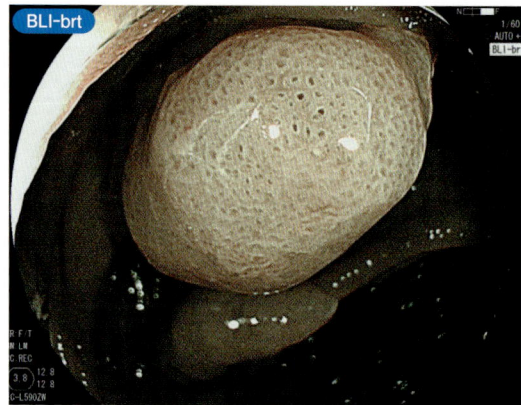

BLI-bright magnifying observation (middle magnification): Type II open-shape pit pattern (Type II-O) is discerned.

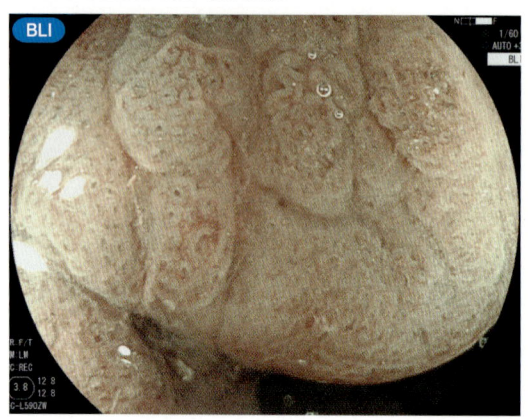

BLI magnifying observation (high magnification): The type II-O pits with asteroid pattern are discerned. Although vascular dilations are visible in the intervening part, the vascular structures are not clearly discernable in most areas.

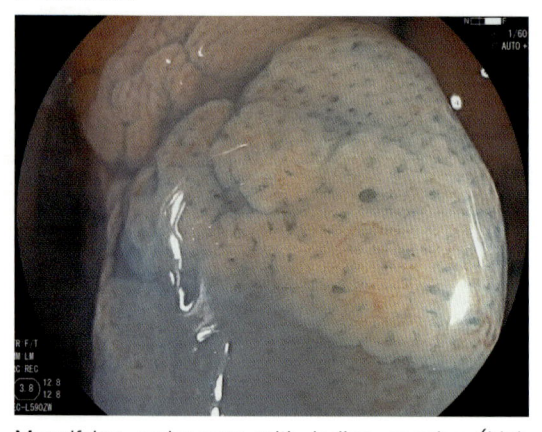

Magnifying endoscopy with indigo carmine (high magnification): Very large pit openings can be seen. However, the dye does not attach to areas coated with a lot of mucus.

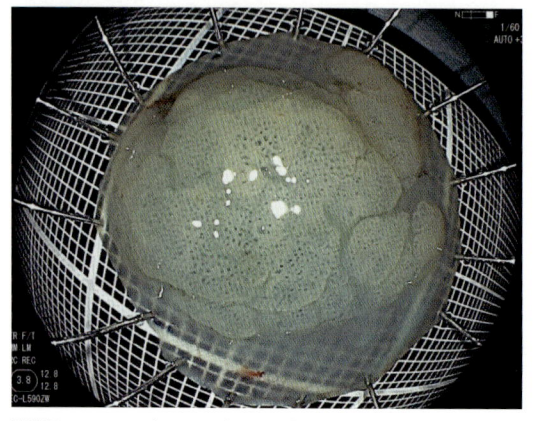

EMR-resected specimen: The lesion surface is coated with a large amount of mucus.

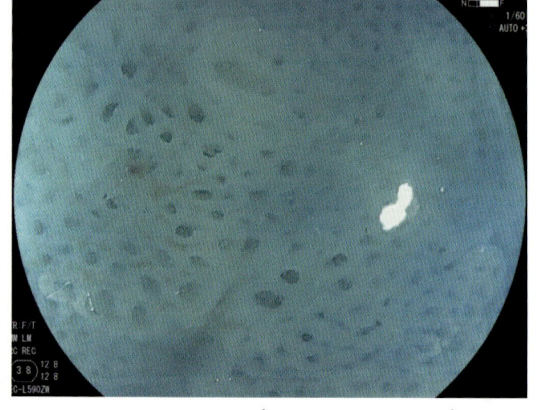

Magnifying observation (high magnification) of resected specimen: An asteroid pattern and large pit openings can be clearly seen.

Endoscope : EC-L590ZW (Fujifilm)　　Light source : LASEREO (Fujifilm)
BLI setup : BLI-bright—Structure enhancement B7, color enhancement C1 ; BLI—Structure enhancement B7, color enhancement C1

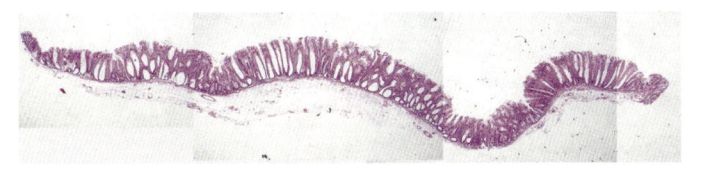

Magnified image

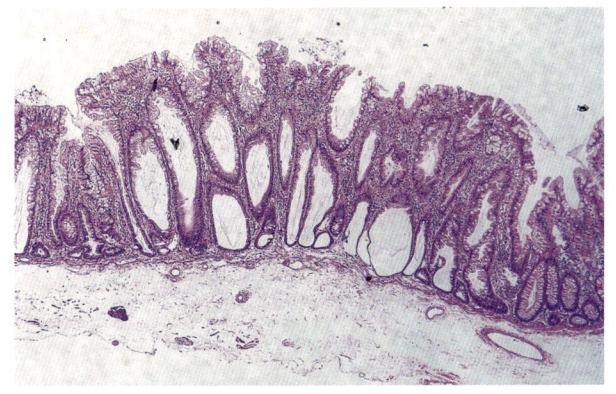

Image with increased magnification : Dilation of crypts, irregular branching of crypts and deformation of crypt bases in the horizontal direction are observed.

Comment

The SSA/P and HP (hyperplastic polyp) resemble each other in many points including macroscopic morphology, color tone and magnified view. Unlike the HP, however, the SSA/P is regarded as a tumorous lesion with a risk of carcinogenesis. SSA/P occurs more frequently on the right side while HP occurs more on the left side.

▶**Observation tips** As an SSA/P often appears as a flat, pale-colored lesion under white light imaging, it is important to differentiate it from a similar-looking HP. Magnifying endoscopy can confirm the asteroid pattern in both lesions. With the SSA/P, however, the pit openings are enlarged to enable production of a large amount of mucus, so magnifying endoscopy can often find the Type II-open shape pit pattern, which is a characteristic feature.

(Hayashi, Y., Yamamoto, H., Fukushima, N.)

Case 51 # SSA/P (sessile serrated adenoma/polyp)

Male in his 40s　*Purpose* Colon polypectomy　*Location* Cecum　*Macroscopic type* 0-Ⅱa

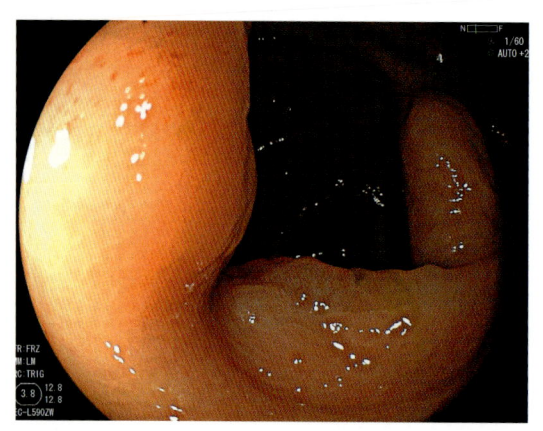

White-light observation: An elevated lesion can be seen in the cecum on the posterior wall side near Bauhin's valve.

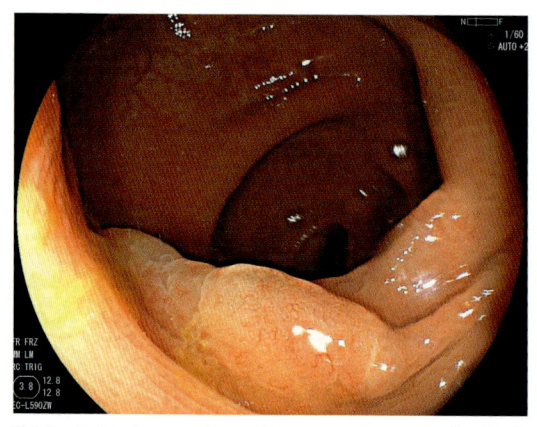

White-light observation: A flat elevated lesion (0-Ⅱa) showed the same color as the surrounding mucosa across the folds. The lesion surface is coated with mucus.

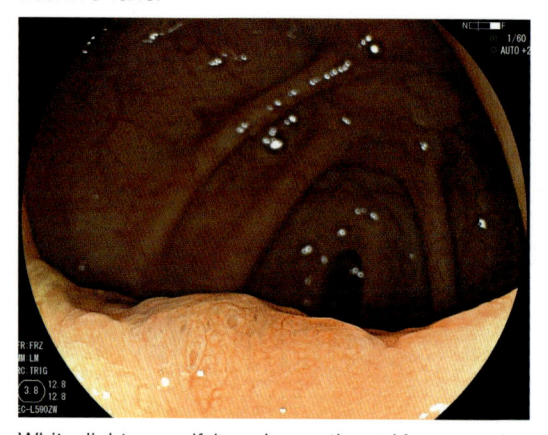

White-light magnifying observation: After removing the mucus, expanded crypt openings and thick and branching vessels that are slightly thicker in size than capillaries can be seen on the lesion.

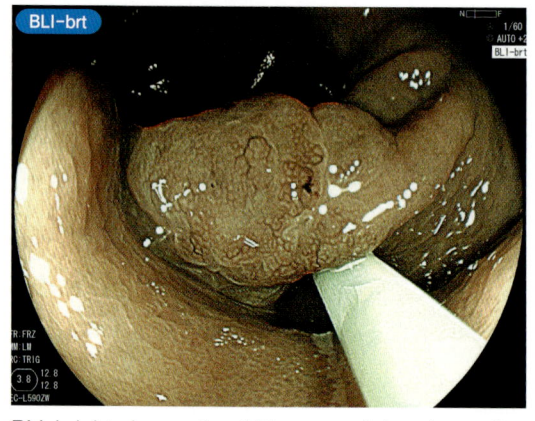

BLI-bright observation: Non-magnifying observation of the overall image shows that the lesion is slightly brownish and that its surface presents networked vessels that are slightly thicker than the vessels on the normal mucosa.

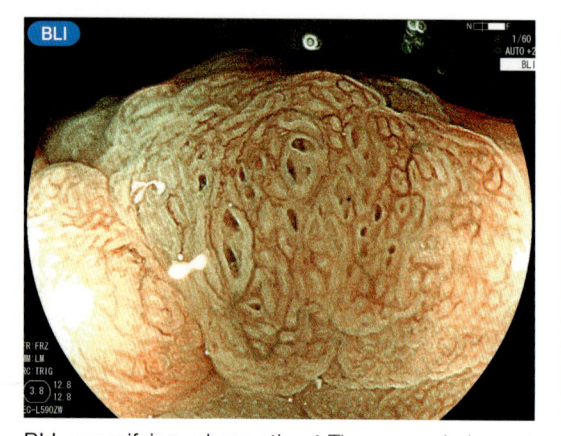

BLI magnifying observation: The expanded crypt openings can be seen clearly, as well as the capillaries around them and relatively thick and branching vessels.

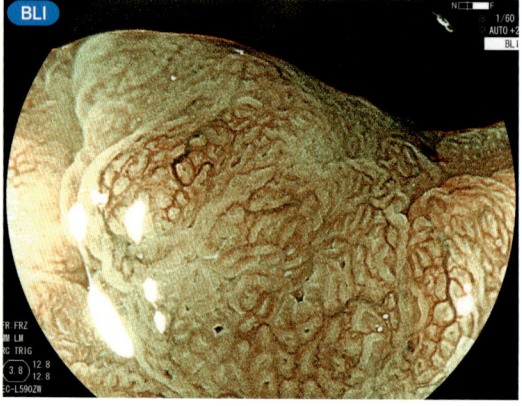

BLI magnifying observation: Several thick and branching vessels thicker than capillaries can be seen which are not observed in normal adenomas.

Endoscope : EC-L590ZW (Fujifilm)　　Light source : LASEREO (Fujifilm)
BLI setup : BLI-bright—Structure enhancement B6, color enhancement C2 ; BLI—Structure enhancement A8, color enhancement C2

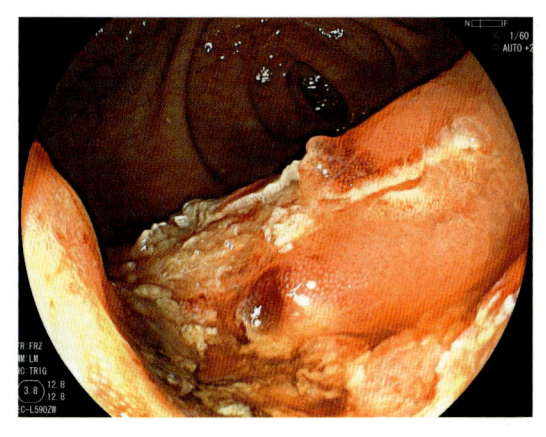

White-light observation : The lesion is resected by piecemeal EMR.

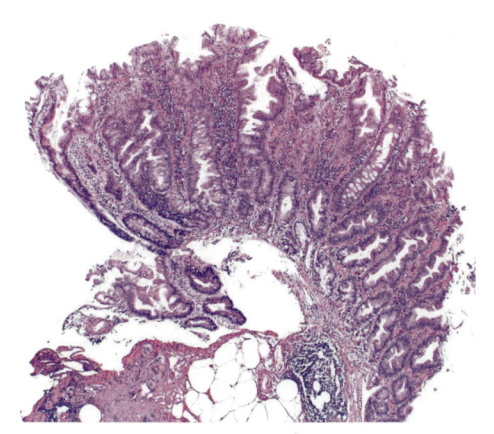

Pathological specimen (low magnification) : The lesion presents serrated structures like a hyperplastic polyp.

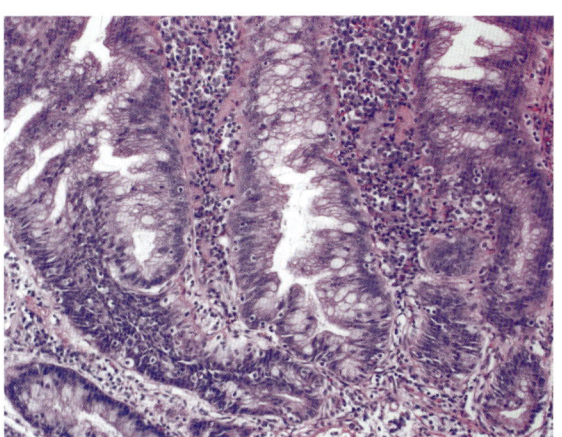

Pathological specimen (high magnification) : Dilation of crypts, irregular branching and deformation of crypt bases allows the lesion to be diagnosed as a sessile serrated adenoma/polyp (SSA/P).

Comment

This is a case of an SSA/P (sessile serrated adenoma/polyp) in the cecum. Thick and branching vessels and expanded crypt openings are characteristic of SSA/P. In a prospective study conducted at our hospital, when these findings are observed with a lesion with NICE Classification Type 1, the diagnosis as an SSA/P is possible with a sensitivity of 98% and specificity of 60%. The diagnostic performance of the expanded crypt openings is better than the finding of thick and branching vessels.

▶Observation tips　As the surface of SSA/P is often coated with mucus, it is helpful to remove as much of it as possible before magnifying observation with dye spraying. However, when using narrowband imaging including BLI, observation is usually possible even with a small amount of mucus coating, so it is not necessary to eliminate all of the mucus.

(Takeuchi, Y., Yamashina, T., Tomita, Y.)

Case 52　Protruding serrated adenoma

Female in her 60s　|Purpose| Screening　|Location| Sigmoid colon　|Macroscopic type| 0-Ｉs+Ⅱa

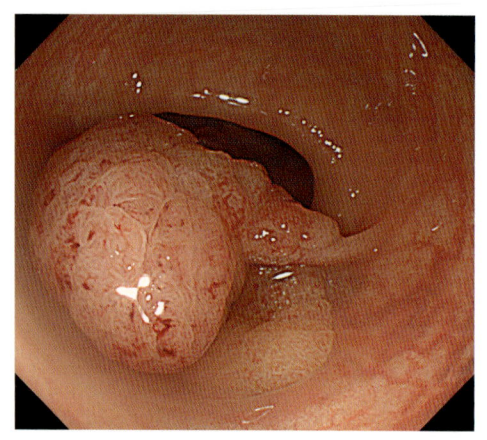

WLI normal observation: A 40 mm lesion composed of an elevated, protruding erythematous component (Ｉs) and a pale-colored slightly elevated component (Ⅱa) is observed.

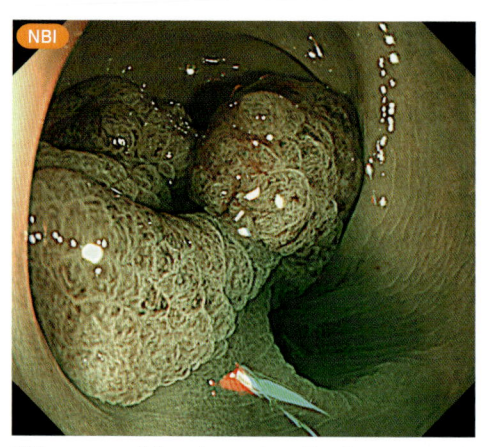

NBI non-magnifying observation: The Ｉs area is freely mobile. The color of the Ｉs area is slightly brownish while that of the Ⅱa area is whitish. The ELITE system of bright NBI makes it possible to assess a relatively large lesion such as this one in a single field of view.

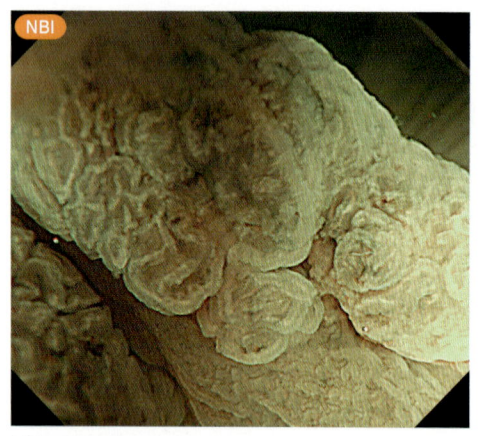

NBI magnifying observation: Although the evaluation of microvessels is difficult, the surface pattern is clearly visible. The visible surface pattern does not present irregularities in the margin, so the presence of type Ⅲ_L or Ⅳ pits is likely.

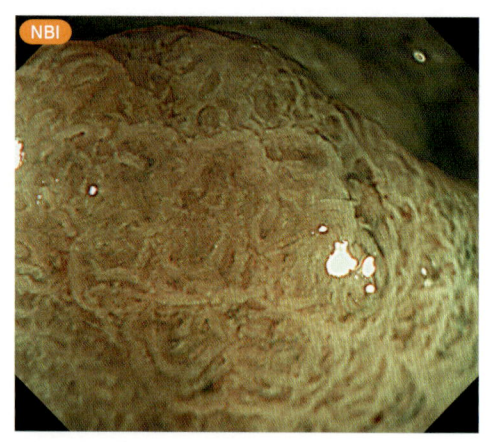

NBI magnifying observation of another area: The microvessels are visible in this region but overall lesion evaluation is difficult. The surface pattern is also visible as in the previous image, but the individual pit-like structures look relatively irregular.

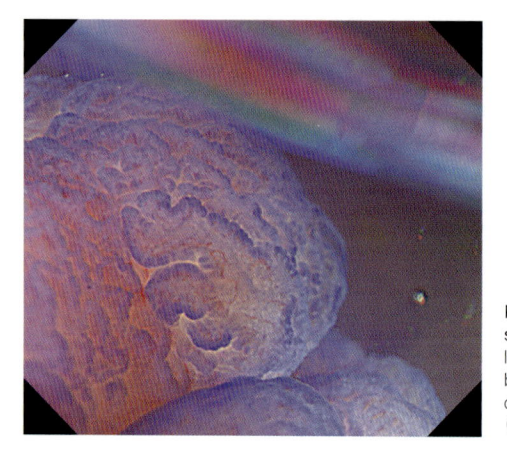

Magnifying observation after crystal violet staining: There is a region in which the pits look like branching type Ⅳ pits at first glance but, because of fine, jagged irregularities found on the margin, the region is a fern-like region (with type Ⅲ_H pits).

182

Endoscope：CF-FH260AZI（Olympus）　　Light source：EVIS LUCERA ELITE（Olympus）
NBI setup：Structure enhancement A8, color mode 3

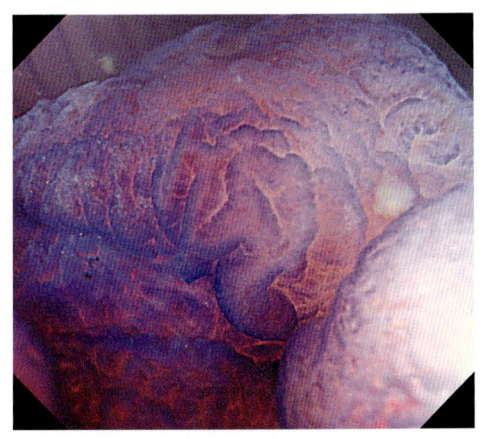

There is another region in which jagged irregularities are found on the margin of the gyrate, or type IV pits. These pits are not typical but judged to be type IV$_H$ pits which are predictive of traditional serrated adenoma.

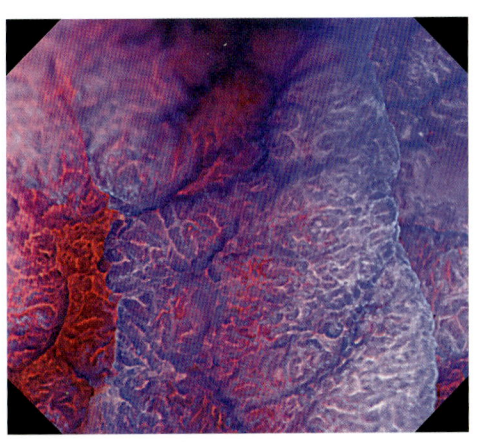

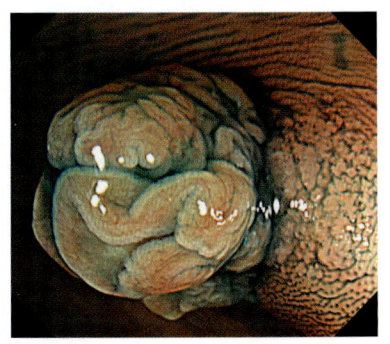

In the II a area, the irregularities similar to those described above are observed with both type III$_L$ type III$_H$ pits present.

[Reference (image of previous system)] With a pineal pattern and fine irregularities observed partially on the margin of the coating epithelium, the pits are judged to be typical type IV$_H$ pits.

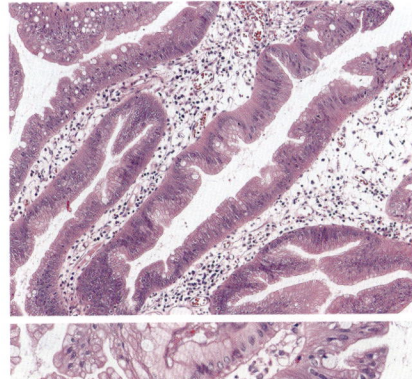

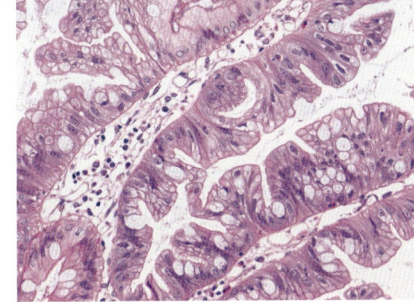

Histopathological image (HE stained)：As interstitial budding is recognized, the lesion is diagnosed as a traditional serrated adenoma (TSA).

Histopathological image (high magnification, HE stained)：The same findings are observed as the reference image.

Comment

The endoscopic assessment of this lesion demonstrates the lesion is composed mainly of branching type IV pits and focally with type III$_H$ or atypical type IV$_H$ pits and that the pathology is predicted to be a TSA. The lesion was treated by en bloc resection by ESD and the final diagnosis was a serrated adenoma.

▶Observation tips　It is hard to diagnose a TSA based only on the microvascular findings in NBI magnifying observation. The surface pattern seems to show that irregularities are observed in the pit-like structure somewhat similar to a typical tubular adenoma. There is currently a lack of evidence to define the typical magnifying NBI findings to establish a diagnosis of traditional serrated adenoma. The diagnosis of a serrated lesion requires detailed assessment of pit pattern. If crystal violet staining is used, it is possible to observe type III$_H$ and IV$_H$ pits. Whilst these patterns may be recognized by with indigo carmine dye spraying, crystal violet staining is recommended for precise diagnosis.

(Sakamoto, T., Nakajima, T., Matsuda, T., Saito, Y.)

Case 53 Elevated tubular adenoma

Male in his 60s Purpose Positive fecal occult blood test Location Sigmoid colon
Macroscopic type 0-Is

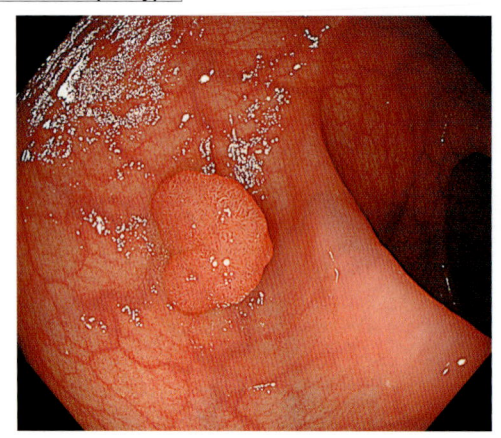

WLI normal observation: An erythematous protruding lesion with a 10 mm size is recognized.

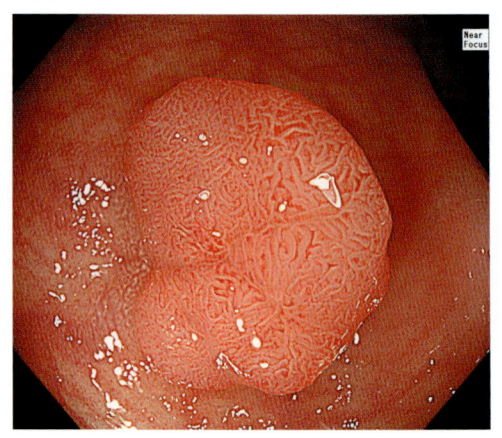

Close-up in the Near Focus mode makes possible recognition of the surface pattern even with the WLI.

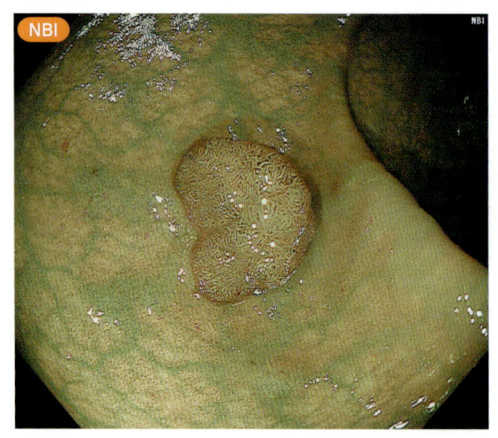

NBI observation: Observation is possible with sufficient brightness.

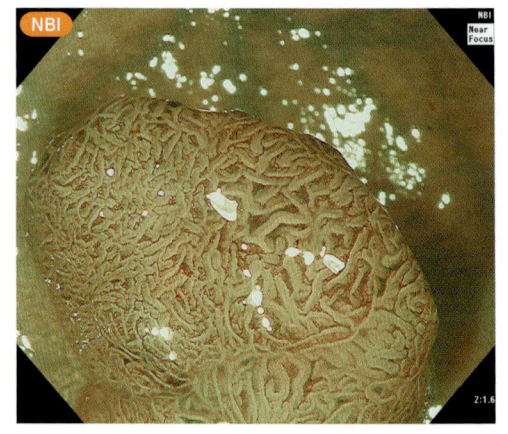

NBI Near Focus+1.6×electronic zoom: The regular surface pattern and the vascular pattern in a regular network shape surrounding the pits are observed.

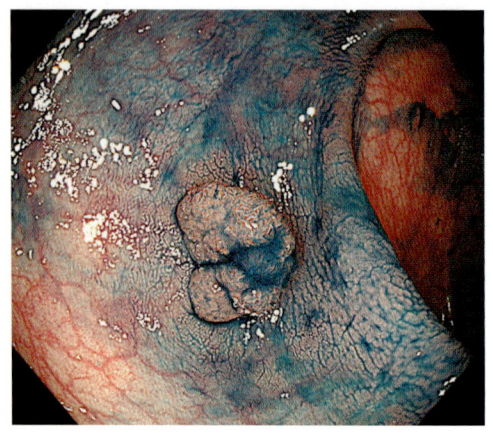

Indigo carmine dye is sprayed to confirm the pit pattern.

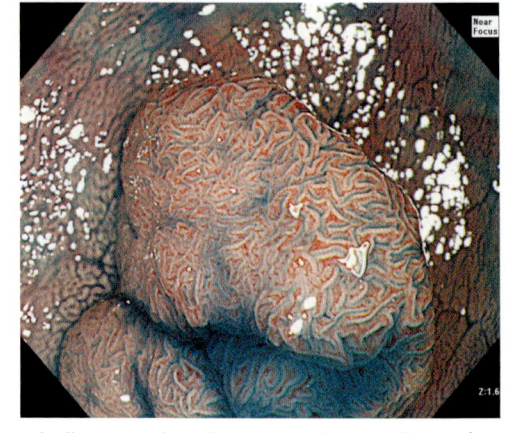

Indigo carmine dye sprayed Near Focus+1.6×electronic zoom: Type III_L-IV pit pattern is observed clearly.

Endoscope：CF-HQ290I（Olympus）　　Light source：EVIS LUCERA ELITE（Olympus）
NBI setup：Structure enhancement B8, color mode 3（Normal observation→Structure enhancement A8, color enhancement 0）

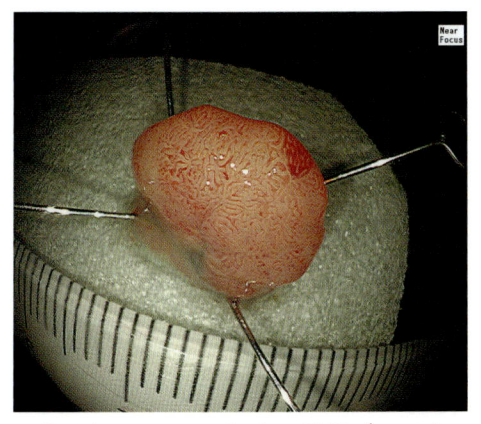

Specimen resected after EMR (normal observation).

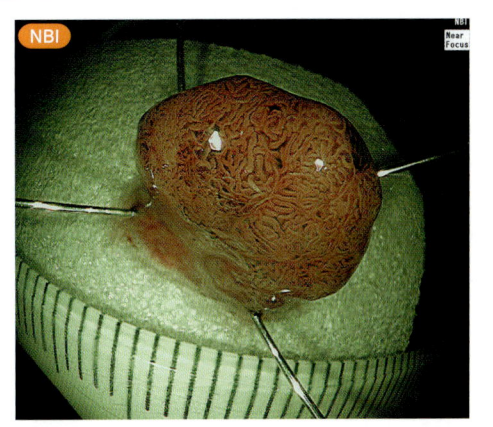

NBI Near Focus mode observation：The regular surface pattern can also be recognized with the resected specimen.

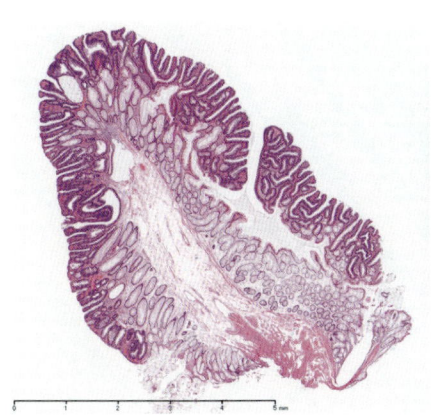

Magnified image.

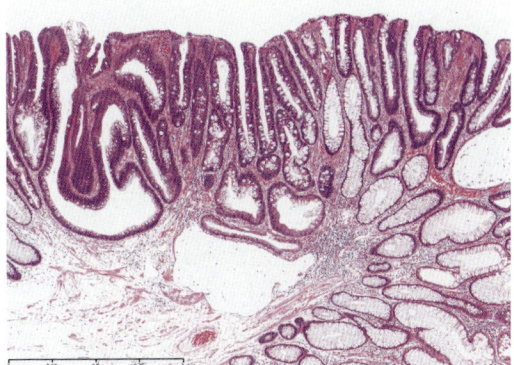

Low-magnification image：The lesion is diagnosed as a tubular adenoma partially accompanied with high-grade atypical changes.

Comment

The protruding adenoma often presents type ⅢL or Ⅳ pit pattern, and close-up in the Near Focus mode can often observe the surface pattern clearly even without using the magnification function. The addition of magnification enables detailed observation with little degradation in image quality, even with electronic zoom. This case was subjected to NBI observation before indigocarmine dye spraying. As a regular surface pattern similar to type ⅢL-Ⅳ was confirmed, it was diagnosed as a tubular adenoma.

▶Observation tips With a protruding tumor like the present case, NBI observation can often confirm a regular surface pattern similar to type ⅢL-Ⅳ and a vascular pattern with a regular network surrounding the pits. In such a case, the pit pattern observation by dye spraying may seemingly be able to be omitted.

(Kawamura, T., Yasuda, K.)

Case 54 Superficial tubular adenoma

Male in his 60s　**Purpose** Prescreening before gastric carcinoma operation
Location Sigmoid colon　**Macroscopic type** 0-Ⅱa

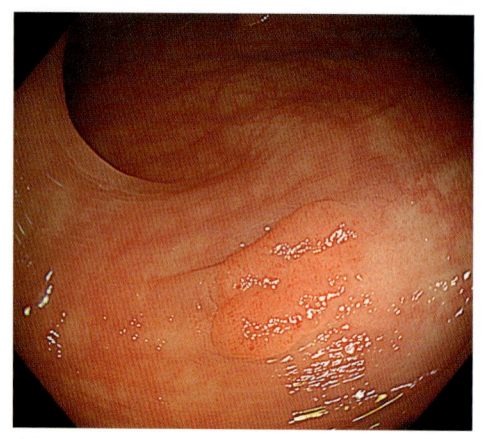

WLI observation : A slightly elevated lesion with a pale erythematous color and 10 mm diameter is observed.

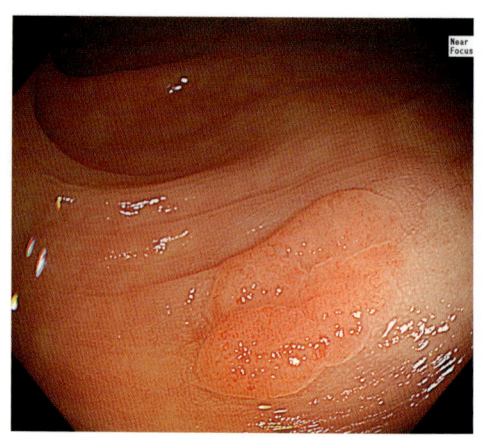

WLI Near Focus observation : The surface properties can be observed even with the WLI.

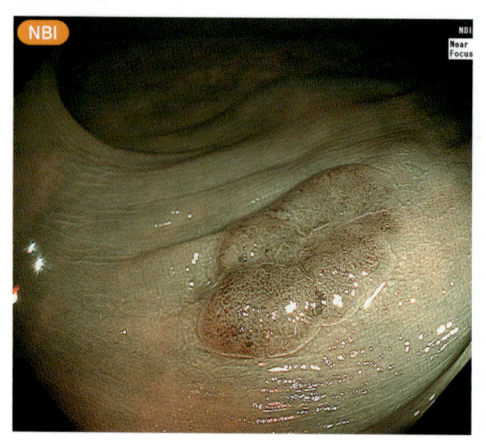

NBI Near Focus observation : The lesion is recognized as a brownish area compared to the surrounding mucosa.

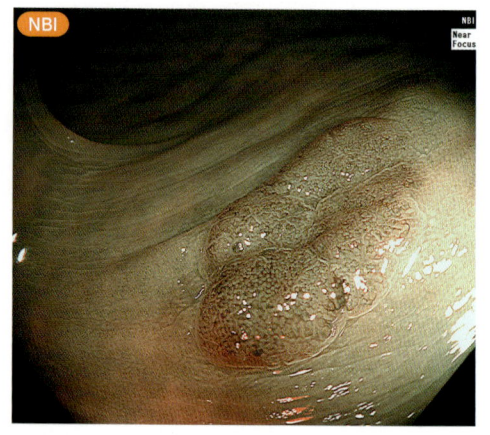

NBI Near Focus observation : Further close-up observed a uniform network of vessels all over the lesion. This finding is equivalent to Sano Classification CP type Ⅱ.

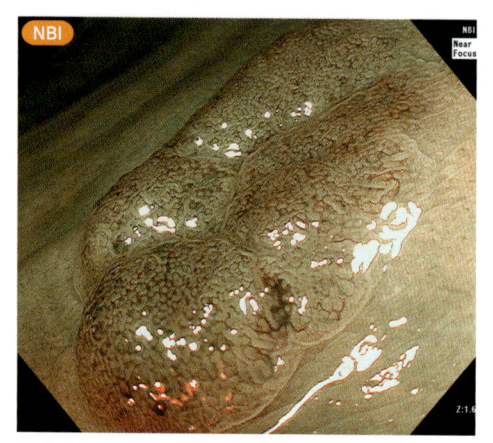

NBI Near Focus+1.6×electronic zoom : The CP type Ⅱ vessels are observed more clearly.

Endoscope：CF-HQ290I（Olympus）　　Light source：EVIS LUCERA ELITE（Olympus）
NBI setup：Structure enhancement A8, color mode 3.

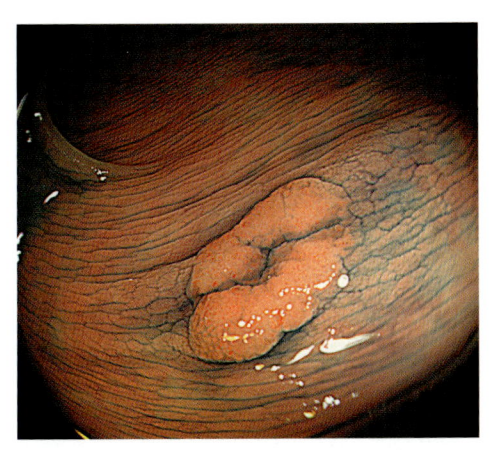

Indigo carmine normal chromoendoscopy：As the indigocarmine is not accumulated in the lesion, it is diagnosed as 0-Ⅱa.

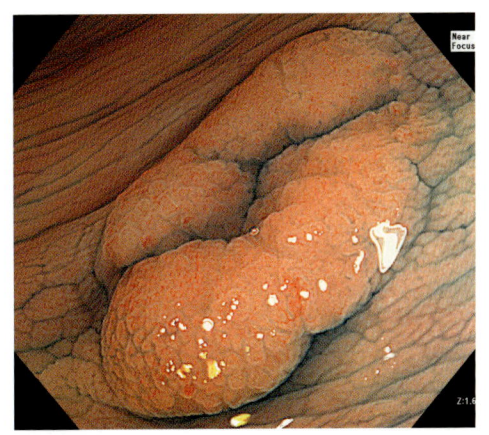

Indigo carmine Near Focus chromoendoscopy：Tubular pits are observed, which is the finding corresponding to the type Ⅲ_L pit pattern.

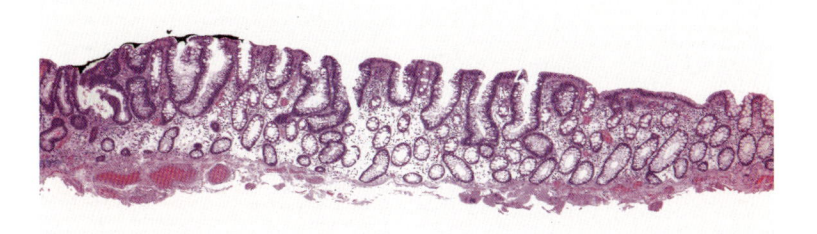

Low-magnification image：The lesion is diagnosed as a tubular adenoma with low-grade dysplasia.

Comment

This case has a pale erythematous elevation with a size of 10 mm in the sigmoid colon. The initial suggestion derived from WLI observation was that it may be a tubular adenoma. In addition, the relatively uniform network of vessels recognized with NBI Near Focus observation suggested that it was a CP type Ⅱ of the Sano Classification. The tubular pits recognized with the indigo carmine dye sprayed in Near Focus observation are a finding of the type Ⅲ_L pit pattern. The lesion was therefore diagnosed as a tubular adenoma and subjected to EMR. The histopathological diagnosis concluded that it was a tubular adenoma with low-grade dysplasia.

▶**Observation tips**　In this region, the overall lesion should first be observed with the non-magnified Near Focus observation and then the details should be evaluated with NBI. Combining 1.6× electronic zoom with the Near Focus mode makes possible clear observation of the vascular pattern.

(Yokoyama, A., Horimatsu, T.)

Case 55 Tubulovillous adenoma

Male in his 60s | Purpose | Further evaluation of the lesion referred from other hospital
| Location | Rectum, Rb (lower rectum) | Macroscopic type | 0-Ⅰs+Ⅱa

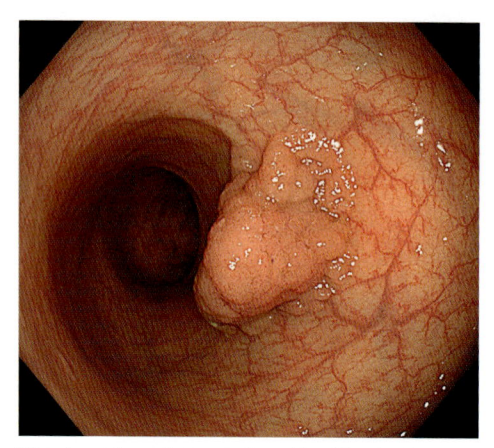

WLI view : A sessile type lesion with mild red color and a size of 30 mm was identified in the lower rectum.

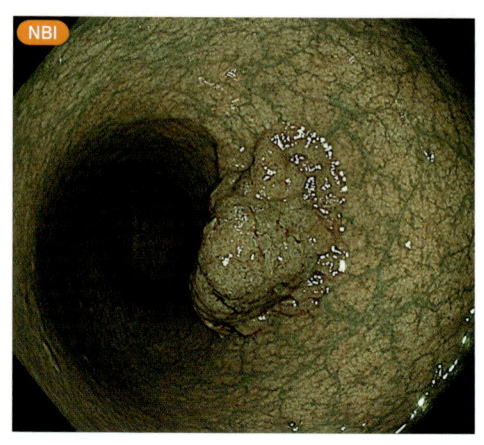

NBI view : The lesion is recognized as a mild brownish area and its border was recognized as disruption of vascular network.

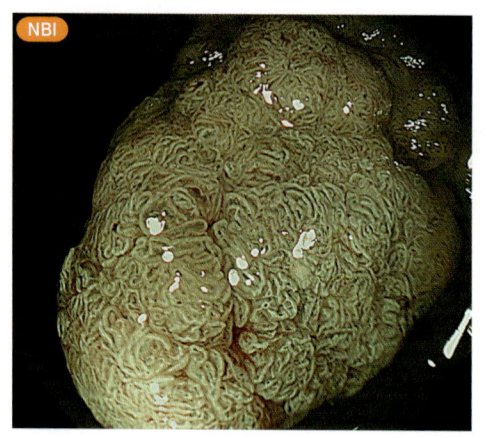

NBI with Near Focus view : Regularly arranged microvessels and surface pattern were identified

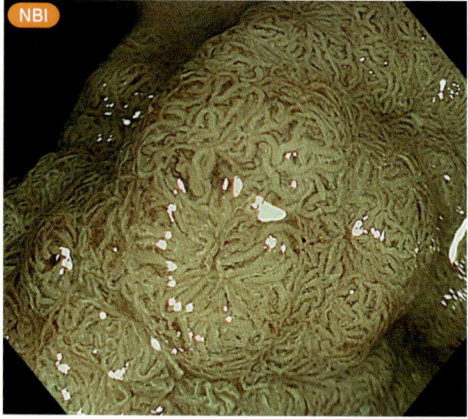

NBI with Near Focus view+1.4×electronic zoom : Regularly arranged microvessels and surface pattern were identified more clearly.

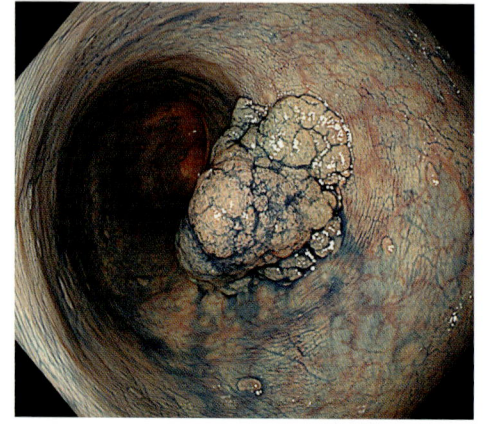

Chromoendoscopy with Indigo carmine dye spraying : The lesion consists mainly of a protrusion, but the 0-Ⅱa was recognized to some extent in the surrounding area. The surface had a lobulated structure.

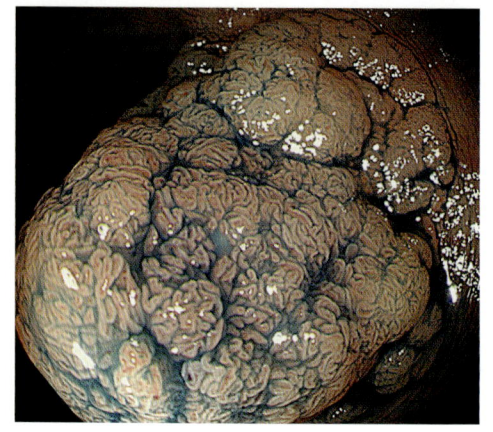

Near Focus view : The Kudo's type Ⅳ pit pattern was identidied.

Endoscope：CF-HQ290I（Olympus）　Light source：EVIS LUCERA ELITE（Olympus）
NBI setup：Structure enhancement function A5（non-maginification view），A7（magnification view），color mode 3

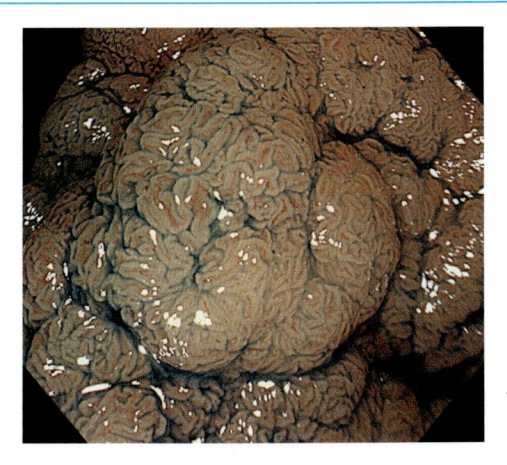

NBI with Near Focus＋1.4×electronic zoom view. The Kudo's type Ⅳ pit pattern was observed clearly.

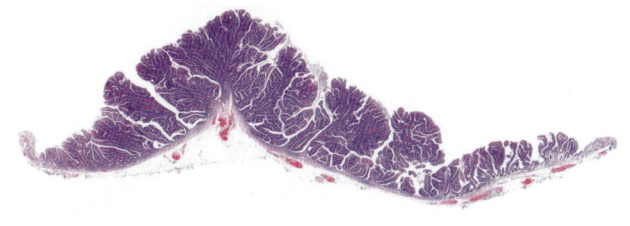

Histopathology of the resected specimen. Magnified image.

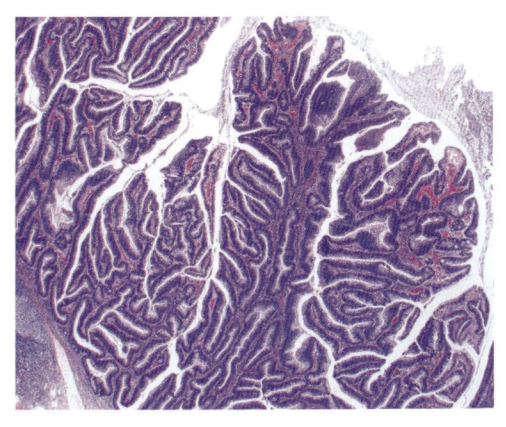

Middle magnified image：The lesion is diagnosed as a tubulovillous adenoma with high-grade dysplasia.

Comment

The first impress was a relatively large protruding lesion like this is the differentiation from early carcinoma. With the WLI observation, the reddening is light and no expansion or depression was recognized, so the lesion was regarded to be intramucosal lesion. NBI magnification view found that the microvessels and surface pattern were regular, so the lesion was endoscopically diagnosed as a tubulovillous adenoma based on the gyrate surface pattern. The Kudo's type Ⅳ pit pattern was composed of branching vessels and gyrate pits, and the gyrate pits often indicates the tubulovillous adenoma.

▶Observation tips　The tubulovillous adenoma surface is more often coated with mucus than the tubular adenoma surface, so sufficient lavage with irrigation is required before the diagnosis. The lesion is diagnosable as an adenoma using NBI with Near Focus view alone, but combining electronic zoom around 1.5× with the Near Focus mode with 40× magnification enables clearer observations of the regular microvessels and surface pattern. The indigo carmine dye spraying is enough for recognizing Kudo's type Ⅳ pit pattern and there is no need of the crystal violet staining for pit pattern diagnosis.

(Uraoka, T., Yahagi, N.)

Case 56 Villous adenoma

Female in her 70s   **Purpose** Detailed examination of colorectal lesion
Location Rectum, sigmoid colon (RS)   **Macroscopic type** 0-Ⅰs

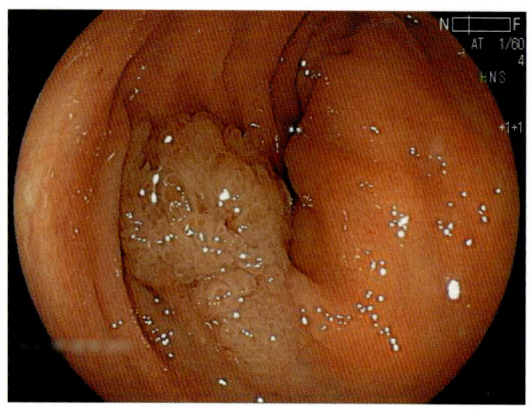

White-light normal observation: A white protruding lesion of around 15 mm is recognized.

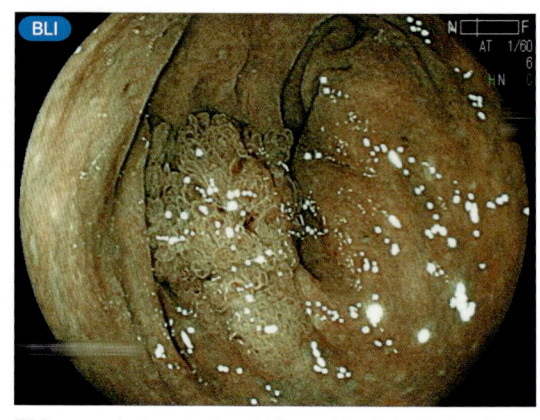

BLI normal observation: The color of the lesion is not much different from the surrounding mucosa.

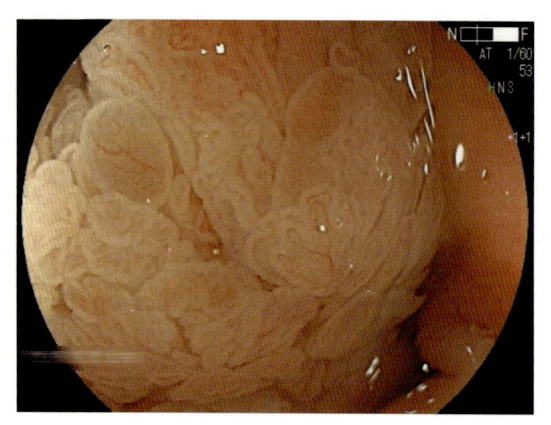

White light low-magnification observation.

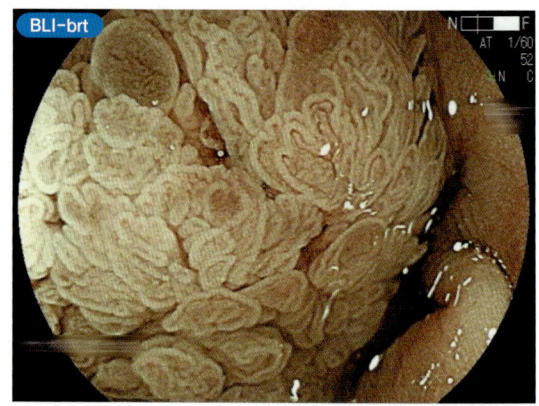

BLI-bright low-magnification observation: Enhancement of the vascular pattern makes the surface structures easier than with the white light imaging.

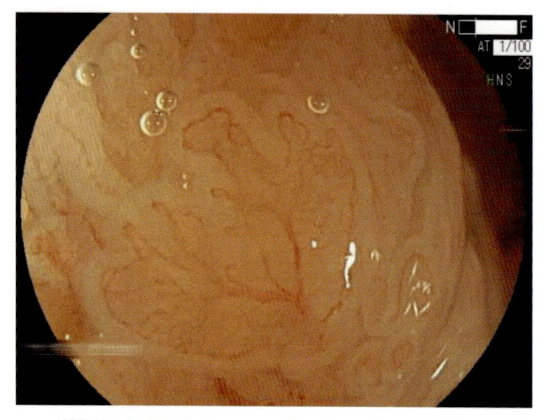

White light high-magnification observation.

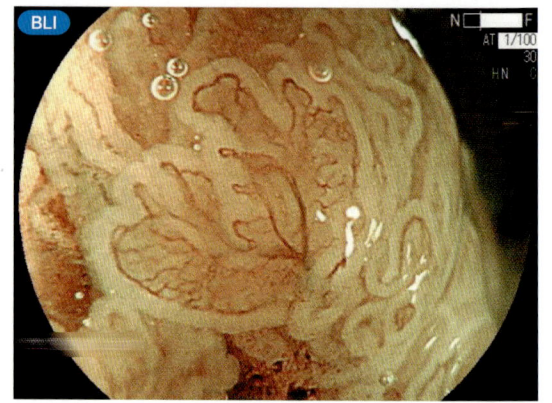

BLI high-magnification observation: Vessels branching as if tracing the inner side of the coating epithelium and a vascular network continued until the deep layer are recognized. The vascular size is not irregular, and the vascular course is also relatively regular.

Endoscope : EC-L590ZW (Fujifilm)　　Light source : LASEREO (Fujifilm)
BLI setup : BLI—Structure enhancement A6, color enhancement C1 ; BLI-bright—Structure enhancement A6, color enhancement C1

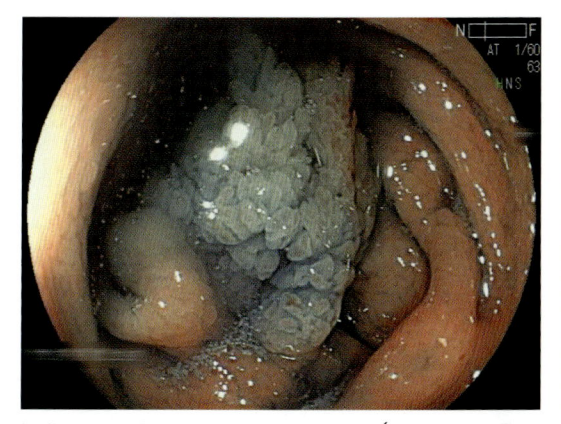

Indigo carmine chromoendoscopy (non-magnification) : Secretion of a large amount of mucus makes the lesion glossy.

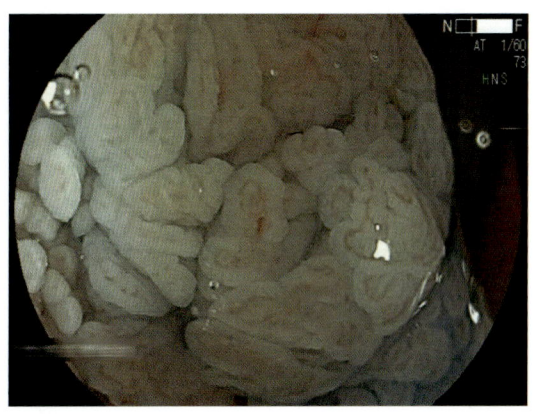

Indigo carmine chromoendoscopy (high magnification) : The villous structures on the surface are enhanced.

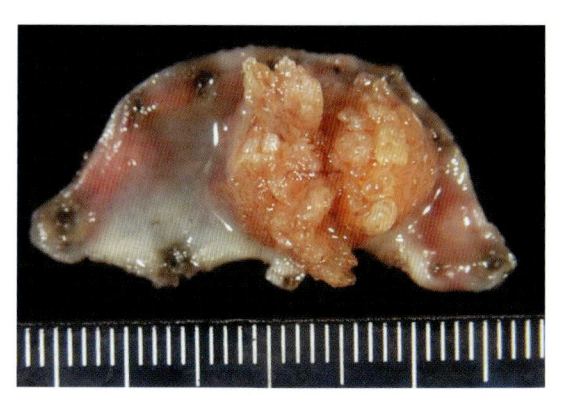

Endoscopically resected specimen : 14×13 mm Is lesion.

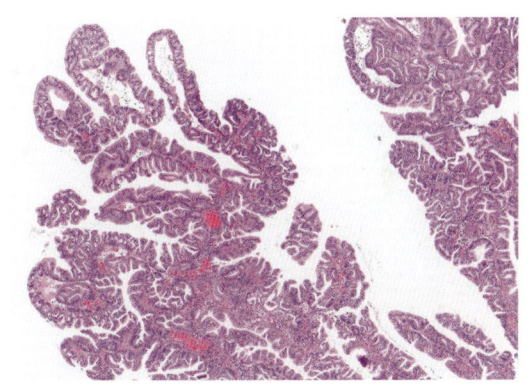

Among the adenomas, those with which the villous component occupies 75% or more are defined as villous adenomas. In the majority of this lesion, the epithelia with light to low grade of atypia present villous or papillary growth, so it is diagnosed as a villous adenoma.

Comment

This is a case of villous adenoma that manifests mainly in the rectum and sigmoid colon. The BLI normal observation renders the lesion in a similar color tone to the surrounding mucosa, but the magnifying observation makes possible clear identification of the microvessels on the tumor surface. The morphology and courses of the vessels of this case makes possible the diagnosis that the tumor has a low grade of dysplasia.

▶**Observation tips** The villous adenoma can be diagnosed by accurate assessment of the surface structures. The conventional contrasting method is an important technique for observing the tumor surface, but the BLI magnifying observation can also enhance the surface structures more clearly than the white-light imaging and offer sufficient information for diagnosis.

(Tominaga, M., Fujiya, M., Kohgo, Y.)

Case 57 Protruding M carcinoma

Female in her 60s **Purpose** Surveillance after colon carcinoma operation
Location Ascending colon **Macroscopic type** 0-Ⅰs

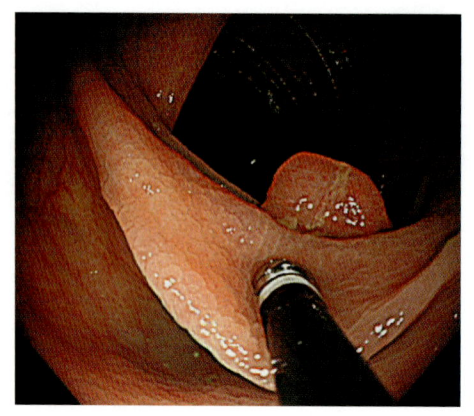

A sessile elevated lesion with a size of 10 mm can be recognized on the backside of a fold on the ascending colon. The lesion was observed using the NT tube.

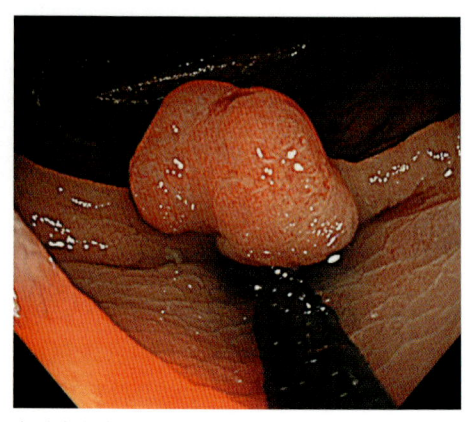

A relatively depressed area can be seen in the center of the lesion. Tension or concentration of folds was not seen under normal observation.

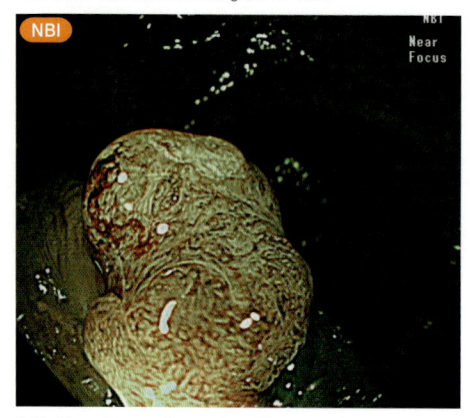

NBI Near Focus observation : The vascular and surface patterns in the relatively depressed area look different from those in the surrounding area.

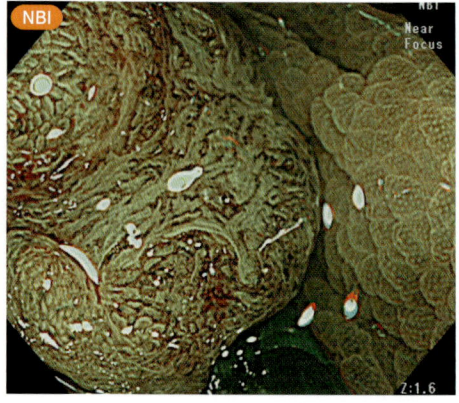

NBI Near Focus+1.6×electronic zoom observation : The findings with the vascular pattern in the relatively depressed area, including irregular sizes, irregular distribution and tortuosity, lead to a diagnosis of Sano Classification Type ⅢA. The surface pattern is obviously irregular compared to the tubular structures in the surrounding area.

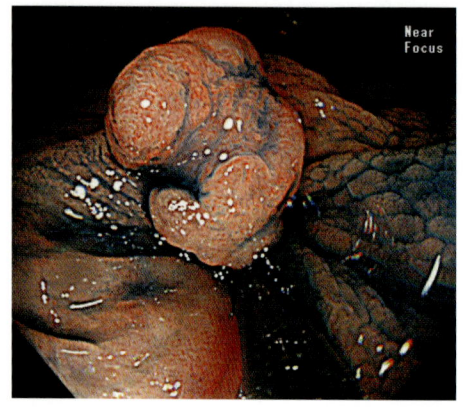

Indigo carmine dye sprayed Near Focus observation : The relatively depressed area is imaged more clearly. A small number of lobulated grooves can be seen in the surrounding area.

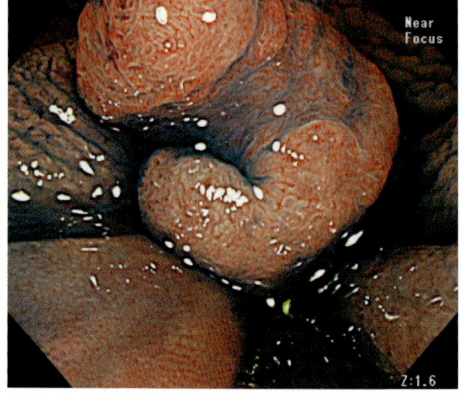

Indigo carmine dye sprayed Near Focus+1.6×electronic zoom observation : The type ⅢL pit pattern in the elevated region around the relatively depressed area is recognizable, but the pit pattern in the relatively depressed area is difficult to discern.

Endoscope : CF-HQ290I (Olympus)   Light source : EVIS LUCERA ELITE (Olympus)
NBI setup : Structure enhancement A7, color mode 3.

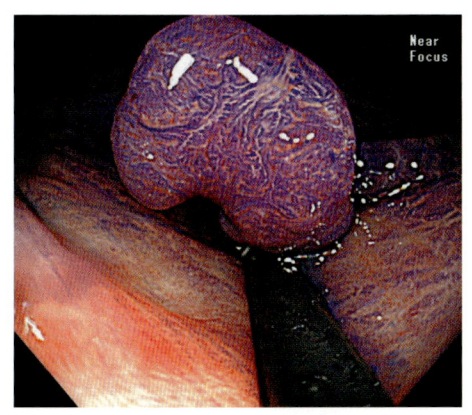

Crystal violet stained Near Focus observation : An irregular pit pattern can be seen in the relatively depressed area.

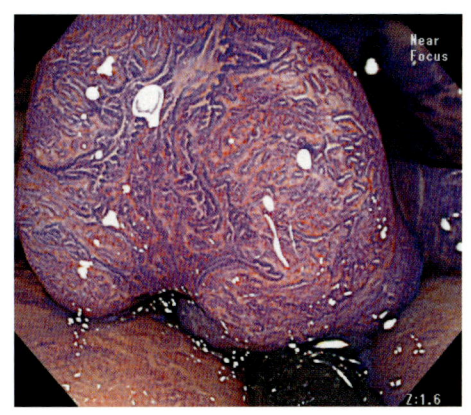

Crystal violet stained Near Focus+1.6×electronic zoom observation : Irregularities in branching and sizes can be seen in the area corresponding to the relatively depressed area, but a relatively clear pit pattern is observed in the contour. The lesion was therefore diagnosed as a V_I lesion with slight irregularity.

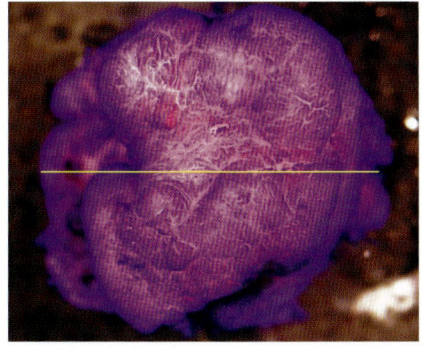

Stereoscopic image : As in endoscopic observation, a pit pattern with more irregularity than the surrounding area can be seen in the relatively depressed area. The pathological specimen of the section indicated by the yellow line is shown on the right.

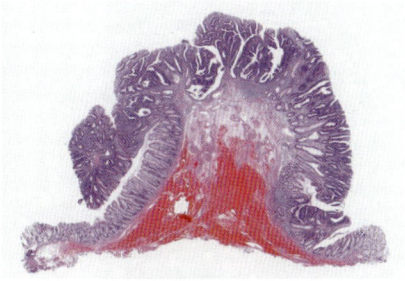

Magnified image : The lesion is an intramucosal well-differentiated adenocarcinoma (cancer in adenoma).

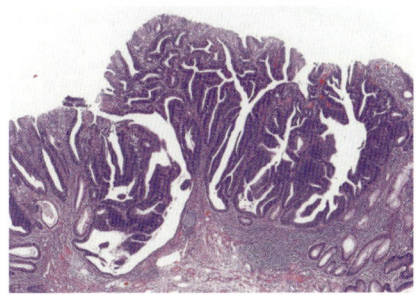

Enlarged view of carcinoma : A well-differentiated tubular adenocarcinoma accompanied with noticeable structural atypia can be seen.

Comment

This is a 10-mm type Is intramucosal carcinoma. In the initial normal observation, attention was paid to the surface irregularities, tensile look and concentration of folds in the surrounding area. As this case existed in a hard-to-observe region, use of an NT tube was helpful. After indigo carmine dye spraying, a relative depression was observed in the center, so an intramucosal carcinoma was suspected. NBI Near Focus observation was performed, concentrating on the vascular and surface patterns of the relatively depressed area. With the addition of an electronic zoom, it was found that the vascular pattern of the relatively depressed area was obviously more irregular than the surrounding area and that it was of Type IIIA of the Sano Classification, so an intramucosal carcinoma or a slightly invasive submucosal carcinoma was suspected. The surface pattern in the relatively depressed area was also found to be more irregular than the surrounding area. In observation following crystal violet staining, the relatively depressed area was found to be a V_I lesion with slight irregularity, while the surrounding area was composed of type IIIL pits, resulting in everything from intramucosal carcinoma to a slightly invasive submucosal carcinoma being suspected. After the lesion was resected en bloc by EMR, the pathological diagnosis concluded that it was an intramucosal well-differentiated adenocarcinoma (cancer in adenoma).

▶Observation tips Accurate endoscopic diagnosis is possible by applying NBI and chromoendoscopy to the regions considered of interest in normal observation.

(Hotta, K., Imai, K., Yamaguchi, Y.)

Case 58 Slightly elevated M carcinoma

Male in his 60s **Purpose** Surveillance after colon cancer operation **Location** Transverse colon
Macroscopic type 0-IIa

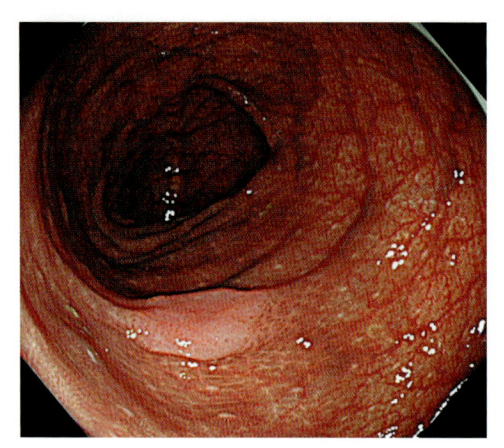

WLI normal observation: A slightly erythematous, flat-elevated lesion, 10 mm in size is recognized.

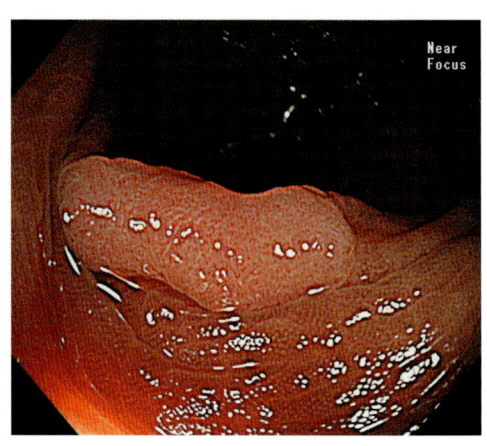

WLI normal Near Focus observation: A coarse mucosal pattern is recognized clearly.

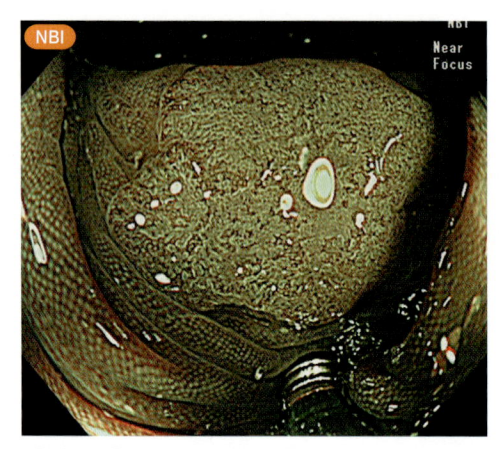

NBI Near Focus observation: The surface structure is imaged more clearly and recognizable as having a surface pattern.

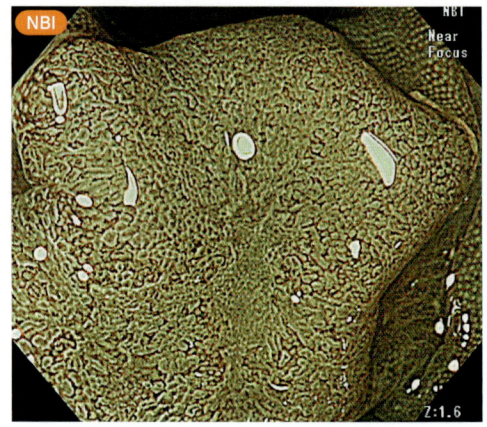

NBI Near Focus + 1.6× electronic zoom observation: Although the morphology of the meshed capillary vessel, such as the size irregularity, is hard to evaluate, the network is retained so the capillary pattern can be diagnosed as belonging to Type II (Sano Classification).

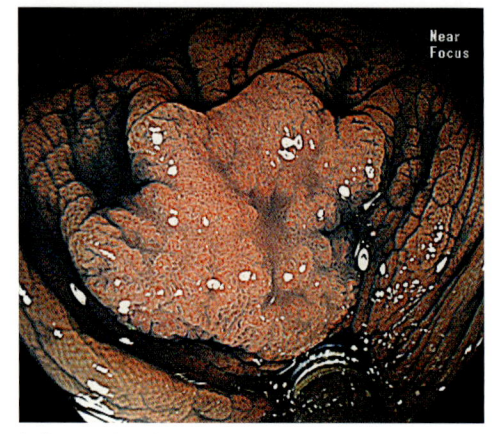

Indigo carmine chromoendoscopy: lobulation is poor but a coarse mucosal structure is observed. A pseudopod-like finding is observed in the margin.

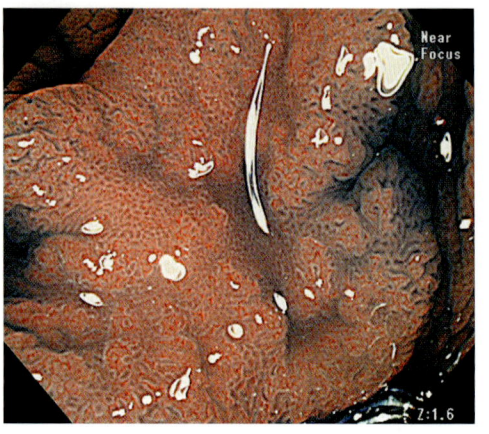

Indigo carmine dye sprayed Near Focus observation: Small tubular pits are recognized but the evaluation of the duct gland morphology is difficult.

Endoscope : CF-HQ290I (Olympus)　　Light source : EVIS LUCERA ELITE (Olympus)
NBI setup : Structure enhancement A7, color mode 3 (Normal observation—Structure enhancement A5)

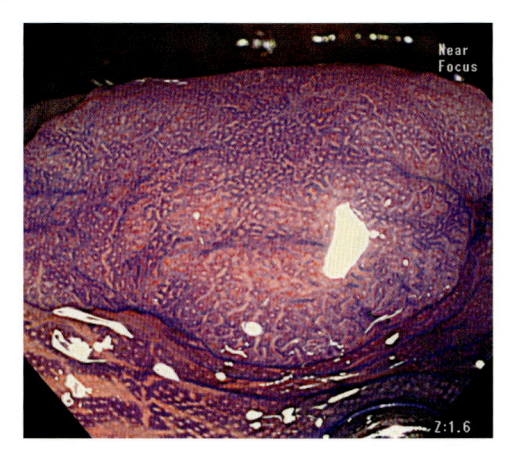

Crystal violet stained Near Focus＋1.6×electronic zoom observation : Tubular (III_L) pits accompanied with minor size irregularities are observed.

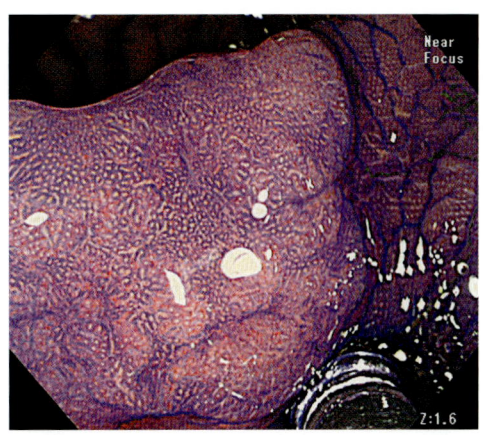

Although the lesion is not interpreted as an obvious type V, it is diagnosed as an early colorectal carcinoma of IIa, cM, 10 mm, because of the irregularities in the gland duct sizes and their arrangement.

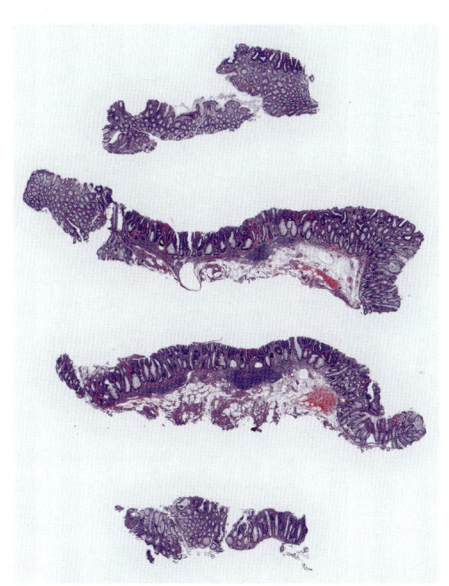

Magnified image of resected specimen : When the specimen is divided into four fragments and examined, tumors are observed in two of them. From the histological viewpoint, they are tumors of almost identical heights to the non-tumorous mucosa.

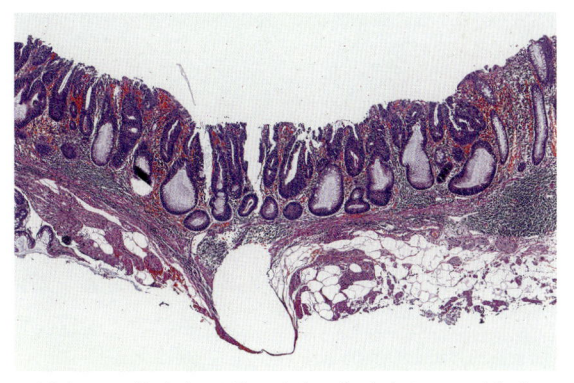

High-magnified view : Though the gland ducts are relatively straight, the irregularities of the sizes and arrangement of pits comply with the endoscopic findings so the lesion is diagnosed as an intramucosal carcinoma (tub 1).

Comment

As this case has fine ductal structures, it has been though that the evaluation of the regularity/irregularity of the surface pattern would be possible before NBI Near Focus observation with electronic zoom. However, detailed evaluation of the capillary vessels is found to be difficult with this method. When the case has small ductal structures, evaluation of the morphology of capillary vessels using NBI can be regarded to be limited with ordinary magnification. Meanwhile, the Near Focus observation after the crystal violet staining is useful because it can observe the pit morphology in details even with this case composed of small gland ducts. As an SM carcinoma presenting the type V pit pattern is negative, this lesion is resected by EMR. The pathological diagnosis concludes that it is an intramucosal carcinoma.

▶**Observation tips** With cases having fine ductal structures like this one, evaluation is sometimes hard even with NBI Near Focus observation. In such a case, it is necessary to consider addition of the crystal violet staining.

(Imai, K., Hotta, K., Yamaguchi, Y.)

Case 59 Slightly depressed M carcinoma

Male in his 60s | Purpose | Positive fecal occult blood test | Location | Transverse colon
| Macroscopic type | Ⅱa+Ⅱc, LST-NG（PD）

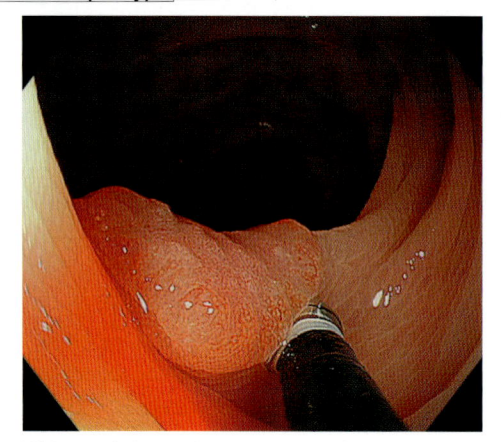

WLI normal observation: A slightly depressed lesion with slightly erythematous color, 15 mm diameter and erythematous margin is recognized as if it is hiding behind the folds on the transverse colon.

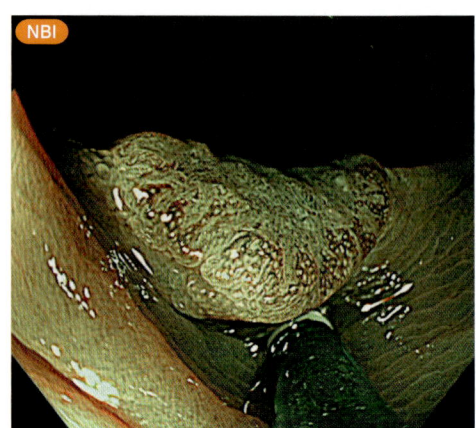

NBI normal observation: The elevated region in the margin is observed as a brownish area.

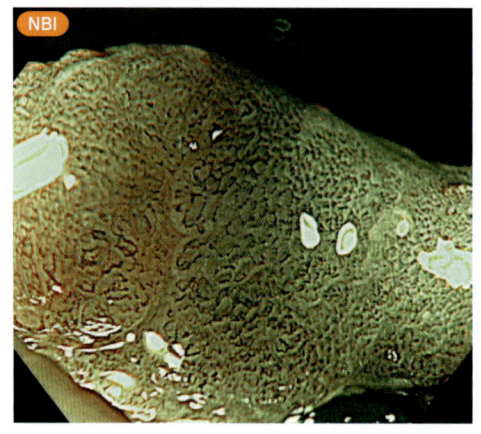

NBI magnified Near Focus observation: Microvessels in the depression present a brownish color tone. The network is disrupted at some regions, but no vessel with noticeable dilation or irregular size is observed, so the lesion can be diagnosed as an intramucosal lesion.

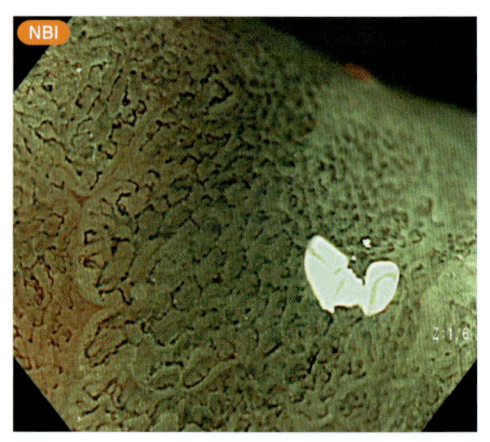

NBI magnified Near Focus+1.6×electronic zoom observation: The microvessels can be observed more clearly. The surface pattern exists, but the view is not clear.

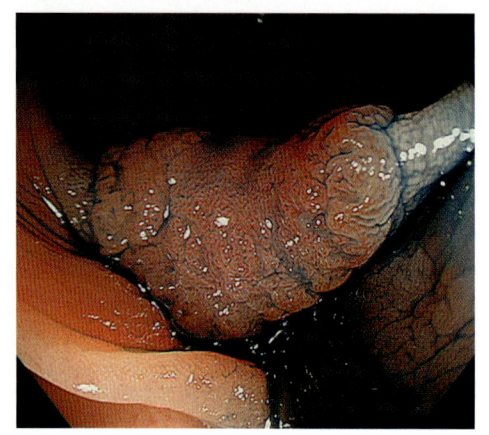

Indigo carmine non-magnifying: Pseudo-depression is observed on the center of the lesion.

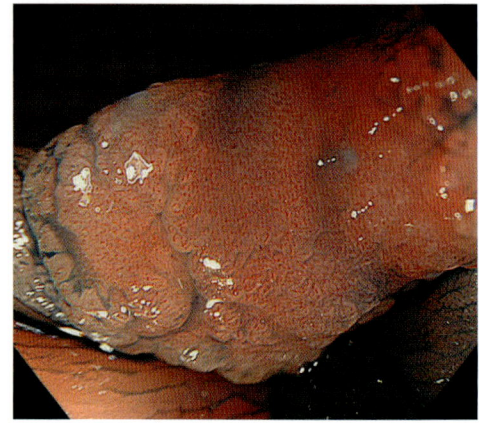

Indigo carmine magnifying chromoendoscopy: No regular pit pattern is observed, so a type V_I pit pattern is suspected. However, detailed diagnosis is difficult.

Endoscope : CF-HQ290I (Olympus)　　Light source : EVIS LUCERA ELITE (Olympus)
NBI setup : Structure enhancement A8, color mode 3

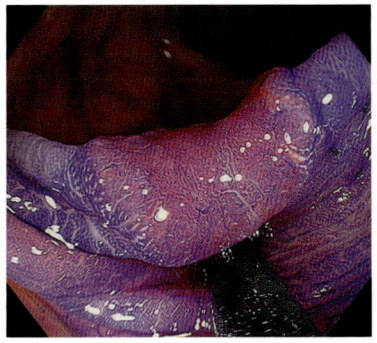

Crystal violet (CV) stained low-magnification observation : The elevation on the margin of the lesion has an open type I pit pattern, which belongs to normal mucosa.

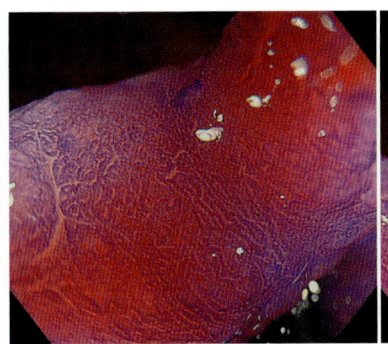

CV-stained high-magnification observation : Dense aggregation of tubular and semi-circular gland ducts with irregular size and arrangement are observed in the depression, presenting a lightly irregular pit pattern of type V_I.
The lesion is diagnosed as an early carcinoma with M to SM1 invasion depth.

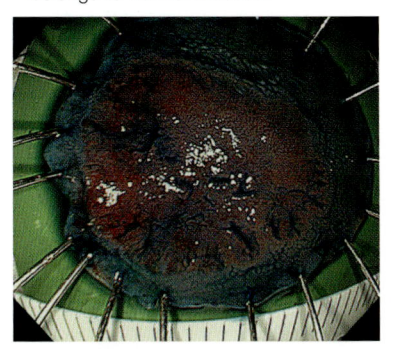

Endoscopically resected specimen.

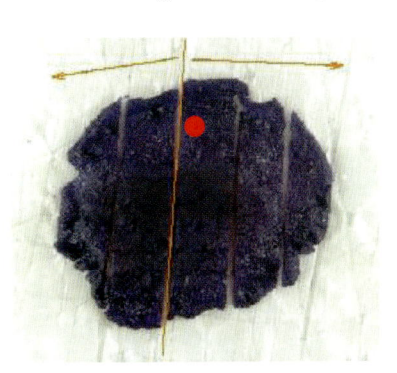

Sectional view.

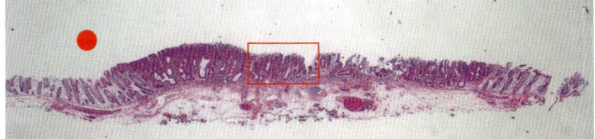

Magnified image.　The lesion is diagnosed as a well-differentiated adenocarcinoma on a background of tubular adenoma localized in the mucosa.

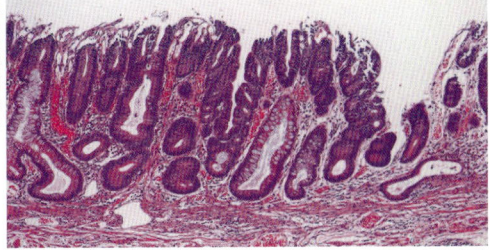

Comment

This case was suspected to be an intramucosal lesion because a partially disrupted vascular network in the depression was recognized with NBI magnifying observation, but microvessels presenting noticeable dilation or size irregularities were not observed. The surface pattern was not clearly observed with NBI magnifying observation, but magnifying chromoendoscopy detected a slightly irregular type V_I pit pattern which led to the diagnosis that the lesion was an early carcinoma with M to SM1 invasion depth. As the lesion was strongly fibrotic and non-lifting, it was dissected en bloc with ESD. The pathological diagnosis concluded that it was an intramucosal carcinoma.

▶Observation tips　It is often difficult to clearly observe the surface pattern of slightly depressed lesions with NBI high-magnification observation. A pit pattern diagnosis based on magnifying chromoendoscopy is indispensable for the diagnosis of slightly depressed lesions because it can enable surface structures to be diagnosed more reliably than with surface pattern observation.

(Wada, Y., Kudo, S., Misawa, M.)

Case 60　Elevated SM carcinoma

Male in his 60s　**Purpose** Detailed examination after blood stool　**Location** Transverse colon
Macroscopic type 0-Ip

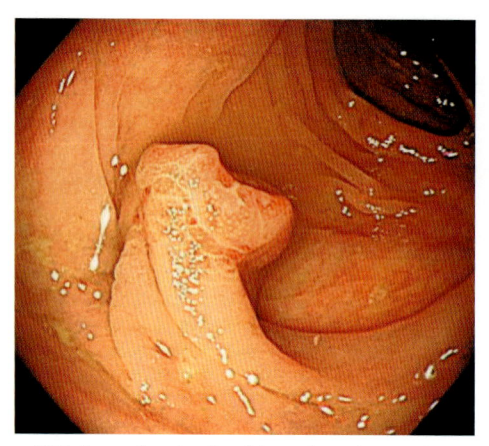

WLI observation, far view : An erythematous pedunculated elevated lesion with a long span of 15 mm in the transverse colon. The peak area is slightly depressed.

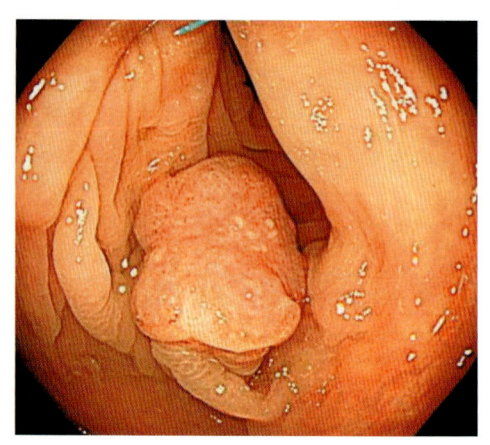

WLI observation, far view : The lesion surface is irregular in height, and the center is slightly depressed.

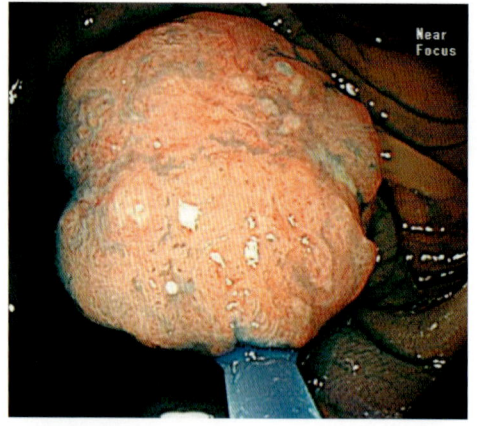

Indigo carmine magnifying chromoendoscopy (Near Focus) : The surface structures can be observed in the margin but are unclear in the center. White areas are partially observed.

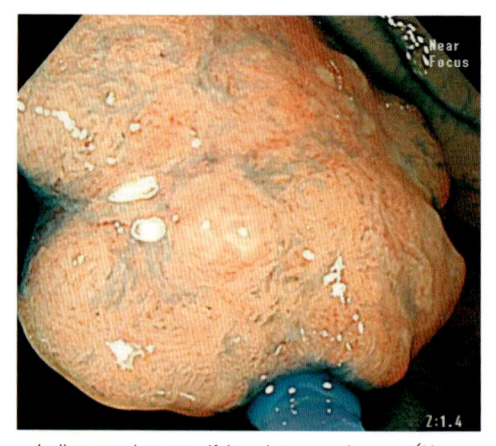

Indigo carmine magnifying chromoendoscopy (Near Focus+1.4×electronic zoom) : As no surface structures are observed in the white areas, the presence of granulation tissues is suspected.

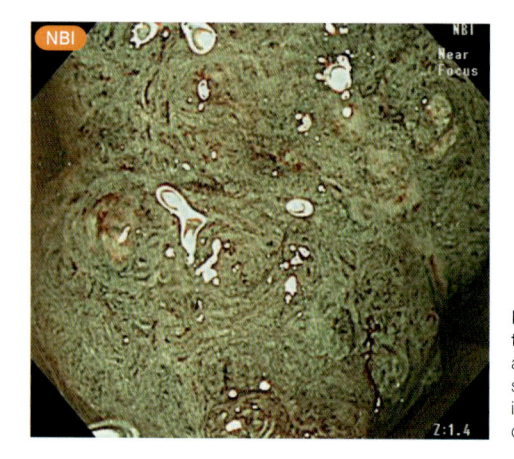

NBI magnifying observation (Near Focus+1.4×electronic zoom) : The microvascular architecture is irregular, and the vascular density is reduced. The surface microstructures are irregular at the margin and unclear or absent in the center. However, it is difficult to make an established diagnosis at this magnification.

Endoscope: CF-HQ290I (Olympus)　　Light source: EVIS LUCERA ELITE (Olympus)
NBI setup: Structure enhancement A8, color mode 1

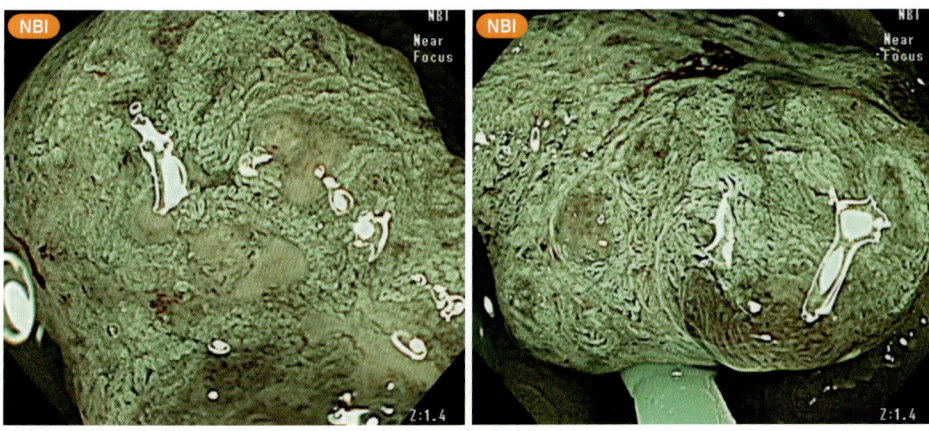

NBI magnifying observation under acetic acid spraying (Near Focus+1.4×electronic zoom): Surface microstructures with variable sizes are observed under acetic acid spraying. No surface structures are observed in the white areas found with WLI observation.

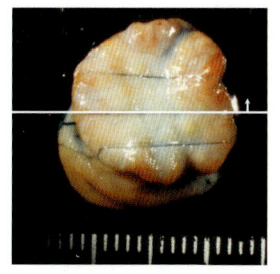

Resected specimen after fixation (EMR): The lesion has a diameter of 14 mm and the center is slightly depressed.

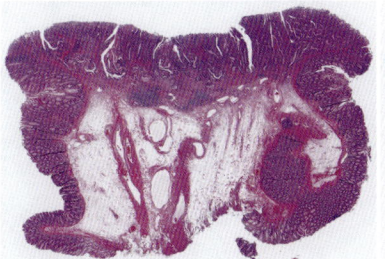

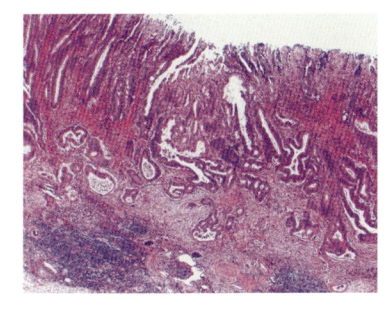

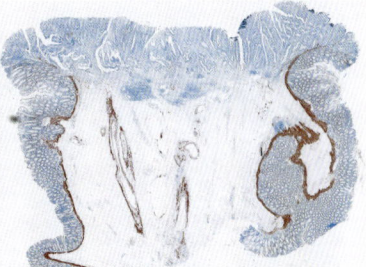

Histopathology of magnified images. (Left: HE stained. Right: Desmin stained.)

Histopathological low-magnification image: The lesion is a well-differentiated tubular adenocarcinoma infiltrating the submucosal layer of T1b, ly0, v0, budding/sprouting Grade 1. The muscularis mucosa has almost disappeared, but desmoplastic reaction is not recognized. The SM infiltration depth is 2,000 μm measured from the surface layer. Granulation tissues are recognized in part of the surface layer.

Comment

In WLI observation, the lesion was recognized as a pedunculated lesion with a long span of 15 mm and shallow depression, and suspected to be a carcinoma. In the indigo carmine-sprayed observation, no surface pattern could be seen in the depressed central part of the lesion, while white areas that seem to be granulation tissues could be seen here and there, so a highly invasive SM carcinoma was suspected. A highly invasive SM carcinoma was also suspected in NBI observation, which showed irregular microvascular architecture, reduced vascular density and unclear or absent surface microstructures. Under acetic acid spraying, irregular surface microstructures were observed. Although this was not enough to establish a diagnosis of a highly invasive SM carcinoma, observation of granulation-like amorphous area like that observed with WLI led to the diagnosis that the lesion was a highly invasive SM carcinoma. Since the lesion was pedunculated, it was subjected to endoscopic en bloc resection aiming at total biopsy. The histopathological image proves that it was a highly invasive SM carcinoma with surface structures almost retained, without desmoplastic reaction, and with an invasion depth of 2,000 μm. The area observed as white areas with endoscopy seem to coincide with the granulation tissue component. A lesion accompanied with such granulations is regarded to have high atypia of carcinoma and high possibility of deep SM invasion. Although additional colectomy is usually indicated for such a case, it is presently under strict follow-up because the patient refused the surgical operation.

(Kawano, H., Tsuruta, O.)

Case 61 Slightly depressed SM carcinoma

Male in his 70s   **Purpose** Positive fecal occult blood test   **Location** Rectosigmoid colon
Macroscopic type 0-IIc

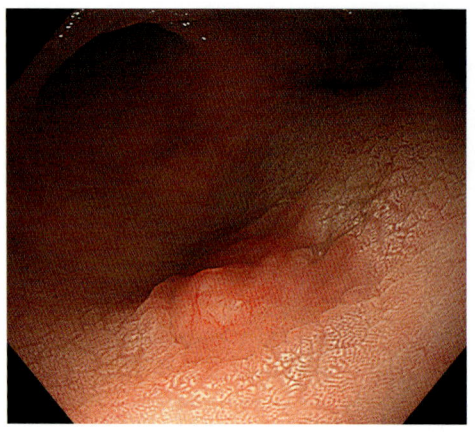

Normal WLI observation : Erythematous slightly depressed lesion 15 mm in size is observed in the rectosigmoid colon. It is accompanied with a slight elevation in the depression.

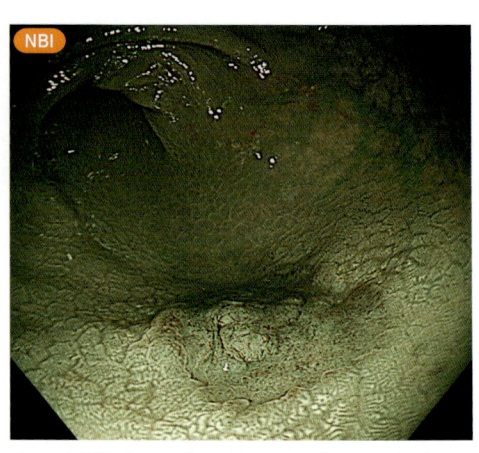

Normal NBI observation : The lesion is recognized as a brownish area.

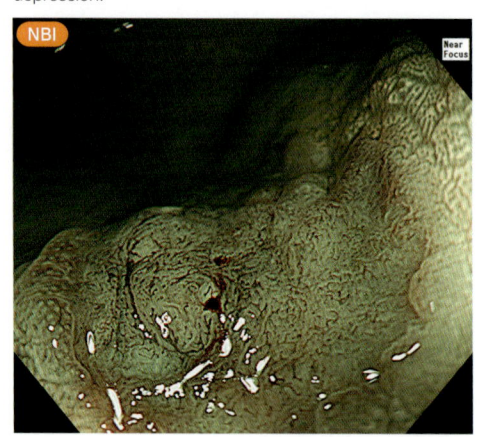

NBI Near Focus observation : The depressed area on the right side of the lesion is primarily composed of regular vessels, but irregular vessels are observed in the elevation in the depression on the left side.

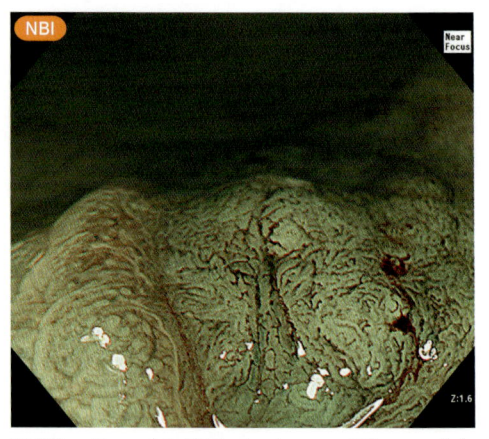

NBI Near Focus+1.6×electronic zoom : The vessels in the protrusion in the depression are irregular and variations in size and tortuosity are noticeable. Although an increase in the distance between vessels—which is usually found with an SM massive—is detected, the vascular density is not sparse, so the lesion is diagnosed as CP type IIIA of the Sano Classification.

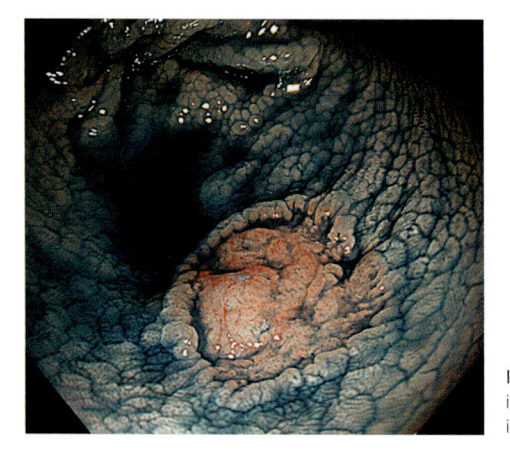

Indigo carmine chromoendoscopy : Indigo carmine spraying has clarified both the depressed area and the raised area inside the depression.

Endoscope : CF-HQ290L/I (Olympus)　　Light source : EVIS LUCERA ELITE (Olympus)
NBI setup : Structure enhancement A8, color mode 3

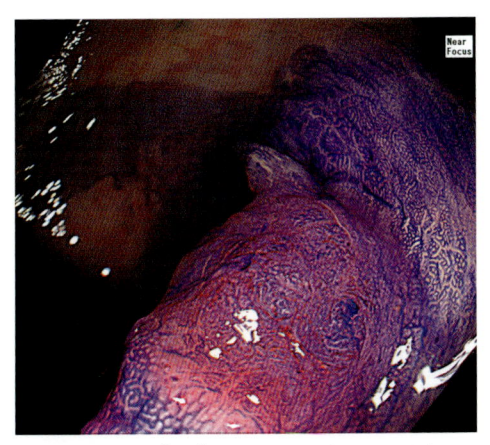

Crystal violet (CV) chromoendoscopy : Irregular pit patterns are observed in areas coincident to the depression with Near Focus observation.

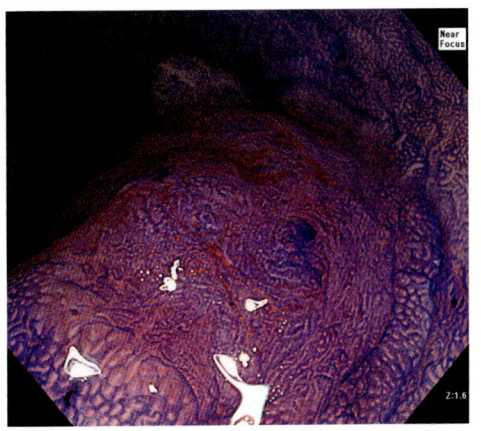

CV chromoendoscopy in Near Focus mode＋1.6×electronic zoom : Highly irregular Ⅴɪ pit patterns with irregular margins are recognized in areas coincident to the elevation in depression. They are diagnosed as invasive patterns.

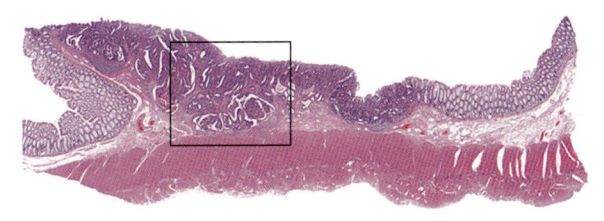

Magnified image : The lesion is a well-differentiated tubular adenocarcinoma presenting irregular tubular structures. The depressed area on the right side could be anything from a lesion to an M carcinoma. The elevated area in the depression suggests SM invasion.

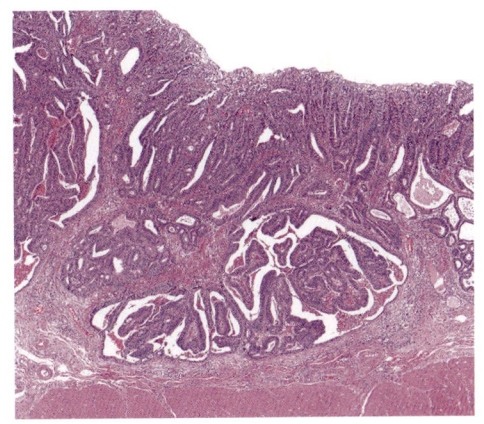

Medium-magnification image : The elevated area in the depression is accompanied with a desmoplastic reaction. The tumor is a highly invasive SM carcinoma infiltrated near the muscularis propria, and the maximum depth is 3,000 μm from the surface layer.

Comment

This is a case of a type Ⅱc SM infiltrated carcinoma in the rectosigmoid colon. Under NBI observation it was diagnosed as CP type ⅢA of the Sano Classification. However, the presence of an elevated area in the depression, as well as highly irregular Ⅴɪ pit patterns, led to a comprehensive diagnosis of highly invasive SM carcinoma. A high anterior resection was performed. The pathological diagnosis was type 0-Ⅱc, well-differentiated tubular adenocarcinoma, pSM (3,000 μm), ly0, v0, pN0, pPM0, pDM0, pRM0. When invasion depth diagnoses derived from normal endoscopic observation and magnifying endoscopic observation do not match as in this case, treatment policy should be based on a comprehensive assessment of the findings.

▶**Observation tips**　In NBI Near Focus observation with electronic zoom, focusing is difficult if the endoscope is too close to the lesion. It is important to maintain sufficient distance to observe the lesion accurately.

(Osera, S., Ikematsu, H.)

Case 62 Composite (Ⅱa+Ⅱc) SM carcinoma

Male in his 50s　*Purpose* Preoperative staging of early colon cancer　*Location* Cecum
Macroscopic type 0-Ⅱa+Ⅱc

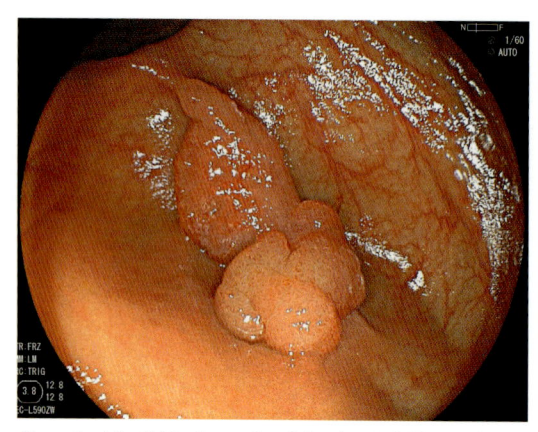

Normal white-light observation: An elevated 20-mm lesion located in the cecum, composed of an elevated nodule-aggregating area and a flat elevated area. At this point, the macroscopic type was classified as 0-Ⅰs (+Ⅱa).

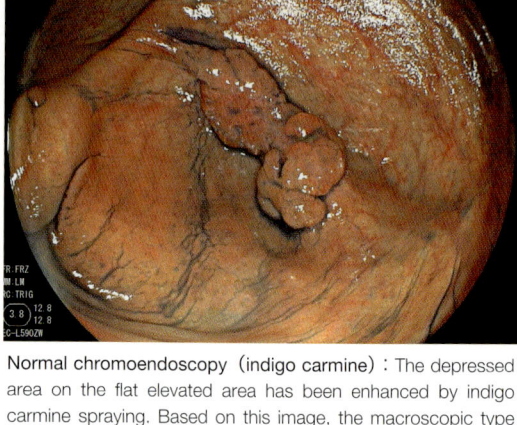

Normal chromoendoscopy (indigo carmine): The depressed area on the flat elevated area has been enhanced by indigo carmine spraying. Based on this image, the macroscopic type was corrected to 0-Ⅱa+Ⅱc.

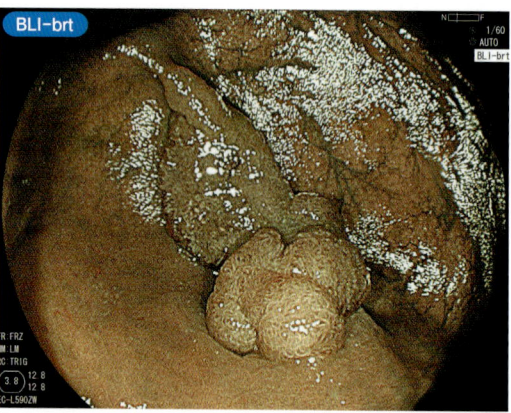

BLI-bright observation: The groove-like surface pattern of the elevated area can be seen even without magnification.

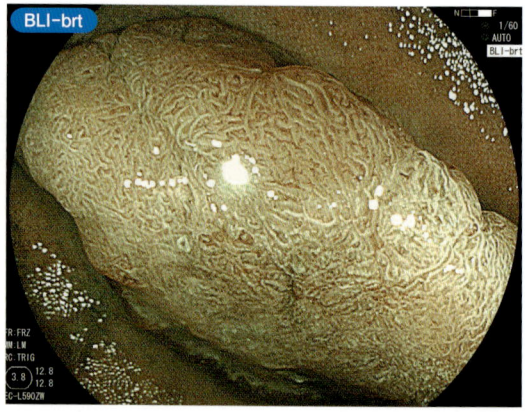

BLI-bright magnifying observation: The surface pattern on the margin of the elevated area presents a branched type Ⅳ-like surface pattern.

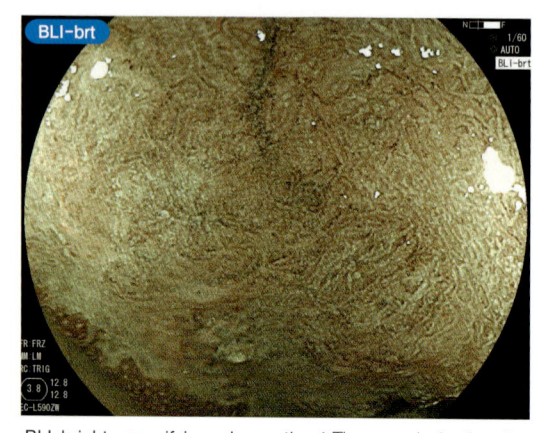

BLI-bright magnifying observation: The vessels in the depressed area are sparse and the remaining ones are fragmented. The surface pattern is unclear, though careful observation indicated that there may still be some surface pattern left.

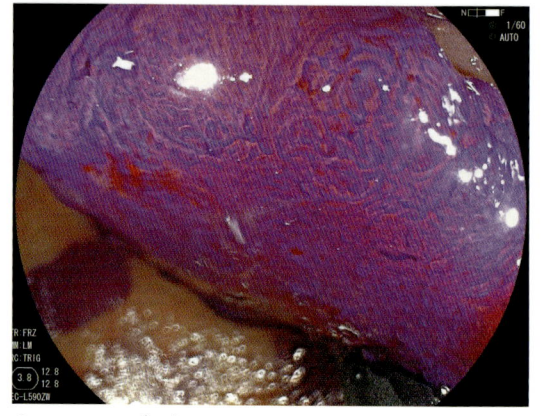

Crystal violet (CV) magnifying chromoendoscopy: The pit pattern on the margin of the elevated region is type Ⅳ or V$_I$ with a low level of irregularity.

Endoscope : EC-L590ZW (Fujifilm)　　Light source : LASEREO (Fujifilm).
BLI setup : BLI-bright—Structure enhancement B6, color enhancement C2.

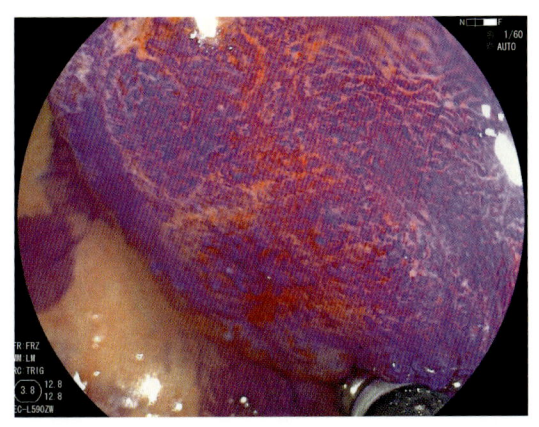

CV magnifying chromoendoscopy : The depressed area includes highly irregular V_I regions composed of pits with highly irregular margins. Some areas in the depressed area look like V_N regions with pits that are almost invisible.

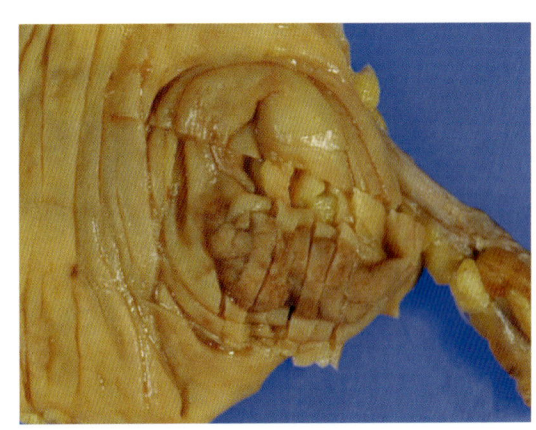

Resected specimen : The lesion was diagnosed as an SM-invading carcinoma and subjected to a surgical operation (ileocecal resection). The lesion size is 25 × 12 mm.

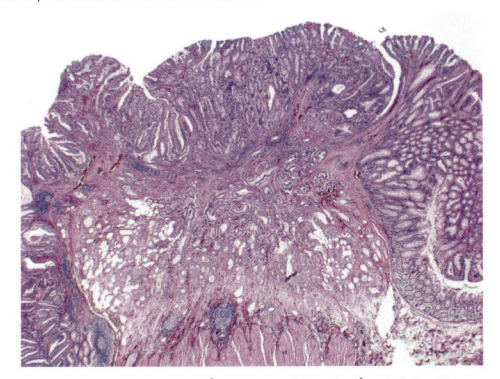

Pathological specimen (low magnification) : Well-differentiated tubular adenocarcinoma invading the deep submucosal layer. A tubular adenoma with low-grade dysplasia can also be seen on the margin of the lesion.
Well to moderately differentiated tubular adenocarcinoma (tub1＞tub2). pSM (2 mm), int, INFb, ly0, v0, pPM0, pDM0, pRM0.

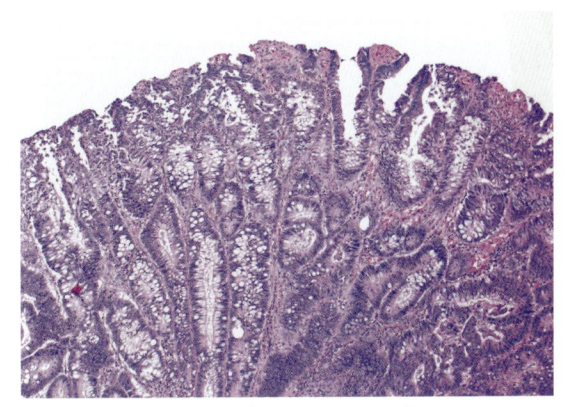

Pathological specimen (high magnification) : The superficial layer of the lesion retains the intramucosal lesion, and no noticeable desmoplastic reaction is observed.

Comment

This case is a deeply invasive cancer in the cecum. Under normal white light imaging, the macroscopic type could be Ⅰs or Ⅰs＋Ⅱa, but it was actually diagnosed as 0-Ⅱa＋Ⅱc because a clearly depressed area was observed after indigo carmine spraying. Under normal observation, the depressed area looks harder than the soft-looking elevated part so an SM carcinoma was strongly suspected, though this diagnosis remains inconclusive. In routine medical practice, the treatment policy (surgery) can usually be decided at this point as the findings on the vessels in the depressed area (NICE Classification Type 3) support the diagnosis in normal observation. The BLI finding that the surface pattern was unclear but recognizable (Hiroshima Classification Type C2) coincided with the CV chromoendoscopy finding of highly irregular V_I, and also corresponded to the histological image which showed an intramucosal lesion on the lesion surface.

▶**Observation tips**　When SM invasion is suspected in the depressed area in normal observation, magnifying observation is usually concentrated solely on the depressed area. However, as an SM-invaded region bleeds easily, care is required to avoid bleeding. Start the endoscope from a certain distance from the lesion and approach the region where SM invasion is suspected while slowly increasing the magnification.

(Takeuchi, Y., Shingai, T., Tomita, Y.)

Case 63 Composite (Ⅱa+Ⅱc) SM carcinoma

Male in his 60s   Purpose Positive fecal occult blood test   Location Rectum
Macroscopic type 0-Ⅱa+Ⅱc

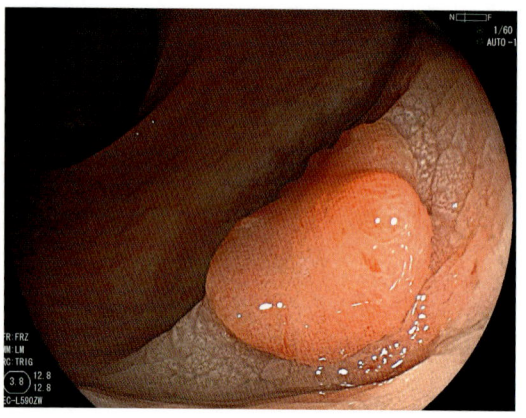

Normal white-light observation: An erythematous elevated lesion with a diameter of 10 mm is observed.

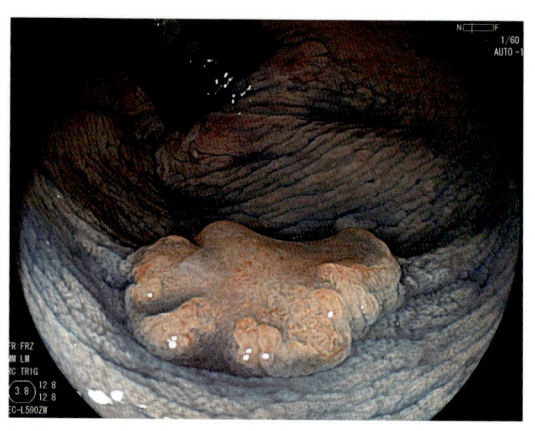

Indigo carmine chromoendoscopy: An irregular depression with clear demarcation is recognized.

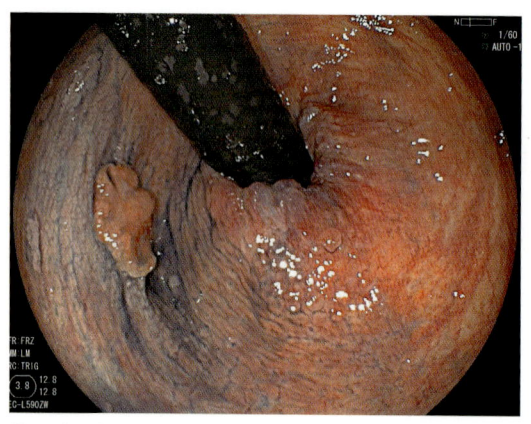

Far-view image with much insufflation: Sclerosis of the arc of lumen is observed and insufficient extension is recognized.

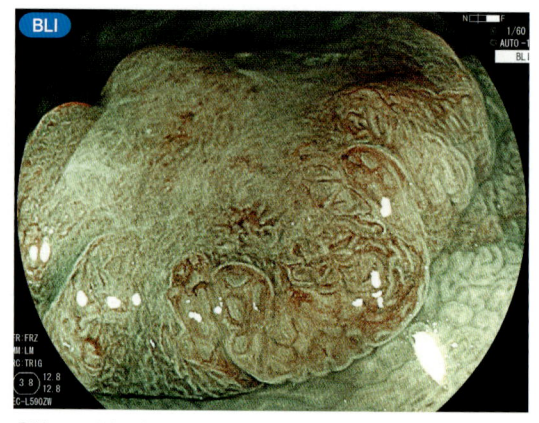

BLI-combined medium-magnification observation: A demarcation line is recognized between the depressed area and the elevated part of the margin.

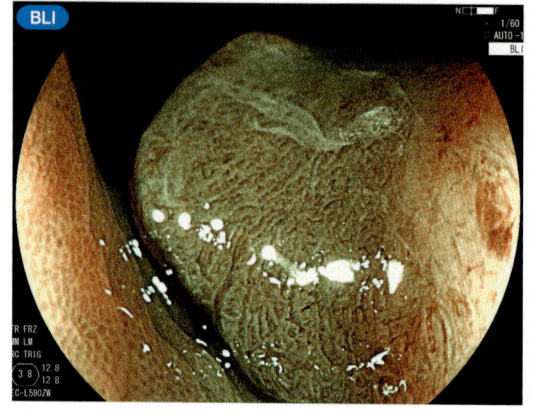

BLI-combined magnifying observation: Regarding the surface pattern, the morphology of the epithelium of crypt margin is irregular. As for the vascular pattern, the vascular morphology is irregular and greatly variable.

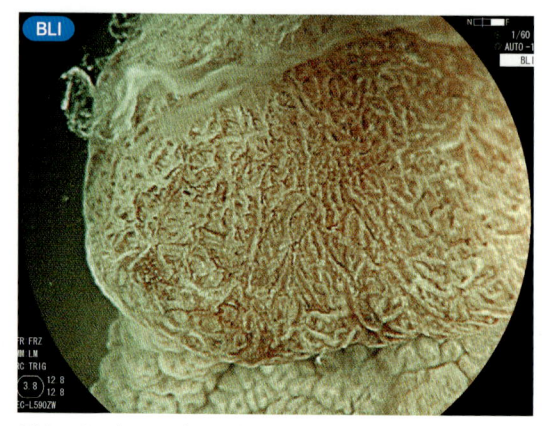

BLI water-immersion colonoscopy: Irregular surface and vascular patterns are observed more clearly. Some parts are harder to distinguish due to the presence of a white opaque substance (WOS).

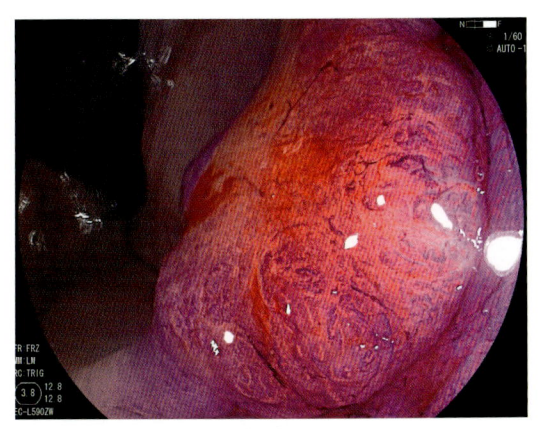

| Endoscope : EC-L590ZW (Fujifilm) | Light source : LASEREO (Fujifilm) |
| BLI setup : Structure enhancement A6, color enhancement C2 |

Crystal violet (CV) stained image.

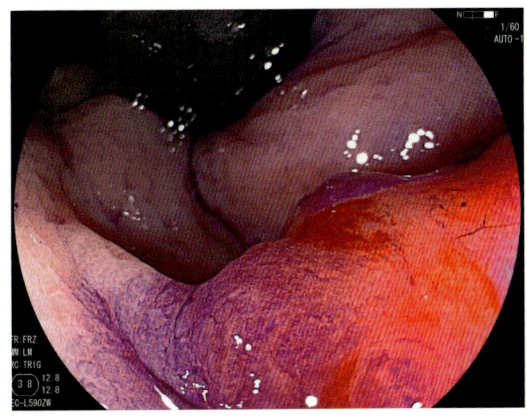

CV chromoendoscopy : An amorphous region is recognized in the irregular gland duct structure with unclear contours and a narrowed lumen. The pit pattern is type V_N.

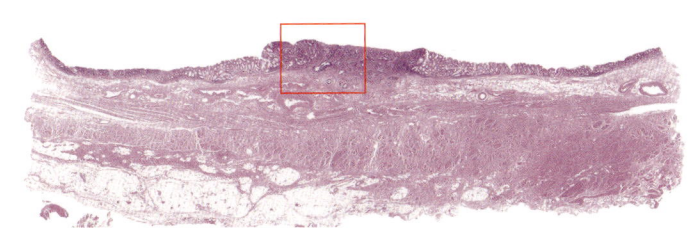

Magnified image of histopathological specimen : The lesion size is 10×10 mm.

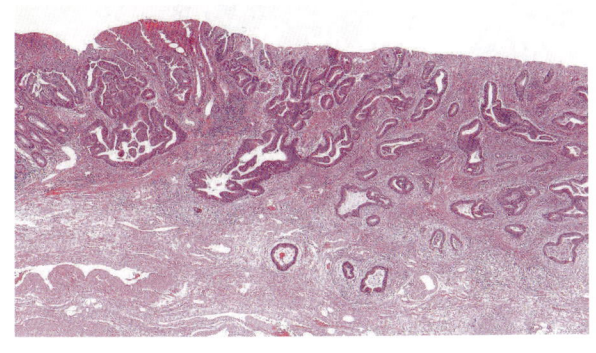

Further magnified observation of histopathological specimen : Well differentiated adenocarcinoma, pT1b (1,850 μm), INFα, ly0, v1, pN0, pPM0, pDM0.

Comment

BLI magnifying observation can diagnose this case as a cancer because both the surface and vascular patterns are irregular. It is more difficult to evaluate SM deep invasion with BLI, but crystal violet chromoendoscopy made it clear that the region with the unclear irregular surface pattern actually presented as a type V_N pit pattern.

▶**Observation tips** Use of the water immersion colonoscopy technique in BLI magnifying observation facilitates more detailed observation. Even if halation or cardiac pulsation interferes with observation, the water immersion technique can make observation easier.

(Hisabe, T.)

Case 64 Composite (Ⅱa+Ⅱc) SM carcinoma

Male in his 50s **Purpose** Positive fecal occult blood test **Location** Rectum (Rb)
Macroscopic type 0-Ⅱa+Ⅱc

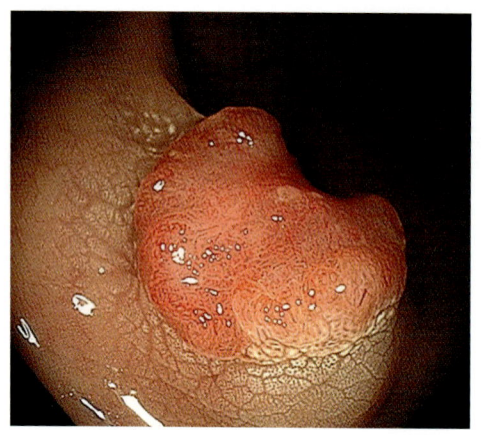

WLI observation: An erythematous elevated lesion with a diameter of 10 mm is recognized. It has a depression inside it.

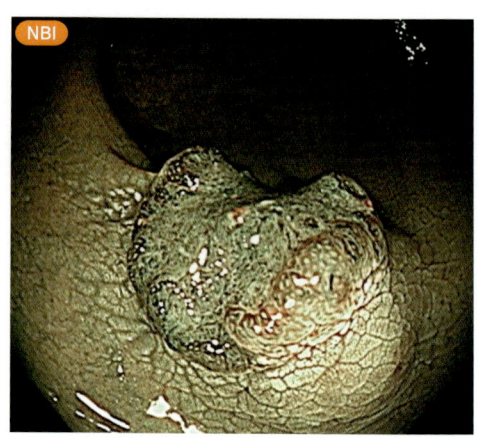

NBI observation: The lesion appears brownish and the internal depression is imaged more clearly.

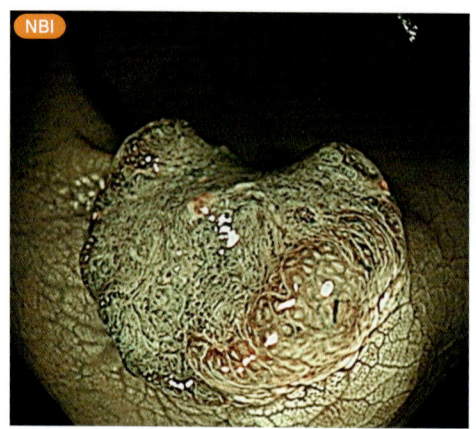

NBI Near Focus observation: A NICE Type 2, capillary pattern Type ⅢA region is found inside the depression. In the center, a capillary pattern type ⅢB region with a diameter of 2 mm that is nonvascular or has a very low vascular density is also recognized.

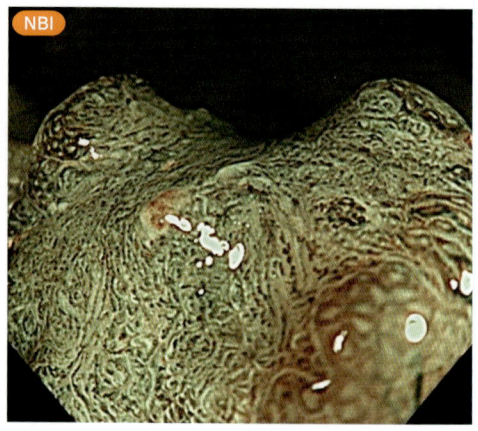

NBI Near Focus+1.4× electronic zoom: The disorganized ductal structure and the irregular sizes, disruption and tortuosity of the vessels are observed more clearly.

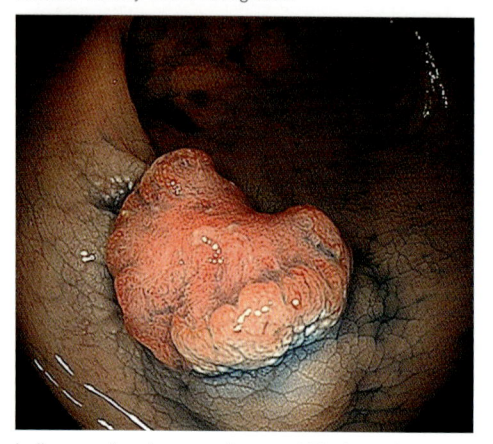

Indigo carmine chromoendoscopy: The inner depression is imaged more clearly.

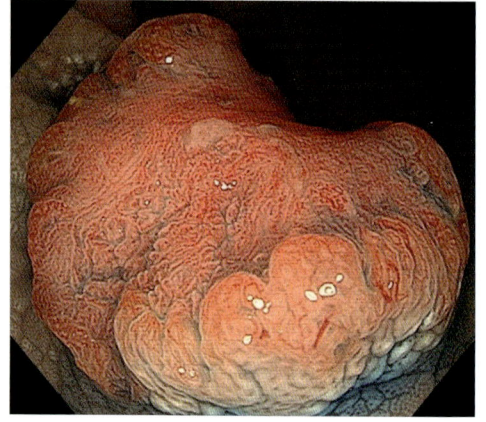

Indigo carmine chromoendoscopy in Near Focus mode: Irregular pits are recognized in the inner depression.

Endoscope : CF-HQ290L/I (Olympus)   Light source : EVIS LUCERA ELITE (Olympus)
NBI setup : Structure enhancement A8, color mode 3.

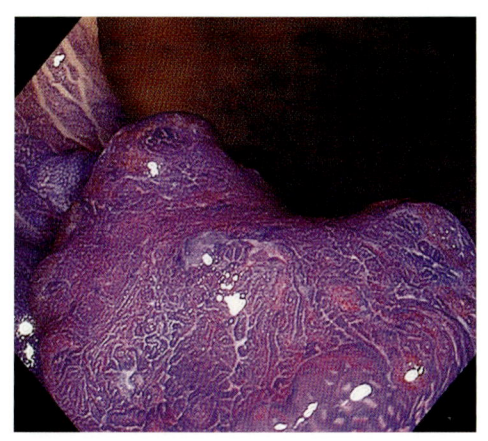

Crystal violet (CV) stained image.
Near Focus observation shows highly irregular type V_I pit pattern.

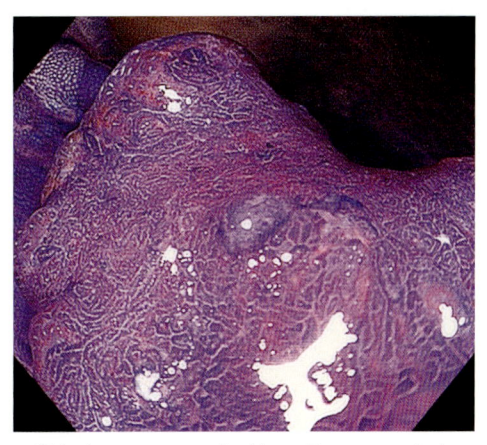

CV chromoscopy in Near Focus mode + 1.4× electronic zoom : The pit pattern is more clarified.

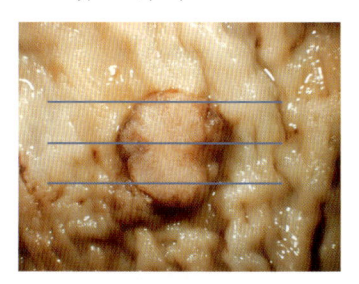

Surgery specimen.

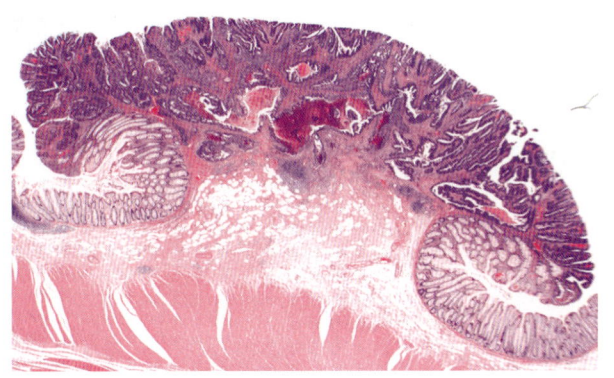

Low-magnification image : The lesion is a tub1+tub2 deep SM invasive carcinoma.

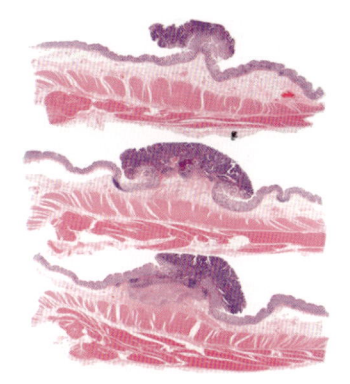

Pathological diagnosis : tub1+tub2, pT1b (SM2, < 3,000 μm), medullary, INFb, pPM (−), pDM (−), pRM (−), ly0, v0, desmoplastic reaction (+), budding/sprouting ; Grade 1.

Magnified image.

Comment

This is a composite lesion composed of an elevated region with a depressed area in it, which is usually called a IIa + IIc lesion. NBI observation of the inside of the depression diagnosed the region as NICE Classification Type 2 or capillary pattern classification (Sano Classification) type IIIA. However, a region with capillary pattern classification Type IIIB was also recognized when crystal violet staining was added. As this showed a highly irregular type V_I pit pattern that suggests a deep SM invasive cancer, surgery was performed.

▶ Observation tips   When a deep SM invasive cancer is suspected in NBI observation, crystal violet staining is absolutely necessary for confirmation.

(Hattori, S., Sano, Y.)

Case 65 Composite (Ⅰs+Ⅱc) SM carcinoma

Male aged 70 *History of present illness* The total colonoscopy after positive fecal occult blood test discovered a colorectal tumor, and the case was referred to our hospital for detailed examination and treatment. *History of previous illness* No appreciable disease *Location* Sigmoid colon *Macroscopic type* 0-Ⅰs+Ⅱc

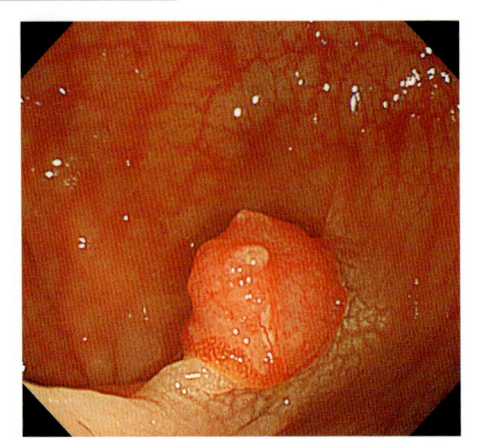

An erythematous protruding lesion is recognized in the sigmoid colon. It is a 0-Ⅰs+Ⅱc lesion with a size of 12 mm, mainly composed of a protruding component with surface irregularities, as well as a well-demarcated depression on the margin.

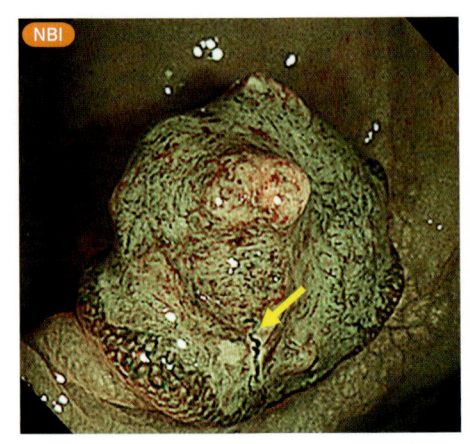

NBI observation: An elevated area of non-neoplastic mucosa is recognized on the tumor margin. The growth pattern seems to be of the NPG type. A thick vessel is recognized inside the depression (arrow).

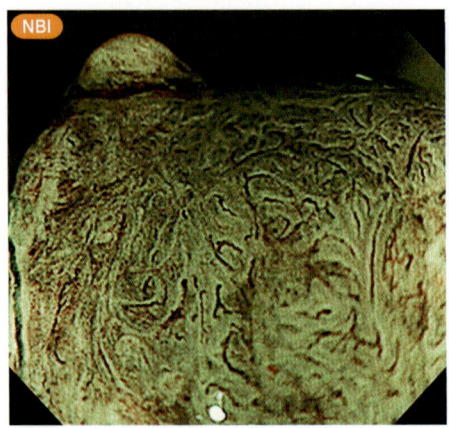

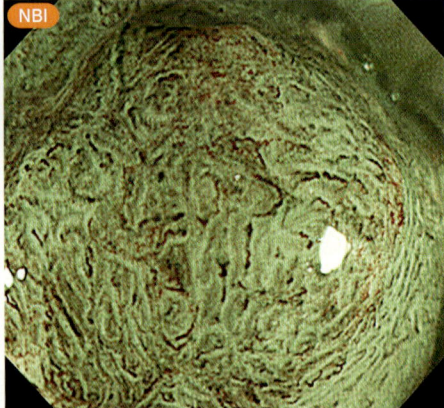

NBI magnifying observation: Microvessels with irregular dimensions are meandering through the area in an irregular pattern. As the vascular arrangement is also irregular and the density is low, the lesion is diagnosed as Sano Classification Type ⅢB.

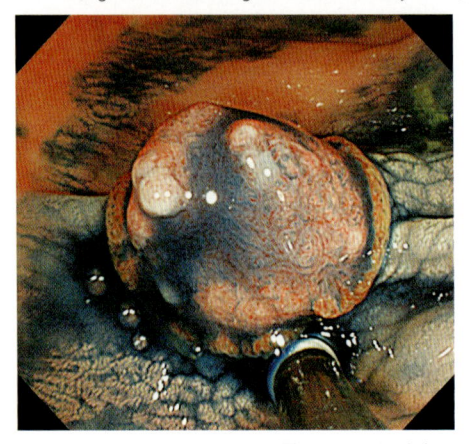

Indigo carmine chromoendoscopy: The depression is imaged more clearly.

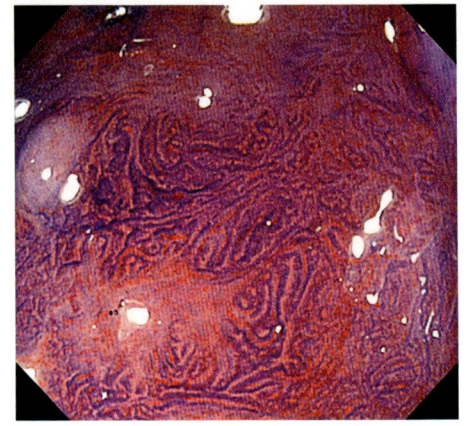

Crystal violet magnifying chromoendoscopy: Pit patterns with irregular margins and variable sizes are observed in the region coincident to the depression. As the arrangement is also irregular, it is diagnosed as a Vı pattern (invasive pattern).

Endoscope ： CF-H260AZI（Olympus）　　Light source ： EVIS LUCERA ELITE（Olympus）
NBI setup ： Structure enhancement A8, color mode 3.

＜Endoscopic diagnosis＞ The lesion is diagnosed as S/C, 0-Ⅰs+Ⅱc（NPG-type）, 12 mm, cT1（SM）, and subjected to surgical resection.
＜Treatment＞ Laparoscopic sigmoid colectomy.

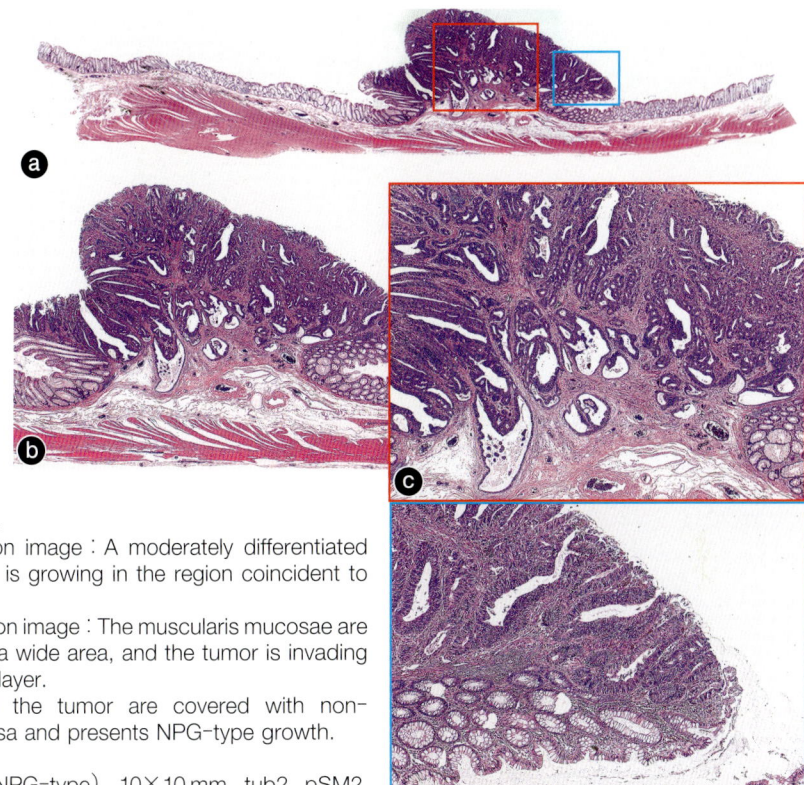

a ： Magnified image.
b ： Low-magnification image ： A moderately differentiated adenocarcinoma is growing in the region coincident to the lesion.
c ： High-magnification image ： The muscularis mucosae are ruptured across a wide area, and the tumor is invading the submucosal layer.
d ： The margins of the tumor are covered with non-neoplastic mucosa and presents NPG-type growth.

＜Diagnosis＞
S/C, 0-Ⅰs+Ⅱc（NPG-type）, 10×10 mm, tub2, pSM2, INFβ, ly0, v0, ne0, pN0（0/5）, pPM0, pDM0, pRM0.

Comment

This case is a 12 mm-sized lesion in the sigmoid colon that consists mainly of a protrusion. It has noticeable height irregularities on the surface and a well-demarcated depression. A steep elevated area composed of non-neoplastic mucosa is recognized on the margins, so the lesion seems to present NPG-type growth. The lesion is suspected to involve deep SM infiltration and exposure of SM carcinoma on the surface based on the surface irregularities observed in the normal observation and the NPG-type growth morphology. As irregular microvessels with irregular arrangement and pit patterns with various sizes and irregular arrangement recognized in NBI magnifying observation and crystal violet magnifying chromoendoscopy are typical findings of the Sano Classification Type ⅢB architecture and the V_I pit pattern（invasive pattern）respectively, a highly invasive SM cancer is suggested.

▶**Observation tips** The Sano Classification Type ⅢB architecture and the V_I pit pattern（invasive pattern）recognized in NBI magnifying observation and magnifying chromoendoscopy respectively convinced us that the lesion was a highly invasive SM cancer, so laparoscopic sigmoidectomy was indicated. With a lesion that has non-neoplastic mucosa on the rising part of the lesion, a depression with localized property and clear elevation of the depression, it is relatively easy to diagnose a highly invasive SM cancer in normal observation（including indigo carmine chromoendoscopy） stage. Even when a protruding lesion looks like a 0-Ⅰs lesion at first glance, it is important to observe the irregularities on the protruding surface and the NPG-type growth pattern accurately to avoid making a mistake with the invasion depth diagnosis.

(Sato, C., Matsuda, T., Saito, Y.)

Case 66 LST-G, homogeneous type

Female in her 50s | **Purpose** Surveillance after polypectomy | **Location** Ascending colon
Macroscopic type LST-G homogeneous type, 0 - Ⅱa

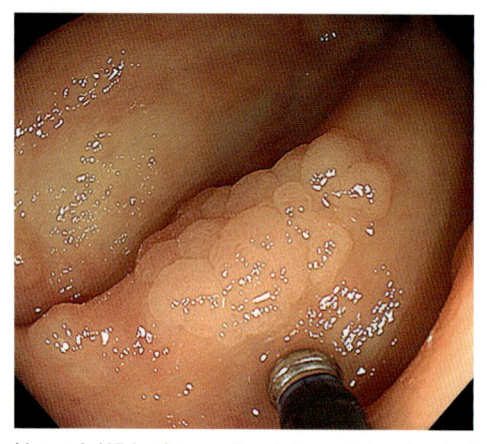

Normal WLI observation: A slightly elevated lesion with normal color tone and 15 mm diameter is recognized in the ascending colon.

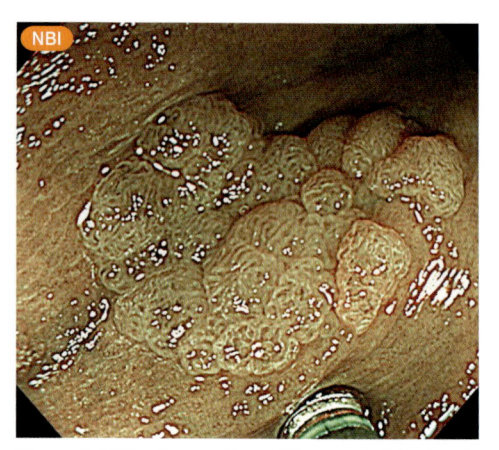

Normal NBI observation: The overall lesion is observed to be pale brownish.

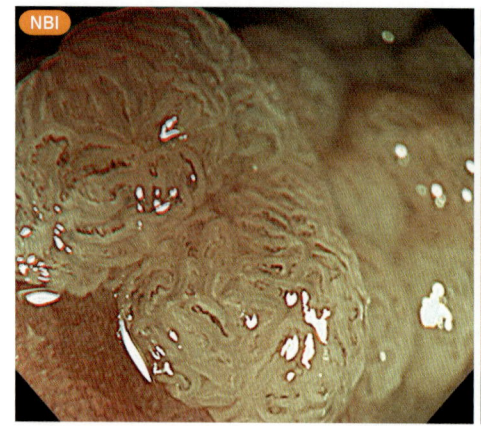

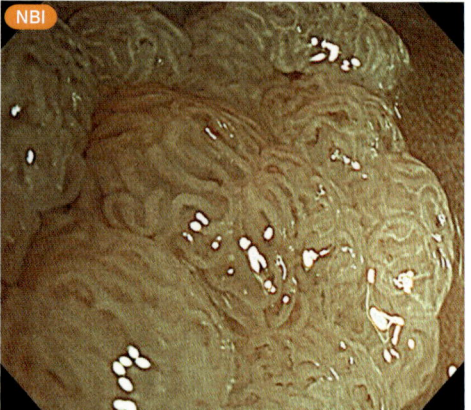

NBI magnifying observation: The microvessels have relatively uniform dimensions. As there is no noticeable dilation or dimensional irregularity, it is considered to be an intramucosal lesion. The surface pattern is recognizable and regular.

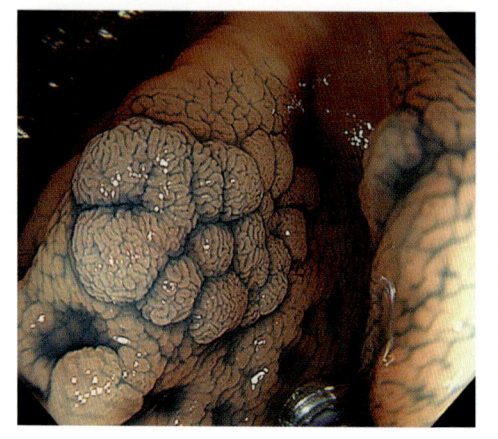

Indigo carmine chromoendoscopy: As the lesion is slightly elevated and composed of almost uniform granules, its macroscopic type can be classified as LST-G homogeneous type (0 - Ⅱa).

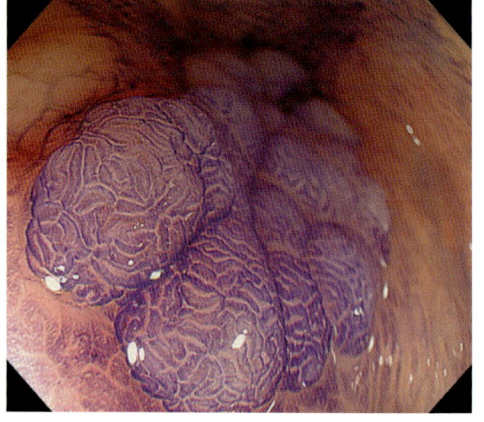

Crystal violet (CV) low-magnification chromoendoscopy: A type Ⅳ pit pattern is observed.

Endoscope : CF-H260AZI (Olympus)　　Light source : EVIS LUCERA ELITE (Olympus)
NBI setup : Structure enhancement A8, color mode 3.

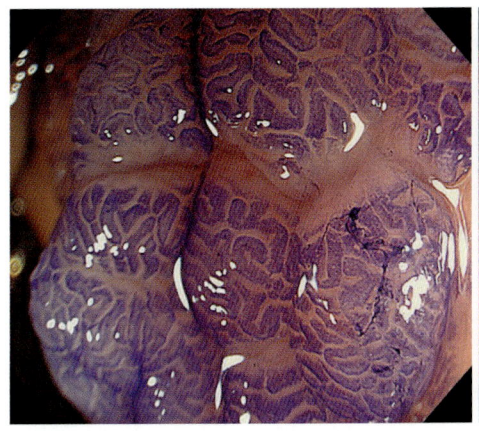

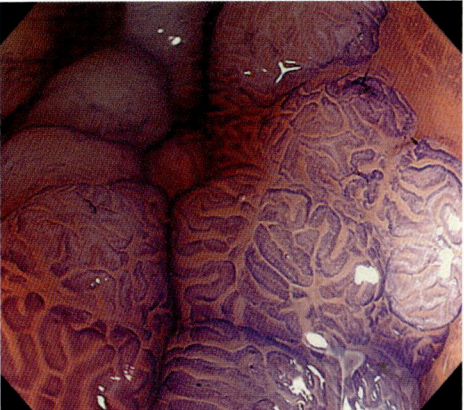

CV high-magnification chromoendoscopy : A surface structure that is more consistent than the surface pattern recognized with NBI magnifying observation can be observed. As the type IV pit pattern is recognized, the lesion can be diagnosed as a tubular adenoma.

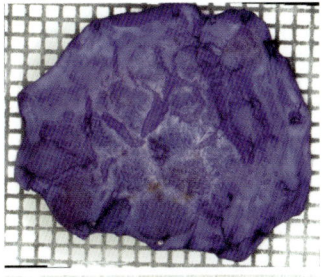

Endoscopically resected specimen.

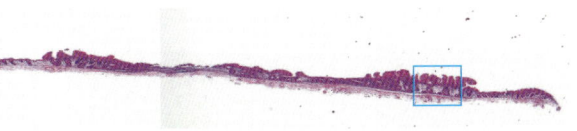

Slicing.

Magnified image.

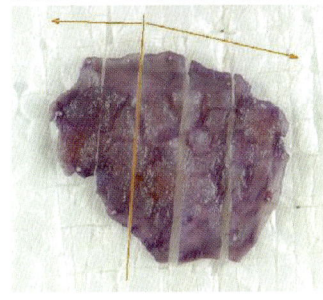

Low-magnification image : Tubular adenoma, low grade, HM0, VM0.

Comment

As no signs of dilation or dimensional irregularity were exhibited by vessels when viewed under NBI magnifying observation and the surface pattern was regular, this case was diagnosed as an intramucosal lesion. Magnifying chromoendoscopy showed a type IV pit pattern, so the lesion was diagnosed as a tubular adenoma and subjected to EMR. The pathological diagnosis concluded that it was a tubular adenoma with low-grade dysplasia.

▶Observation tips　(1) Although this case has a relatively small tumor diameter of 15 mm, observations at high magnification of large-diameter tumors with lateral growth/extension take a long time and can often be made more difficult by peristalsis of intestinal tract. Accurate diagnosis is possible by checking for the presence of coarse nodules and localized depressions with normal endoscopy and indigo carmine chromoendoscopy, and then focusing on important findings with magnifying observation. (2) Most typical LST-G homogeneous type lesions are adenomas, which are relatively easy to diagnose even with NBI magnifying observation alone. NBI magnifying observation is basically used to observe the vascular pattern, but it can also image the surface pattern clearly if the lesion is an intramucosal lesion with a type IV pit pattern. Nevertheless, if it is hard to determine whether the pit pattern is clear or not, then chromoendoscopy should be performed without hesitation.

(Misawa, M., Wada, Y., Kudo, S.)

Case 67 LST-G, nodular mixed type

Male in his 40s Purpose Detailed examination of tumor Location Rectum (Ra)
Macroscopic type 0-Ⅱa+Ⅰs, LST-G, nodular mixed type

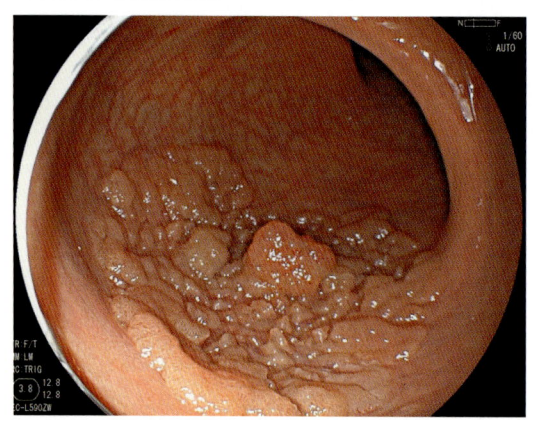

Normal white-light observation: A flat elevated lesion 50 mm in diameter, nodules in the center, and granules on the surface is recognized.

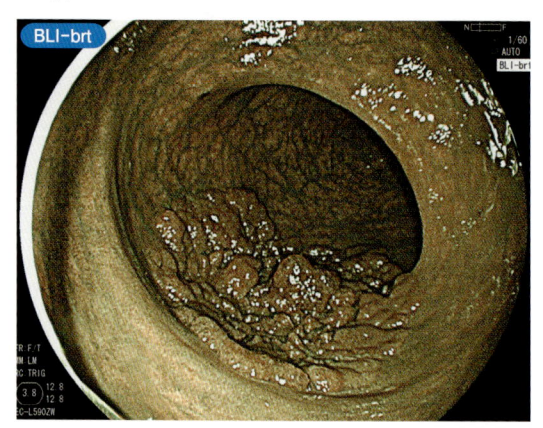

BLI-bright distant observation: The tumor is clearly visible with the bright field of view. The normal vascular patterns in the surrounding area are disrupted in the tumor region.

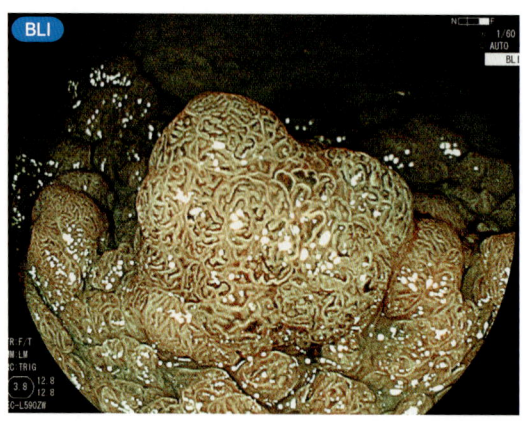

Low-magnification BLI observation: The nodule area in the center has a type Ⅳ-like pit pattern with slight irregularities, and the vascular pattern is tortuous.

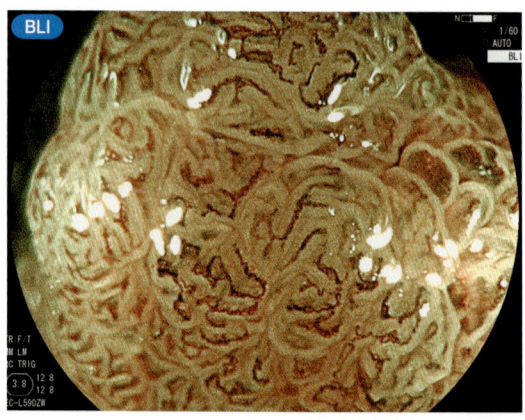

High-magnification BLI observation: The nodule area in the center shows a type ⅤⅠ pit-like surface pattern with a somewhat irregular margin. The vascular pattern presents dilation and tortuosity.

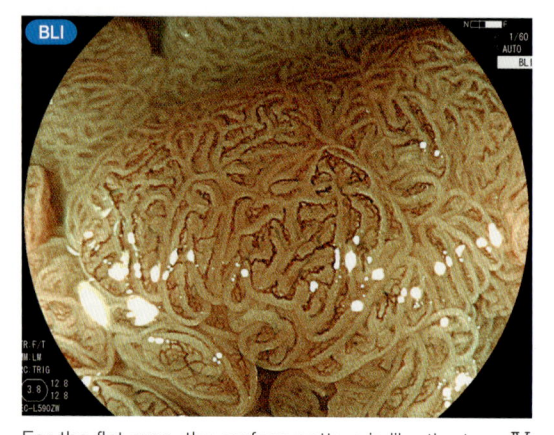

For the flat area, the surface pattern is like the type Ⅳ pit, and the vascular pattern is not irregular but presents slight dilation and tortuosity.

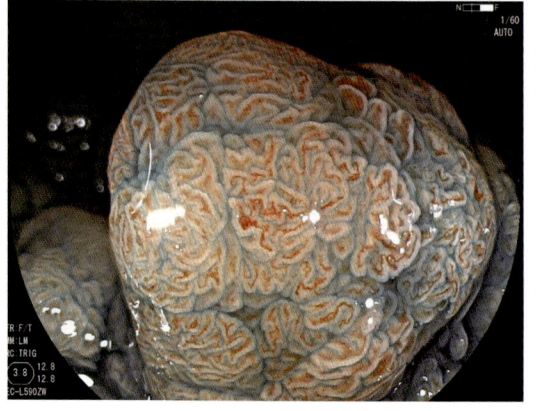

Indigo carmine magnifying chromoendoscopy: The nodule area has high-density pits with slight irregularity.

Endoscope: EC-L590ZW (Fujifilm)　　Light source: LASEREO (Fujifilm)
BLI setup: BLI-bright—Structure enhancement A6, color enhancement C2; BLI—Structure enhancement A6, color enhancement C2.

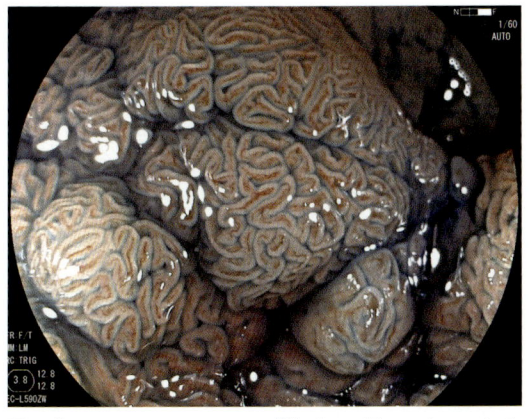

The flat area presents type IV pits with no irregularities.

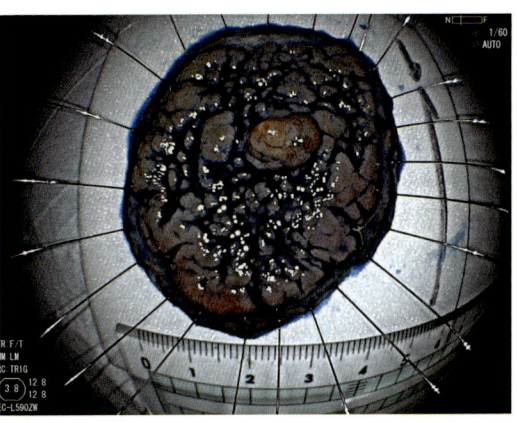

ESD-resected specimen: Resected size is 50×35 mm.

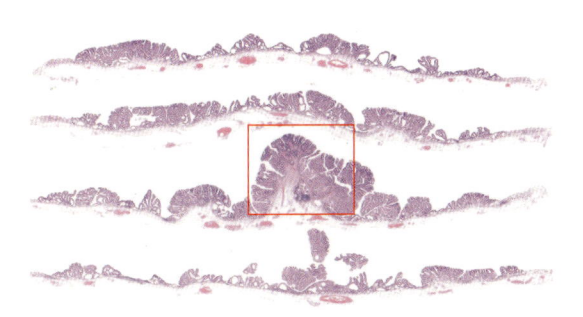

Magnified image: The lesion is a carcinoma in adenoma. Most of it consists of an adenoma, but the nodule area presents structural atypia and cellular atypia. Slight submucosal invasion is also recognized in the nodule area.

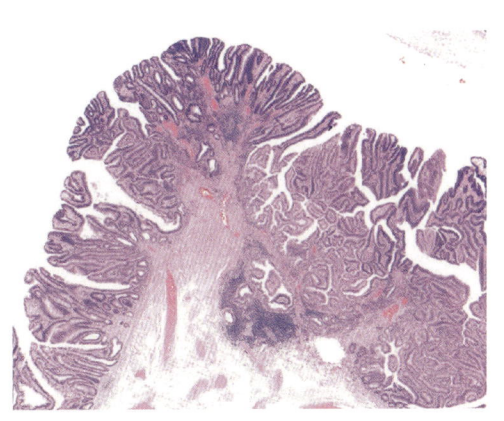

Low-magnification image: The submucosal layer has been invaded to a depth of 600 μm and is accompanied with lymphoid infiltration. No vascular invasion is observed.

Comment

It is best to use the BLI-bright mode for distant BLI observation because its bright field makes it possible to clearly distinguish the lesion. The BLI mode is used with close-up or magnifying observation. In this case, BLI observation found that the entire flat area was composed mainly of type IV pits like structure. While the vascular pattern of such a lesion is often accompanied with tortuosity and dilation, you have to be careful not to diagnose them as irregularities. The surface pattern of the nodule area presented type V_I pits like structure with slight irregularities so it was diagnosed as Hiroshima Classification Type C1. The vascular pattern of the same area showed advanced dilation, but caution is required before coming to any conclusions because many papillary lesions present serious irregularities even when they are not SM-invaded. En bloc resection was performed on this lesion using ESD, a procedure which took about 60 minutes. The histopathological diagnosis concluded that it was a slightly invasive submucosal carcinoma accompanied with adenoma (SM invasion depth 600 μm), vascular invasion negative, negative margin.

▶Observation tips LST-G nodular-mixed type lesions often present a type IV pit-like surface pattern. As a vascular pattern accompanied with dilation and tortuosity proper to papillary lesion is recognized with this lesion, caution is required when making a diagnosis.

(Yoshida, N., Yagi, N., Naito, Y.)

Case 68 | **LST-NG, pseudo-depressed type**

Female in her 80s　Purpose Positive fecal occult blood test　Location Sigmoid colon
Macroscopic type 0-Ⅱa（LST-NG, PD）

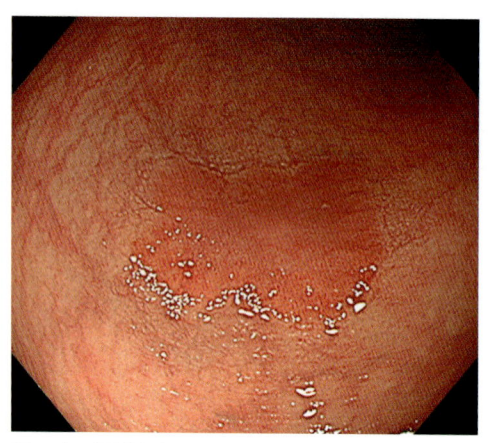

Standard WLI observation : A slightly reddish flat elevated lesion with a diameter of 20 mm is recognized.

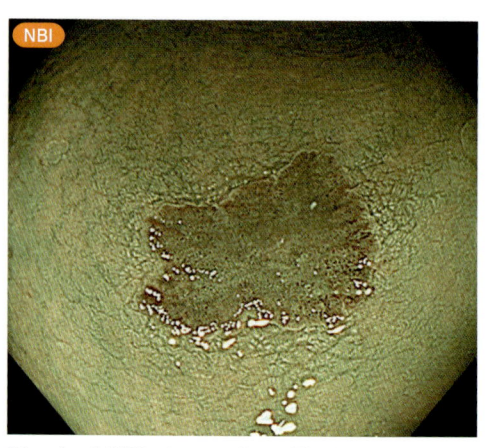

Standard NBI observation : The lesion appears brownish.

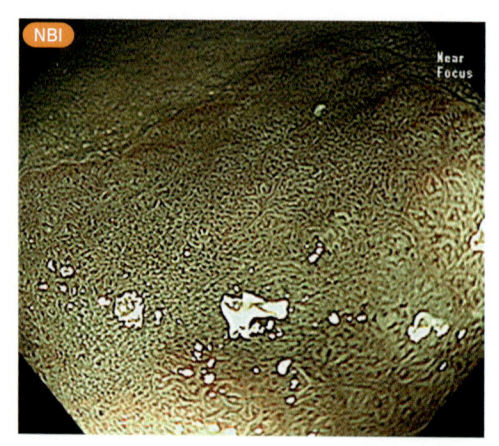

Near Focus NBI observation : A regular surface pattern is recognized.

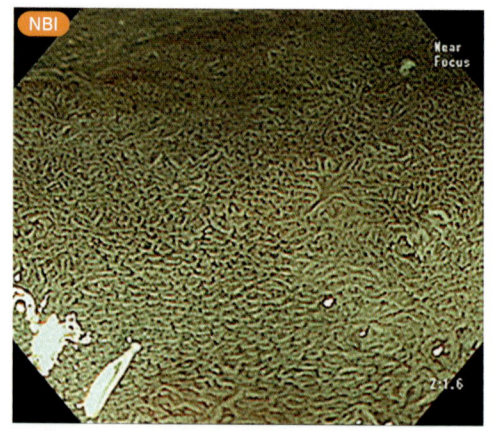

Near Focus NBI＋1.6×electronic zoom : The regular surface pattern can be seen more clearly.

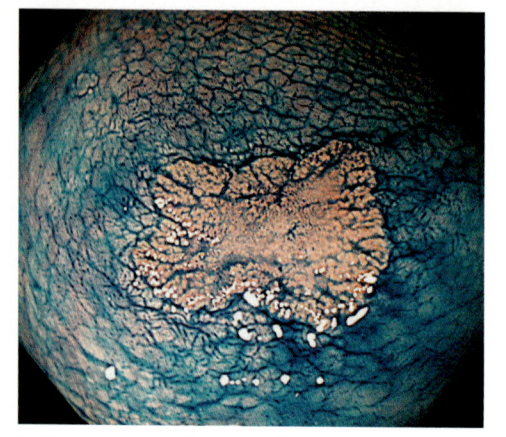

Indigo carmine dye spraying view : The presence of a gently sloping tray-shaped depression is made clear

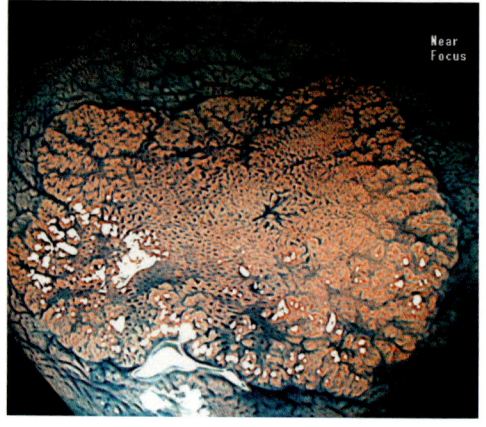

Indigo carmine dye spraying view in Near Focus mode : Small regular pits are recognized.

Endoscope：CF-HQ290L/I（Olympus）　　Light source：EVIS LUCERA ELITE（Olympus）
NBI setup：Structure enhancement A8, color mode 3.

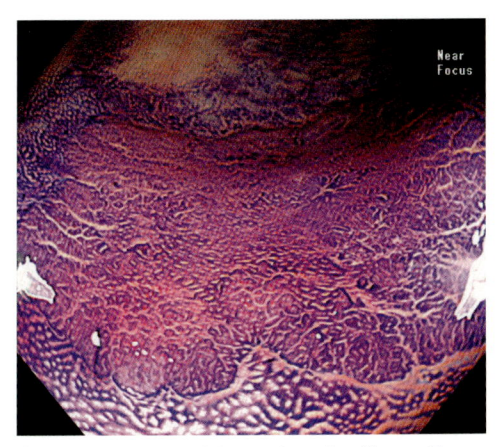

Crystal violet staining view in Near Focus mode：A type Ⅲ_L pit pattern is recognized.

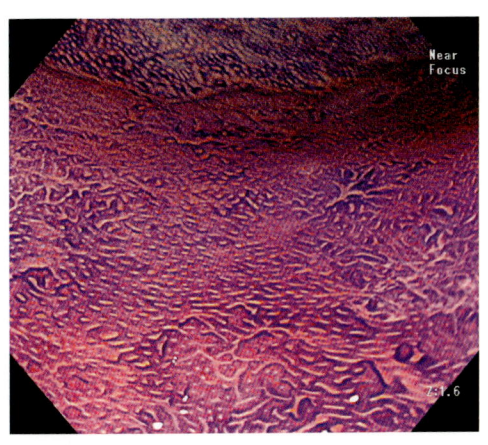

Crystal violet staining view in Near Focus mode ＋1.6×electronic zoom：The pit pattern is made clearer.

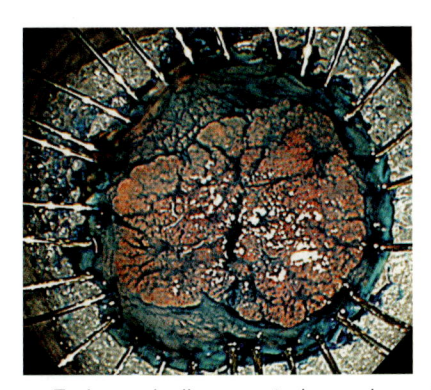

Endoscopically resected specimen.

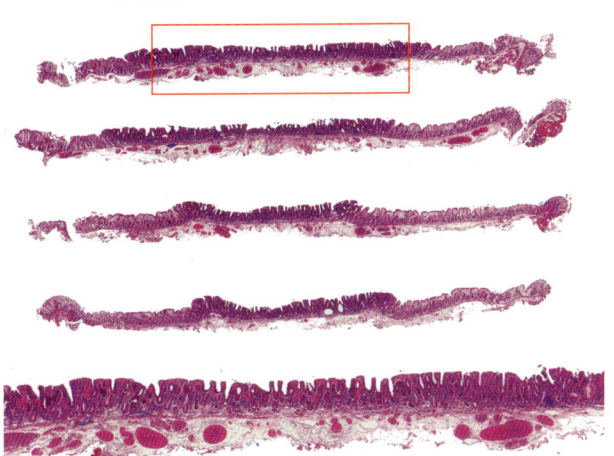

Cross section and Magnifying image（HE staining×40）.

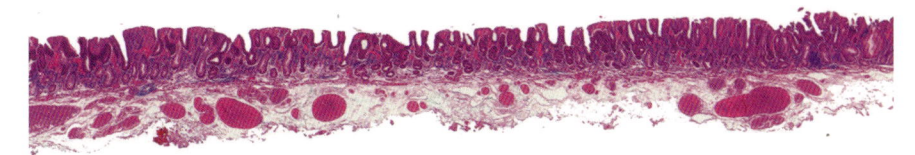

Low-magnification image of ☐：The lesion is diagnosed as a tubular adenoma with low-grade dysplasia.

Comment

Both the surface pattern and vascular pattern are important when evaluating findings from NBI magnifying observation. Since, in this case, NBI magnifying observation in the Near Focus mode recognized a regular surface pattern, it was diagnosed as a Hiroshima Classification Type B lesion. As the vascular pattern was hard to evaluate as in this case, we found it helpful to evaluate the surface pattern with NBI magnifying observation-based diagnosis. Crystal violet staining was also applied, revealing that the pit pattern was type Ⅲ_L. No findings suggesting SM invasion were observed in either standard or magnifying observation. The lesion was subjected to endoscopic treatment（ESD）. Histopathological diagnosis concluded that it was a tubular adenoma.

▶Observation tips　It is important to correctly evaluate both the surface pattern and the vascular pattern.

（Hayashi, N., Tanaka, S.）

Case 69 LST-NG, pseudo-depressed type

Female in her 70s | Purpose | Voluntary health checkup | Location | Transverse colon
Macroscopic type | 0-Ⅱa, LST-NG (PD)

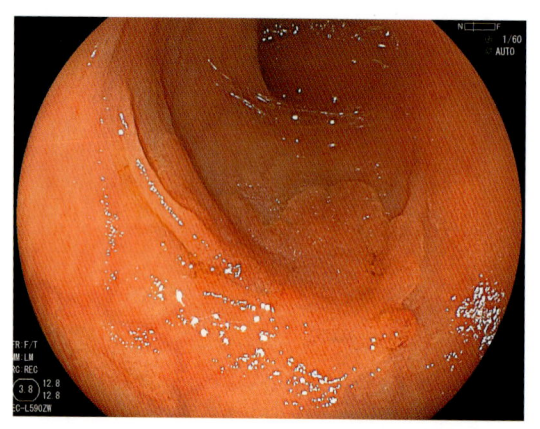

White-light non-magnifying observation: A low lesion with a size of about 3 cm and amoeboid extension can be seen. Accurate judgment of the lesion's demarcation using only white light imaging is difficult. The entire lesion is slightly elevated and an erythematous small elevation can be seen on the proximal side. The case does not have a history of biopsies, but tightening of folds toward the same region is observed. The morphology of the lesion varied depending on the amount of air and no rigidity was noted in endoscopy.

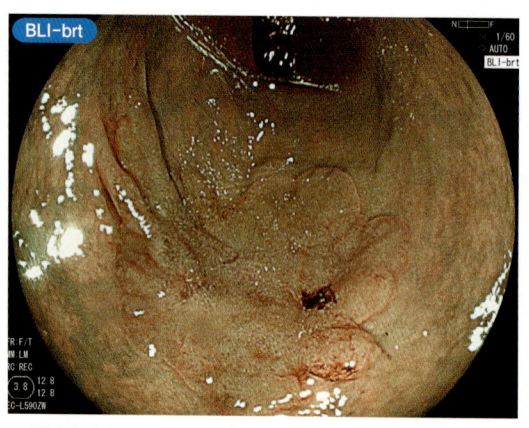

BLI-bright non-magnifying observation: Even in the far view, it can be clearly seen that microvessels are distributed more densely than in the surrounding normal mucosa. This makes it possible to identify the lesion's borders.

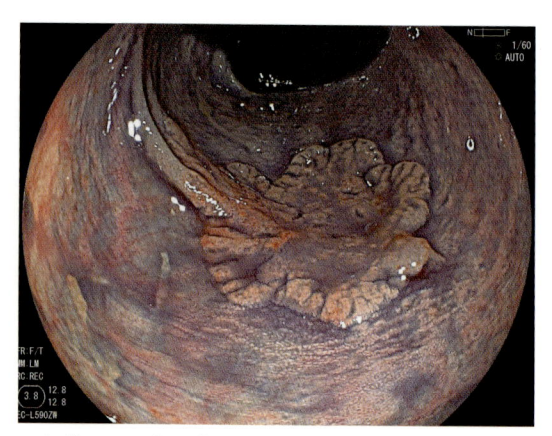

Indigo carmine chromoendoscopy: The minor depression is imaged clearly. The morphology indicates a laterally spreading tumor, non-granular type, pseudo-depressed type [LST-NG (PD)].

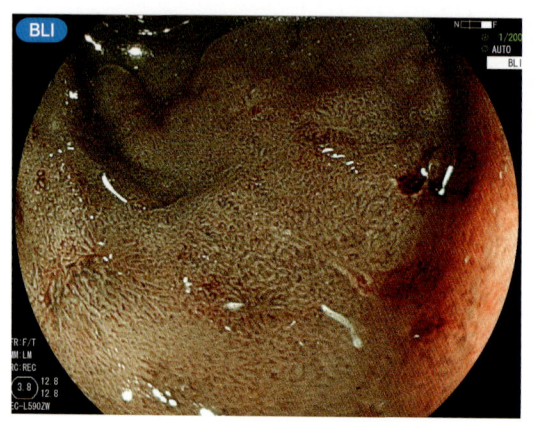

Low-magnification BLI observation: The surface pattern and vascular pattern can be identified clearly and the field is bright even in the far view.

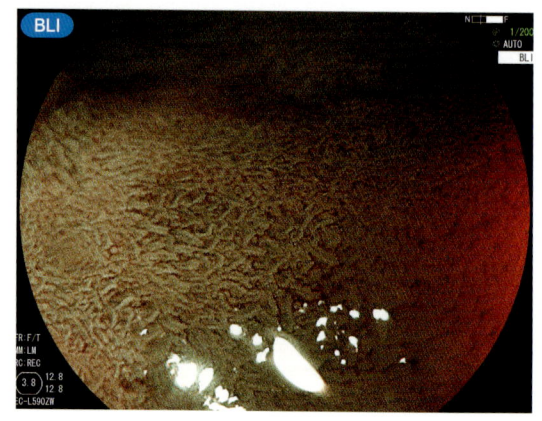

BLI magnifying observation: The surface pattern and vascular pattern are irregular but the degree of vascular irregularity is low. The lesion was diagnosed as corresponding to Hiroshima Classification type C1.

Endoscope : EC-L590ZW (Fujifilm)　　Light source : LASEREO (Fujifilm)
BLI setup : Structure enhancement B6, color enhancement C1

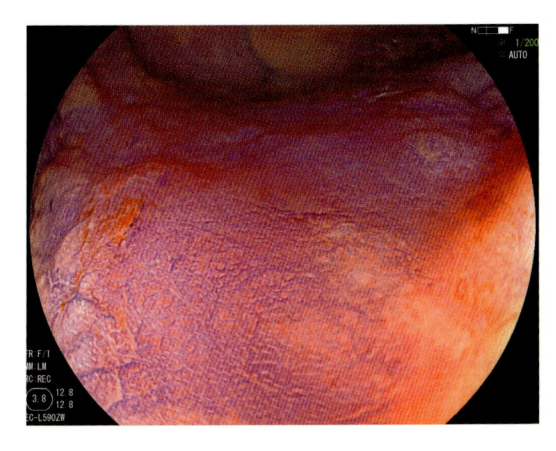

Crystal violet (CV) chromoendoscopy : Pits ranging from tubular to circular are arranged irregularly. They are mainly type V_I pits with slight irregularities.

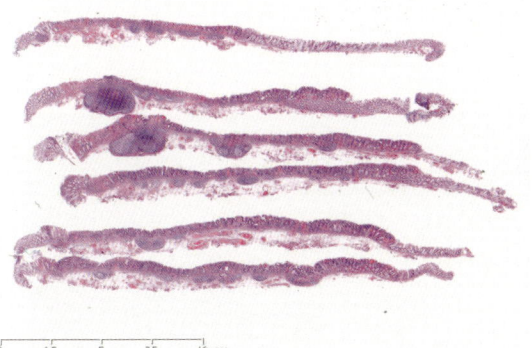

Cross section image : The lesion is slightly elevated but a slight depression can be seen in the center. On the lesion margin, what is called a double-layer development can be seen, in which neoplastic ducts are distributed on the superficial layer. Development of lymphoid follicles is also noticeable.

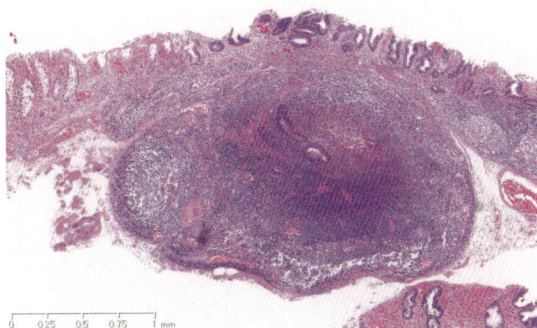

Histology : With lymphoid follicles observed in the erythematous elevated region, an invasion of well-differentiated carcinoma is recognized in this region. Similar cancerous invasions are found in four locations, and the maximum SM invasion depth from the muscularis mucosae is 680 μm. No vascular infiltration or tumor budding is recognized. Histopathological diagnosis : Well-differentiated adenocarcinoma, pSM (680 μm), ly0, v0, budding 1, pVM0, pHM0.

Comment

This is a typical case of depressed LST-NG with a maximum diameter over 3 cm. The lesion's borders were not clear under white light observation, but a clear demarcation line was visible under BLI-bright observation. Based on the surface pattern and vascular pattern findings with BLI magnifying observation, the lesion was recognized as a carcinoma with little or no SM invasion.

▶Observation tips　The BLI system has a BLI-bright mode suitable for detection and a BLI mode suitable for detailed magnifying observation. It is important to match the mode and application properly. Begin with overall observation of the lesion using the BLI-bright mode without magnification. The extent of the lesion should be evaluated also at this time. Then, use the BLI-bright mode to identify the region with advanced histological atypia based on changes in color tone and superficial structure. Finally, apply BLI mode to get magnified images of the surface pattern and vascular pattern by focusing on the region identified above.

(Nemoto, D., Endo, S., Togashi, K.)

Case 70 LST-NG, pseudo-depressed type
—Comparison of NBI/BLI observations

Female in her 70s **Purpose** Detailed examination after epigastric pain and body weight loss
Location Sigmoid colon **Macroscopic type** 0-Ⅰs+Ⅱa, LST-NG (PD)

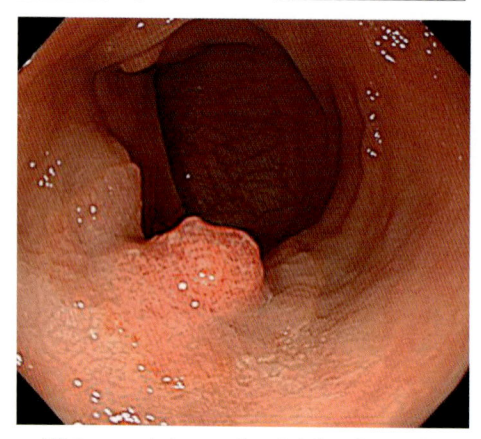

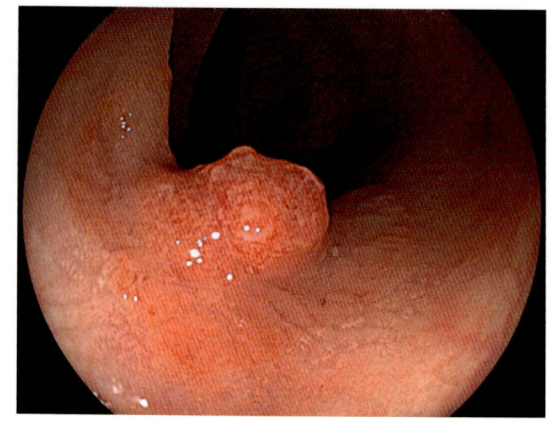

WLI normal observation: A flat elevated lesion with a size of 35 mm is recognized. In the center of the lesion, an erythematous nodule taller than the surrounding area is observed. White dots are found on the lesion margin.

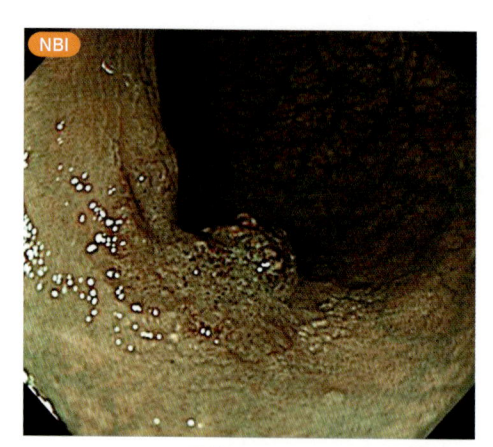

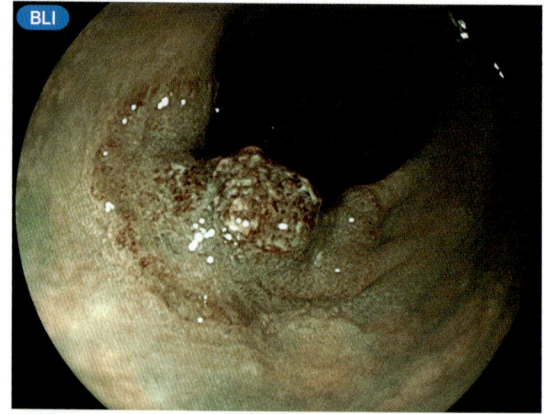

NBI/BLI normal observations: The lesion is imaged as a brownish area.

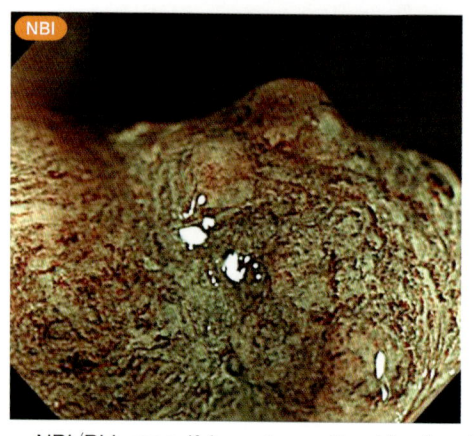

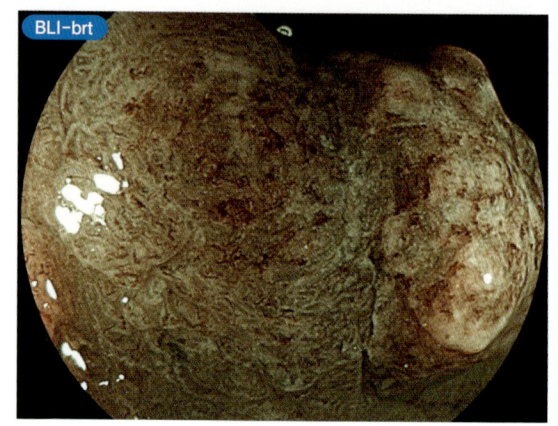

NBI/BLI magnifying observation: In the flat elevated region on the margin, the mesh-like microvascular architecture is maintained but some microvessels are disrupted or branched. As the erythematous elevation is approached, the size irregularity, tortuosity and disruption of vessels become more noticeable.

218

Endoscopic image（left）
　Endoscope：CF-FH260AZI（Olympus）　　Light source：EVIS LUCERA SPECTRUM（Olympus）
　NBI setup：Structure enhancement A8, color mode 3
Endoscopic image（right）
　Endoscope：EC-L590ZW（Fujifilm）　　Light source：LASEREO（Fujifilm）
　BLI setup：BLI—Structure enhancement A3, color enhancement C2；BLI-bright—Structure enhancement A4, color enhancement C2

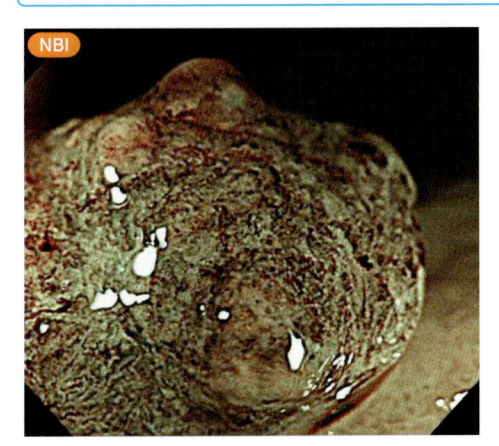

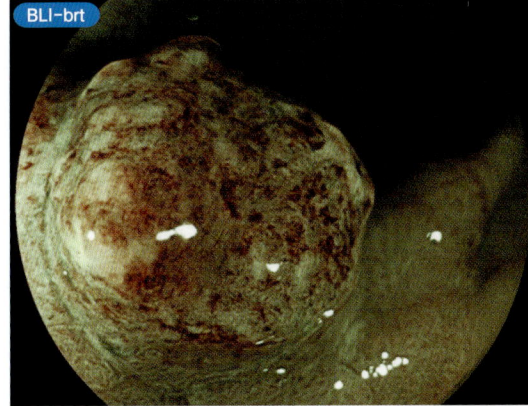

Magnifying observation of erythematous nodule：An area can be seen in which the mesh-like microvascular architecture has been destroyed and the vascular density is low.

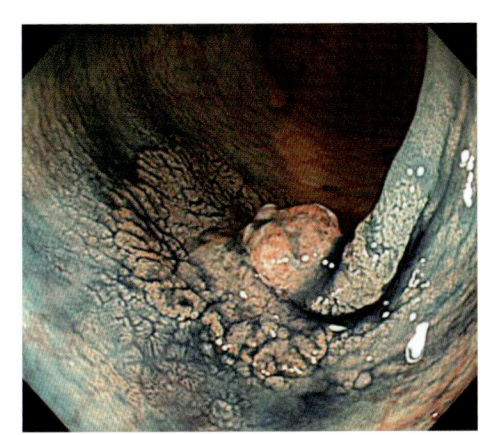

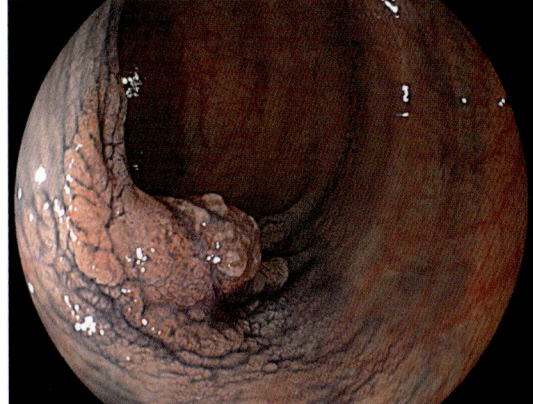

Indigo carmine chromoendoscopy：The lesion borders can be seen clearly and pseudopodial findings are observed on them. A gently elevated region is observed around the erythematous nodule.

219

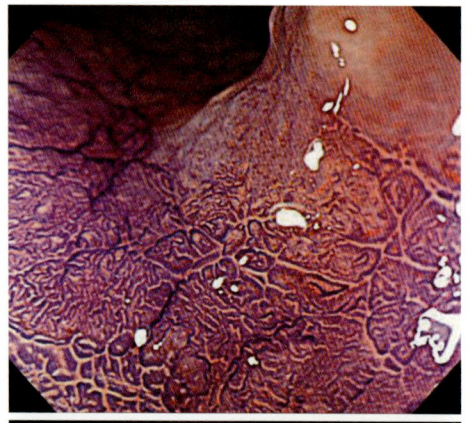

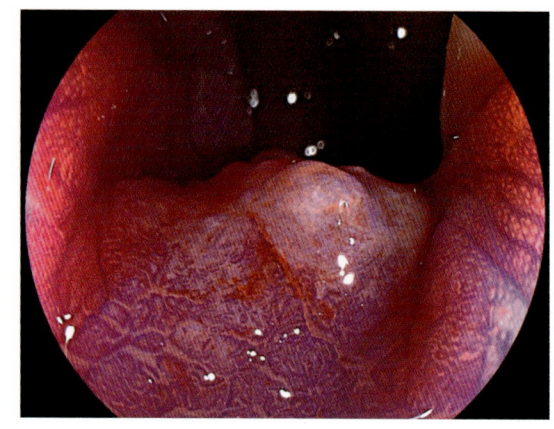

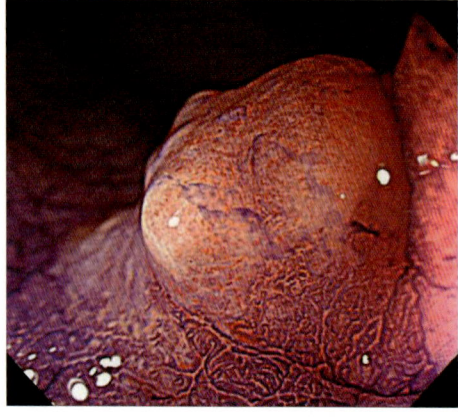

Crystal violet magnifying chromoendoscopy : The pit pattern in the flat elevated region in the margin is diagnosed as a mild irregular type V_I and that in the gentle elevation around the erythematous nodule as sever irregular type V_I. As the erythematous nodule itself is diagnosed to have a V_N pit pattern, the lesion is eventually diagnosed to have a V_N pattern (invasive pattern)

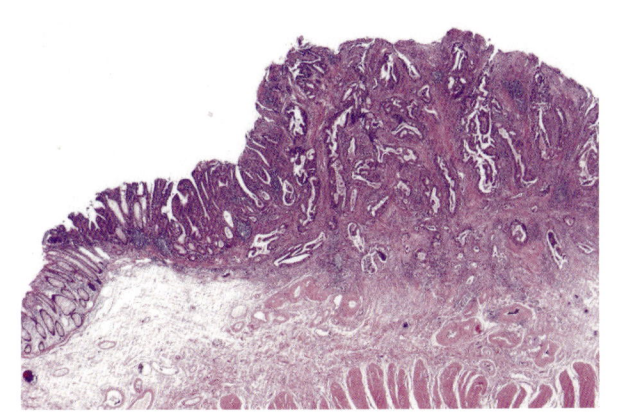

A well-differentiated adenocarcinoma with low-grade atypia is recognized in the marginal elevated region where the mild irregular type V_I pin pattern is present. SM invasion of a moderately differentiated adenocarcinoma is observed in the erythematous nodule where the V_N pit pattern is present.

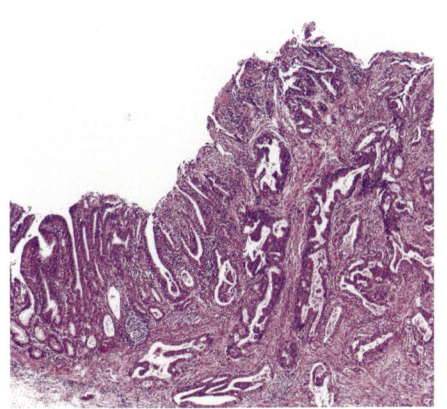

In the slightly elevated region around the nodule where the severe irregular type V_I pit pattern is present, a well-differentiated adenocarcinoma with low-grade atypia has been pushed up by the moderately differentiated adenocarcinoma below it.

Comment

In this case, the authors were able to observe the same lesion using both the NBI and BLI systems on the same day. Although we know that simple comparison of the two systems is difficult because changes in shooting conditions can result in significant variations in how the images look, we decided to show the images of the two systems side by side in this article.

As an erythematous elevated region that appeared the firm consistency was recognized under macroscopic observation, the lesion was suspected to present deep SM invasion from the initial stage. Subsequently, in both NBI and BLI magnifying observation, magnified views of the erythematous nodule showed an area in which the mesh-like microvascular architecture has been destroyed and the vascular density is low. Similarly, a V_N pattern (invasive pattern) was recognized on the erythematous nodule. Based on the findings of both macroscopic and magnifying observation, the lesion was comprehensively diagnosed to have deep SM invasion and subjected to sigmoidectomy. The histopathological diagnosis concluded that the lesion was a moderately to well-differentiated adenocarcinoma with an SM invasion (depth 3,000 μm), with no vascular invasion or lymph node metastasis.

▶**Observation tips** It is important to start with macroscopic observation to identify regions of interest such as areas with erythema or depressions and then apply the NBI/BLI and crystal violet magnifying chromoendoscopy. The NBI settings used at our hospital are as reported above, but BLI permits more precise settings of structure enhancement and color enhancement. As our impression is that microvessels observed with BLI sometimes look clear and sometimes blurred depending on the settings, it is important to determine the settings that best facilitate observation according to the needs of each endoscopist in advance.

(Haruyama, S., Saito, Y., Kushima, R.)

Case 71 LST-NG, pseudo-depressed type

Male in his 60s | Purpose | Positive fecal occult blood test | Location | Sigmoid colon
Macroscopic type | 0-Ⅱa+Ⅱc (LST-NG, PD)

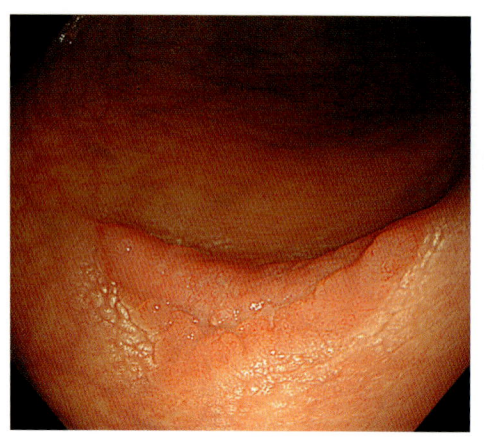

Standard WLI observation: An slightly reddish flat elevated lesion 25 mm in diameter and accompanied with depression is recognized.

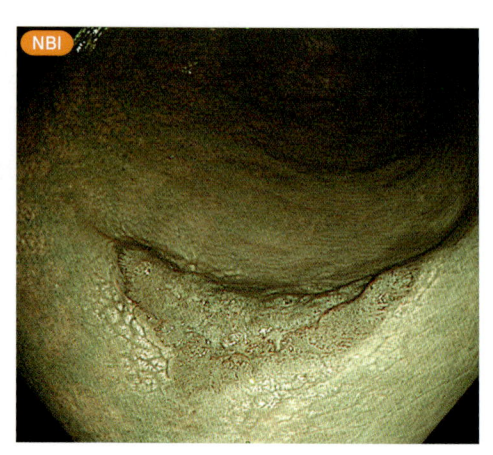

Standard NBI observation: The lesion appears brownish.

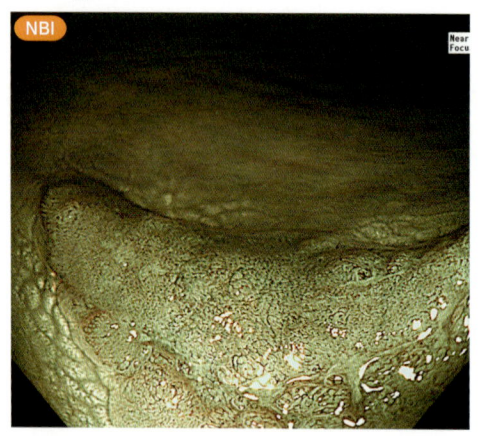

NBI Near Focus observation: A slightly irregular surface pattern is recognized.

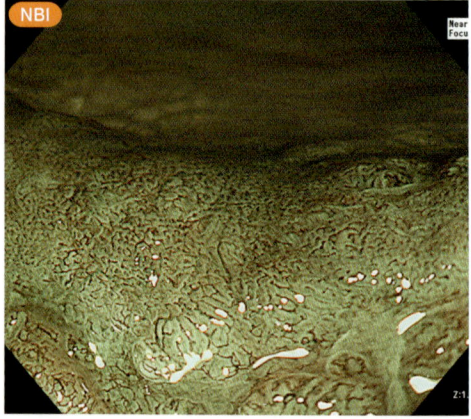

NBI Near Focus observation+1.6×electronic zoom: The surface pattern is clarified.

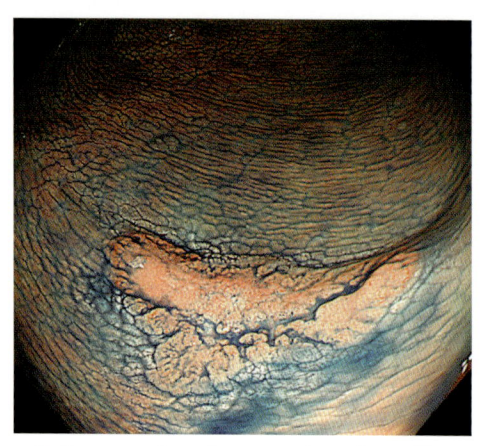

Indigo carmine dye spraying view: The depressed area is imaged clearly.

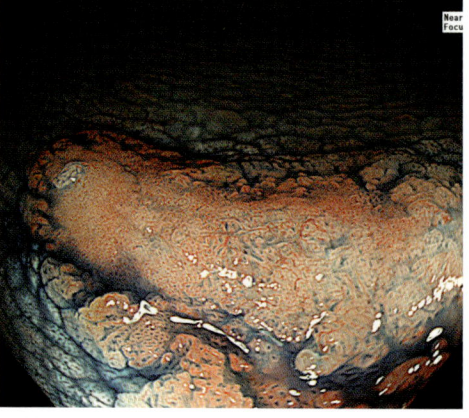

Near Focus observation+1.6×electronic zoom: Slightly irregular pits with variable sizes are observed in the center.

222

Endoscope : CF-HQ290L/I (Olympus)　　Light source : EVIS LUCERA ELITE (Olympus)
NBI setup : Structure enhancement A8, color mode 3

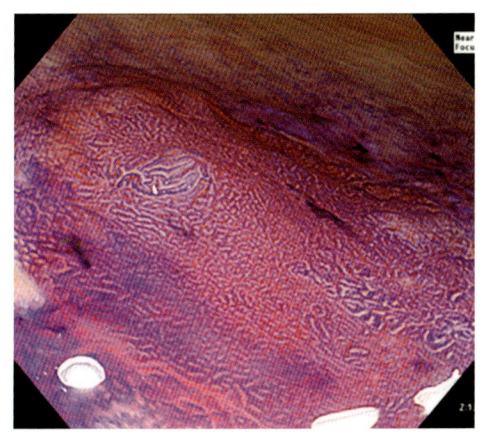

Crystal violet staining view in Near Focus mode+1.6×electronic zoom : Type III_L pits are observed on the margin.

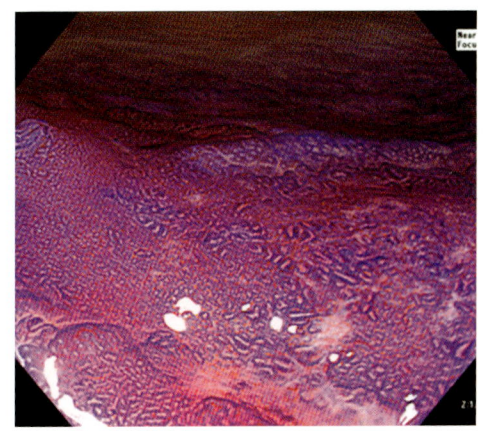

Crystal violet staining view in Near Focus mode+1.6×electronic zoom : Slightly irregular type V_I pits are recognized in the center area.

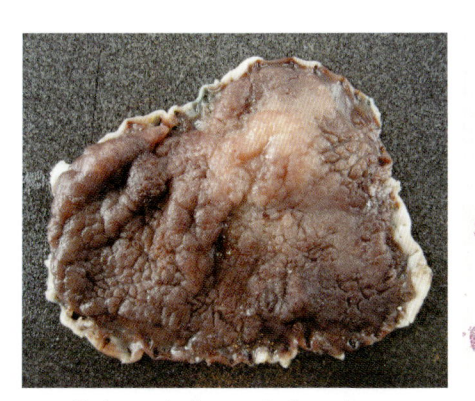

Endoscopically resected specimen.

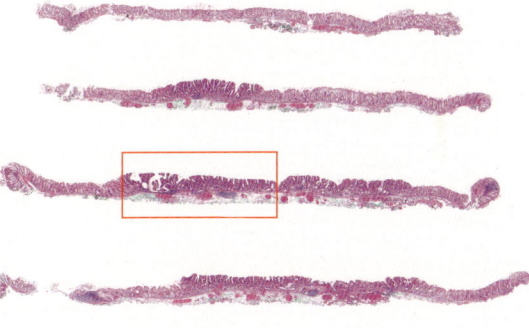

Cross section and Magnifying image (HE staining×40).

Low-magnification image of □ : The lesion is diagnosed as a well-differentiated carcinoma, tub1, SM 120 μm.

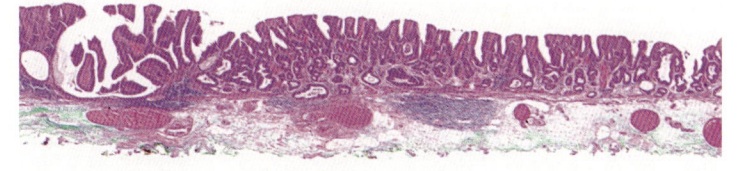

Comment

In many cases, mucus adhered to the tumor surface cannot be eliminated completely by water lavage, and as a result there is insufficient staining in the chromoendoscopy. However, NBI observation is still possible even when some mucus is left on the tumor. In this case, the stained region could only be recognized partially after the Crystal Violet staining, but the same region was clearly observable with NBI. Although there was no finding suggesting SM invasion in the magnifying observation, the fact that an LST-NG of the pseudo-depressed type (PD) with a tray-shaped depression as in this case frequently causes multicentric SM invasion regardless of the pit pattern, en bloc resection was necessary in order to obtain an accurate pathological diagnosis. ESD was performed and the pathological diagnosis result showed tub1 with 120 μm SM invasion.

▶Observation tips　Even a thin layer of mucus can interfere with diagnosis for Crystal Violet staining findings, but NBI observation enables diagnosis even when mucus is adhered to the lesion.

(Hayashi, N., Tanaka, S.)

Case 72 LST-NG, pseudo-depressed type

Male in his 60s   **Purpose** Detailed examination of tumor   **Location** Transverse colon
Macroscopic type 0-Ⅱa, LST-NG (PD).

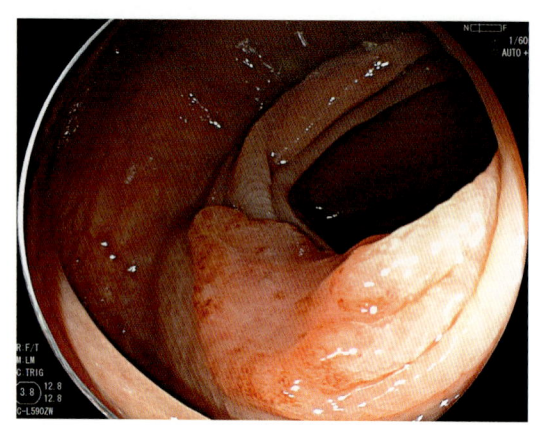

Normal white-light observation: A flat lesion 20 mm in diameter is recognized. The lesion is positioned across folds and accompanied with a low reddish elevation on the margin and a depression in the center.

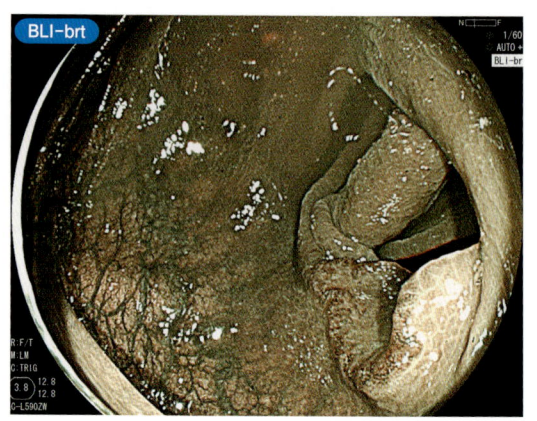

Distant of BLI-bright observation: The low elevated area on the tumor margin is imaged in dark brown and is clearly visible.

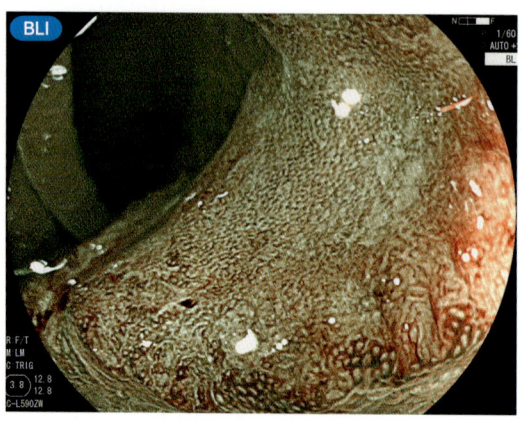

Low-magnification BLI observation: The depression in the center maintains both the surface pattern and vascular pattern. No obviously amorphous areas can be seen.

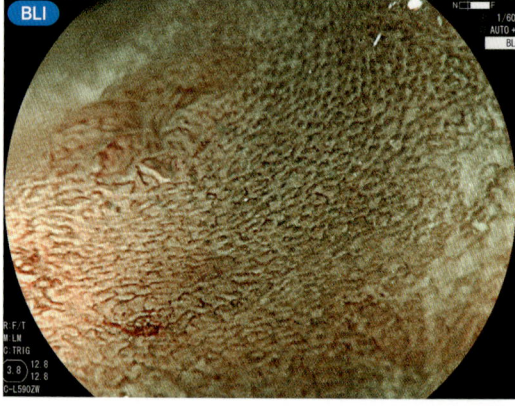

The surface pattern on the depression in the center is small round pit-like and slightly irregular, while the vascular pattern is partially unclear but does not present dilation or tortuosity.

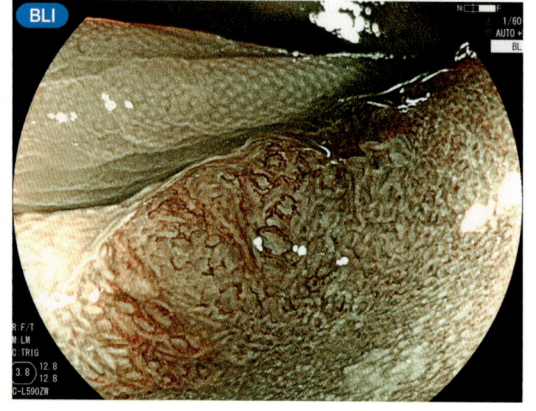

The surface pattern on the elevated area in the margin is slightly irregular, and the vascular pattern presents dilation and tortuosity. Non-neoplastic findings are partially mixed in.

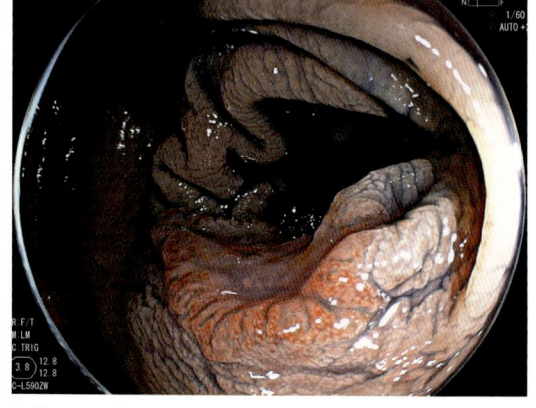

Indigo carmine chromoendoscopy: The tumor margin and the central depression are clearly visible.

Endoscope：ECL-590ZW（Fujifilm）　　Light source：LASEREO（Fujifilm）
BLI setup：BLI-bright—Structure enhancement A6, color enhancement C2；BLI—Structure enhancement A6, color enhancement C2

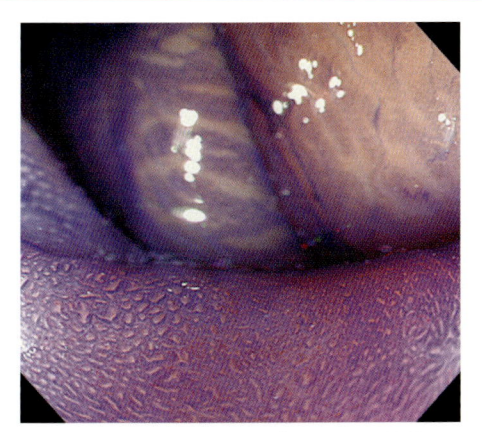

Magnified pit pattern（Olympus PCF-Q260AZI）：As there are irregular pits on the depression in the center, the pit pattern is diagnosed as slightly irregular type V$_I$.

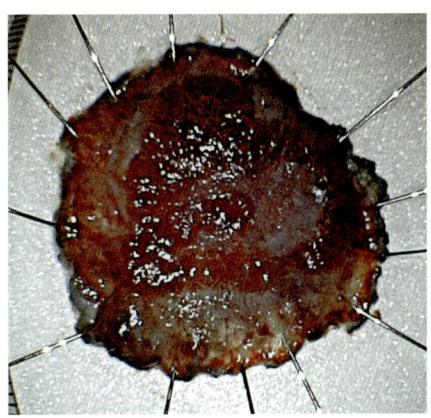

ESD-resected specimen：Resected size 30×28 mm.

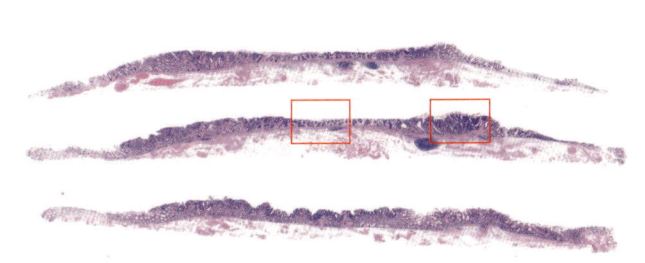

Magnified image：As there is no apparent submucosal invasion, the lesion is a mucosal lesion. The central part is composed of low gland ducts.

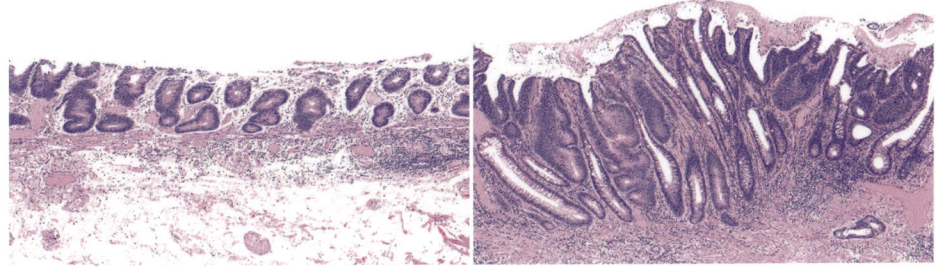

Low-magnification image：As gland ducts with medium to advanced structural atypia are recognized, the lesion is diagnosed as a highly atypical adenoma.

Comment

For distant BLI observation, it is best to use the BLI-bright mode as it can offer a bright view, which enables clear identification of the lesion. The BLI mode should be used for close-up and magnifying observation. With an LST-NG（PD）, start observation at low magnification because the remaining structures in the central area can be evaluated best at low magnification. In this case, when high magnification was used, a small round surface pattern accompanied with slight irregularities was observed, so the lesion was diagnosed as Hiroshima Classification Type C1, while pit pattern observation showed that the central part had a slightly irregular V$_I$ pit pattern. Since it is not unusual for LST-NG（PD）to cause multifocal SM invasion, the lesion was subjected to en bloc resection by ESD, which took 118 minutes due to respiratory variations and a moderate degree of fibrosis. The histopathological diagnosis concluded that the lesion was an adenoma with high-grade atypia and negative margin.

▶**Observation tips** With an LST-NG（PD）, it is important to check that there is no residual mucosa by observing the vascular pattern and surface pattern with low-magnification BLI observation.

（Yoshida, N., Yagi, N., Naito, Y.）

Case 73　Ulcerative colitis

Female in her 30s　**Purpose** Detailed examination after mucous and bloody stool
Location Sigmoid colon, rectum

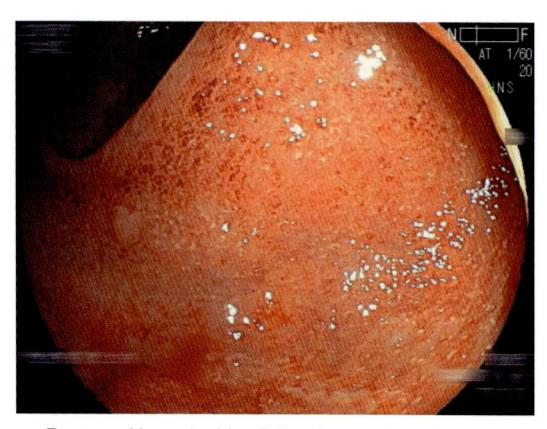

Rectum. Normal white-light observation : The visibility of the vascular pattern in the intestinal mucosa has deteriorated, and brownish color tone changes are recognized in spots.

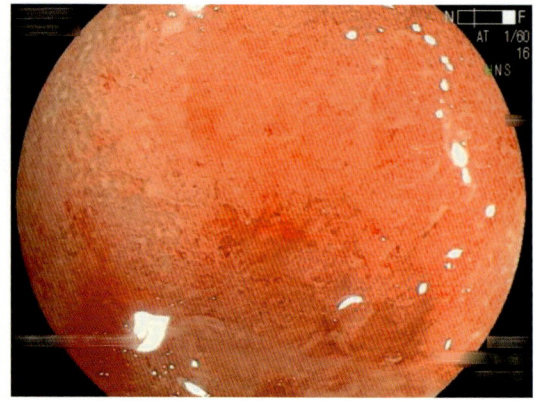

Rectum. Low-magnification white-light observation : The mucosa is rough, and detailed observation of the surface is difficult due to the large amount of mucus.

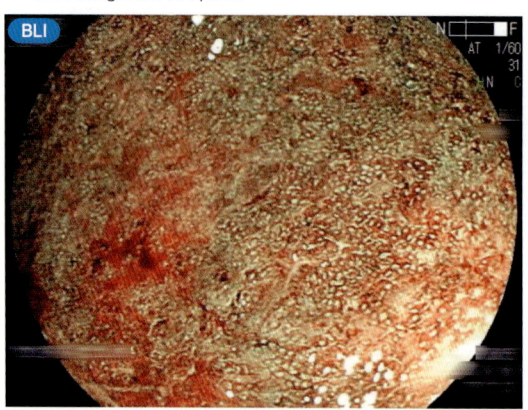

Rectum. Low-magnification BLI observation : The mucosal pits are imaged more clearly than with the white-light normal observation. The absence of pits suggests mucosal defects.

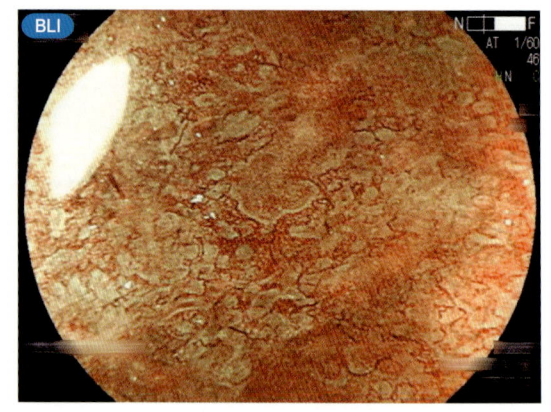

Rectum. High-magnification BLI observation : The microvessels in the lamina propria mucosae can be recognized clearly. The mucosal defect regions can be identified by disappearance of visible vascular patterns.

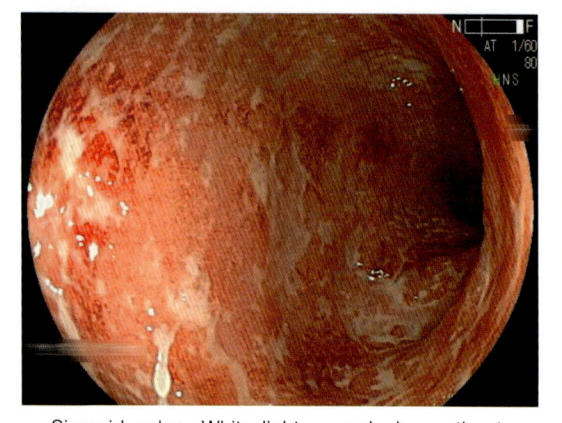

Sigmoid colon. White-light normal observation : The visibility of the vascular pattern in the intestinal mucosa has deteriorated, and irregularly shaped ulcers are scattered.

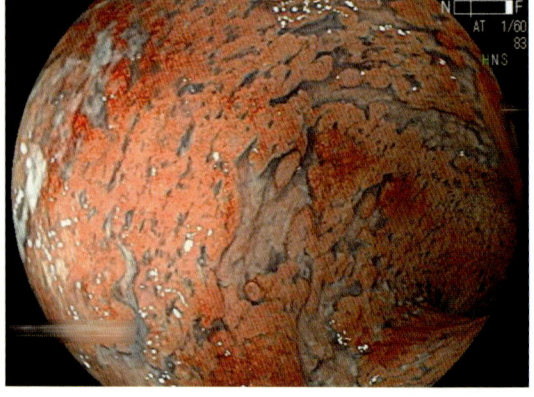

Sigmoid colon. Indigo carmine chromoendoscopy (non-magnification) : The morphology of the ulcers is clearer than in normal observation. Even small ulcers can now be identified.

Endoscope: EC-L590ZW (Fujifilm) Light source: LASEREO (Fujifilm)
BLI setup: Structure enhancement A6, color enhancement C1

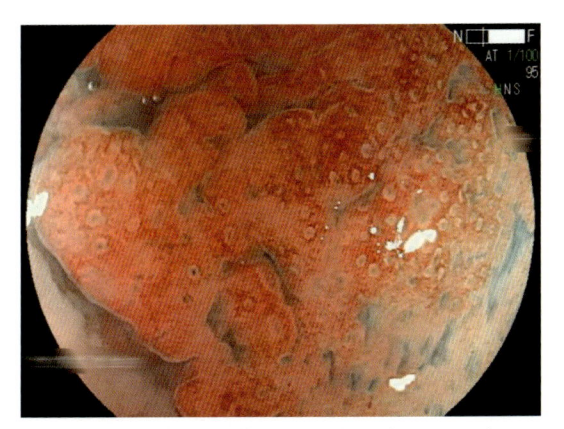

Sigmoid colon. Indigo carmine chromoendoscopy (high magnification): Even pit openings can be recognized on the mucosae around small mucosal defects.

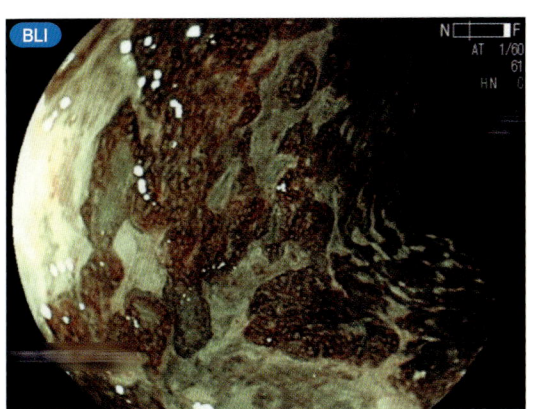

Sigmoid colon. BLI normal observation: The ulcer floor is whitish green while the mucosa looks brownish.

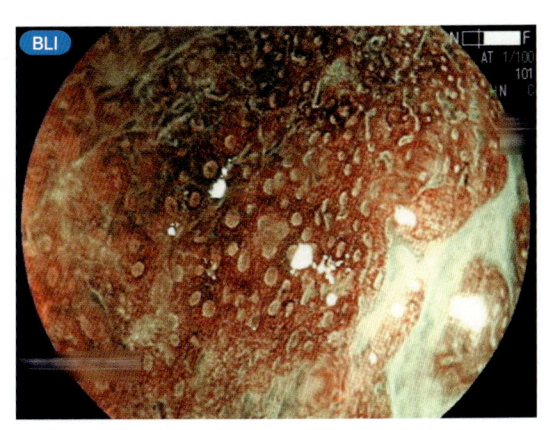

Sigmoid colon. High-magnification BLI observation: The mucosa of the erythematous region looks brownish, but the vascular structure is not recognizable.

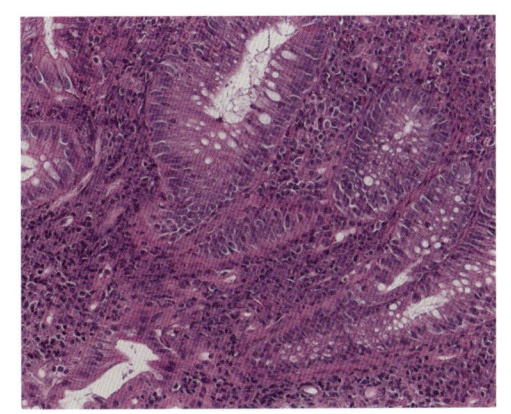

Sigmoid colon. Biopsy from ulcer margin: Infiltration of inflammatory cell mainly composed of plasmacytes accompanied with neutrophil invasion and advanced cryptitis are observed in the stroma.

Comment

This case is an ulcerative colitis of the left-side colitis type. Indigo carmine chromoendoscopy and magnifying endoscopy make clear the presence of minor ulcers and minor epithelial defects. The surface structure is hard to recognize with white-light observation due to secreted mucus, but BLI observation makes possible clear recognition of the pit structure and microvascular pattern.

▶ **Observation tips** BLI enhances the blood vessels. When combined with a magnifying endoscope, BLI enables recognition even of very fine vessels. The ability to recognize vessels in the shallow mucosal layer makes it possible to evaluate very small erosions and ulcers and collect useful findings for the diagnosis of ulcerative colitis.

(Tominaga, M., Fujiya, M., Kohgo, Y.)

Case 74

Tumor associated with inflammatory colon diseases (carcinoma/dysplasia)

Male in his 30s　*Purpose* Surveillance of an ulcerative colitis　*Location* Rectum, upper　*Macroscopic type* 0-IIc

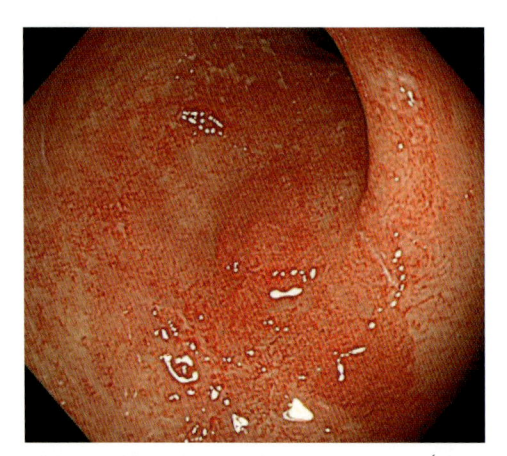

WLI view : Ulcerative colitis in the active phase (Matts Grade 3). Recognition of the tumor was not easy.

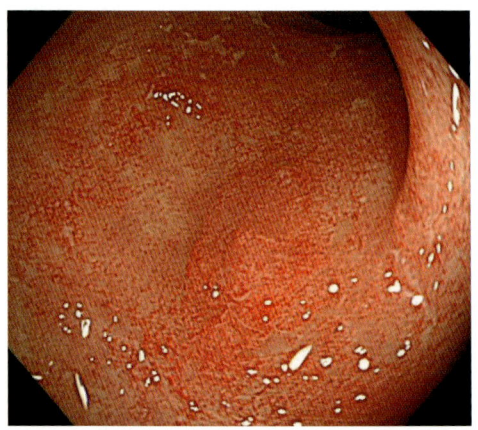

Close-up view : Slight mucosal irregularities were found in the erythematous area.

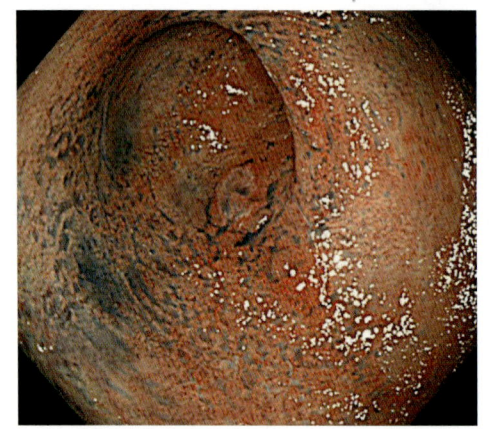

Chromoendoscopy with Indigo carmine dye : In the conventional view, the lesion was identified as a semicircular lesion with thin mucus on its surface in the erythematous area.

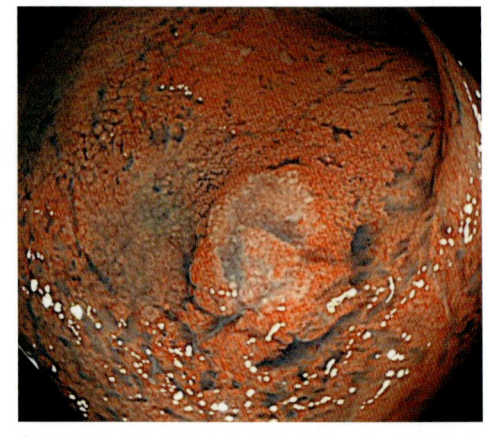

Close-up view : The lesion size was 6 mm in diameter. It was recognized as a depressed lesion accompanied by a very slight reactive elevation, clear demarcation and thin whitish mucus on the lesion surface.

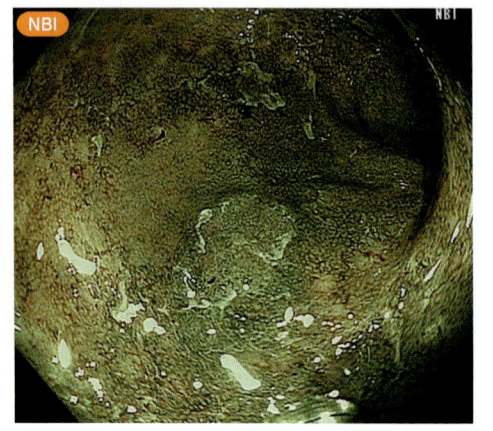

NBI view ; The superficial mucus wass partially removed by repeated irrigation, but recognition of the lesion was still difficult.

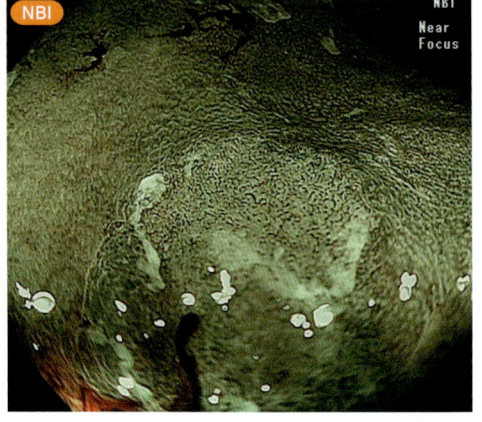

NBI with Near Focus view : Irregular vessels was observed in the depressed area.

Endoscope：CF-HQ290L/I（Olympus）　　Light source：EVIS LUCERA ELITE（Olympus）
NBI setup：Structure enhancement A5（no magnification view），A8（magnification view），Color mode 3

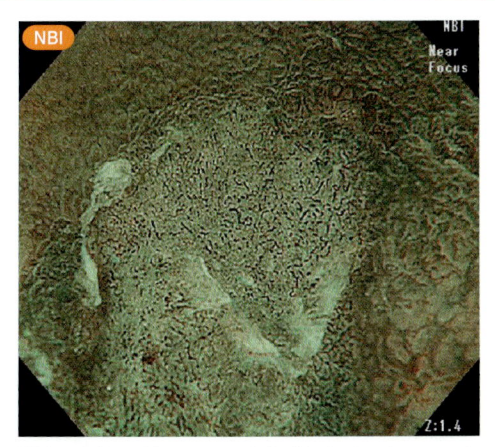

NBI with Near Focus view＋1.4×electronic zoom：Irregular vessels of various sizes were clearly visible. No decrease in vascular density is observed.

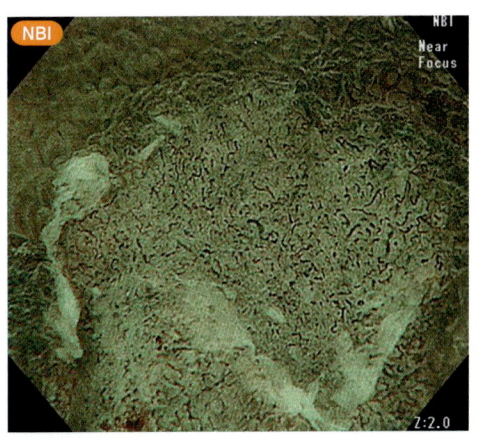

Increasing the electronic zoom ratio to 2.0× makes the irregular vessels more clearly visible.

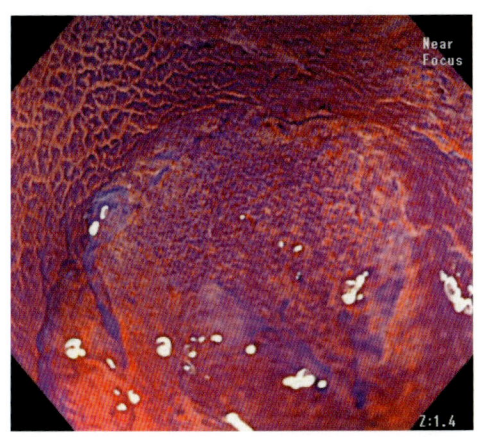

Chromoendoscopy after crystal violet staining with Near Focus mode＋1.4×electronic zoom.

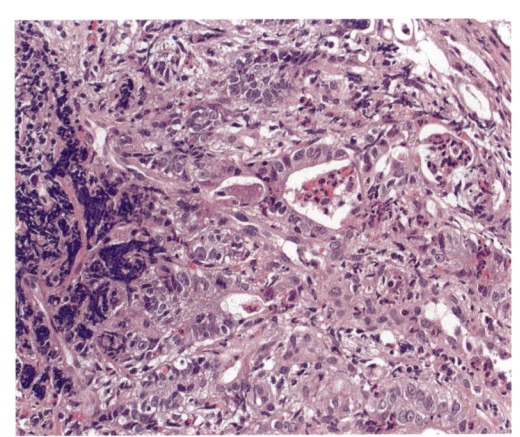

Histopathological diagnosis of biopsy specimen：Atypical ducts accompanied with cellular atypia and structural atypia were revealed. The p53 staining result was positive.

Comment

This was a small depressed lesion found in surveillance of an ulcerative colitis case with a 10-year history. Based on the conventional and magnification endoscopic findings, histopathological findings and p53 stain positivity, the lesion was comprehensively diagnosed as an early carcinoma associated with ulcerative colitis. Total coloectomy was recommended.

▶**Observation tips** Detection of flat and depressed lesions in an ulcerative colitis like this case is generally not easy. Especially, in a case with a long history of disease, careful observation considering the incidence of dysplasia/carcinoma is important. Through preparation is indispensable. The lesion should be lavaged sufficiently by water irrigation. Should a slight mucosal irregularity be found, perform NBI magnification endoscopy and chromoendoscopy with indigo carmine dye spraying as these are helpful for early detection and diagnosis of the lesions. The Dual Focus function makes it easy to obtain a magnification view up to 40×, but an electronic zoom of at least around 1.5× should be added for detailed observation.

（Uraoka, T., Iwao, Y.）

Featured Article

Magnification in Near Focus electronic zoom observation of the LUCERA ELITE system

The main areas where the EVIS LUCERA ELITE CF-HQ290L/I have been improved relative to their predecessors, the EVIS LUCERA CFH-H260AZI, are image quality and brightness (thanks to the increase in light intensity and exposure time). Additional improvements include the incorporation of the Dual Focus function and the expansion of the field of view from 140° to 170° (already available on the EXERA III in Europe and North America).

To support magnifying observation, Olympus provided the Dual Focus function, which makes possible instant switching of two focus ranges at the touch of a button (**Fig. 1**). The Normal Focus mode (suitable for mid- to far-view observation) offers magnification of about 20× when the image is displayed on a 26-inch monitor, and the Near Focus mode (suitable for close-up observation) offers magnification of about 45×. These magnified views can be magnified still more by adding electronic zoom, which produces low-noise magnified images with quality almost as good as those produced by the optical zoom thanks to the overall improvements in image quality. The electronic zoom can be

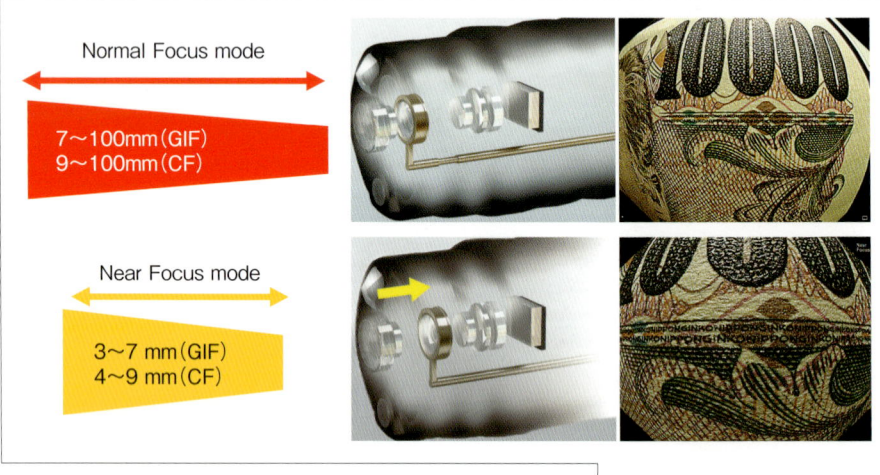

Fig. 1 Dual Focus Function of new Olympus CF-HQ290L/I Colonoscope

The Dual Focus function makes it possible to switch instantly between the two focus ranges at the touch of a button. In addition to the two modes of : ①Normal Focus mode suitable for mid- to far-view observation (approx. 20× on a 26-inch monitor) and ② Near Focus mode suitable for close-up (approx. 45×) ; ③ electronic zoom can instantaneously magnify the image further by 1.2× (total approx. 54×), 1.6× (total approx. 72×) or 2.0× (total approx. 90×). The total magnification of approx. 72× that can be obtained with the Near Focus mode (approx. 45×) + electronic zoom (1.6×) is almost identical to the optical full-zoom ratio available with the CF-Q260AZI.

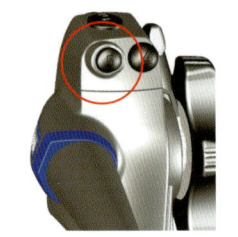

(Source : Olympus Medical Systems Corp.)

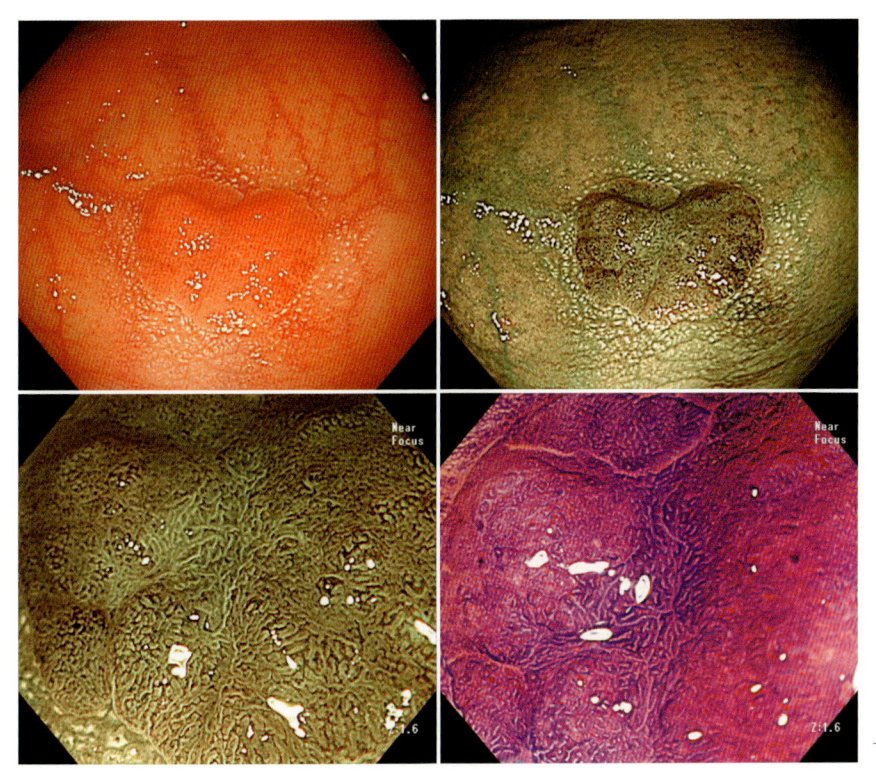

Fig. 2 Endoscopic Image Obtained Using Dual Focus Function of New Olympus CF-HQ290L/I Colonoscope (8 mm in diameter, type 0 - IIa lesion)

a : Standard observation image in Normal Focus mode.
b : NBI observation image in Normal Focus mode.
c : NBI observation image in Near Focus mode＋1.6×electronic zoom (total approx. 72×).
d : Crystal violet chromoendoscopy image in Near Focus mode＋1.6×electronic zoom (total approx. 72×).

Both NBI magnifying observation and crystal violet magnifying chromoendoscopy are able to support satisfactory diagnoses.

switched in three steps of 1.2×, 1.6× and 2×, and the total magnification ratios are approximately 54×, 72× and 90× respectively.

The optical zoom ratio of the EVIS LUCERA CF-H260AZI is slightly below 80×. Since it is rare that observation is conducted at full zoom, actual magnifying observation is usually done at magnifications of about 60× to 70×. The EVIS LUCERA ELITE CF-HQ290L/I can provide a magnified image of about 72× with the combination of the Dual Focus function and 1.6× electronic zoom, which means that a single touch of a button makes it possible to obtain an image almost equivalent to the optical zoom image available with the EVIS LUCERA CF-H260AZI (**Fig. 2**). As an optical zoom function is expected to be available with the EVIS LUCERA ELITE CF-HQ290L/I in the near future, we are interested in any future developments in this line of products.

(Tanaka, S., Hayashi, N.)

Featured Article

Importance of structure enhancement in NBI magnifying observation

Magnifying observation based on Narrow Band Imaging (NBI) is useful for qualitative diagnoses of colorectal tumor. What is most important is a comprehensive diagnosis with proper balance between the vascular pattern and surface pattern observations. A dark-brownish vessel can be recognized even when it is not focused precisely, but the surface pattern cannot be evaluated unless it is focused precisely. Being unable to evaluate the surface pattern due to inaccurate focusing can easily lead to an erroneous diagnosis. The importance of accurate focusing in magnifying observation is exactly the same as in pit pattern diagnosis using chromoendoscopy. However, many colorectal lesions involve more elevations and height unevenness than early carcinomas in the esophagus or stomach, so it is hard to focus on the entire image in magnifying observation. A lesion with big differences in height requires different focal lengths to be used according to the heights, making it necessary to separately capture the images of the lesion at different positions.

In addition to the issue of focusing, it is critical to set the structure enhancement to A8 in order to evaluate the surface pattern (for color enhancement, it is usually recommended to set "3" in ordinary colorectal examinations). It is only under this condition that the surface pattern can be diagnosed in accurately focused magnifying observation.

The figure below shows the NBI magnifying observation images of the same part of the same lesion under the structure enhancement settings of A3, A5 and A8. These images show that the visibility of the surface pattern clearly differs depending on the structure enhancement setting. Setting the structure enhancement too high clarifies the surface pattern, but causes interference of electrical noise in the vascular pattern. It is therefore important to modify the settings according to the conditions of the target lesions when evaluating the vascular pattern. Changing settings can easily be done at the touch of a button because three presets can be specified by the user, including default settings for WLI and NBI as desired. Once the default settings have been set up, the one-touch button operation is much simpler than preparing a dye and spraying it on the lesion or staining the lesion with it.

As described above, the important thing for accurate qualitative diagnosis is to set up the video endoscopy system (particularly the structure enhancement) correctly and evaluate both the surface pattern and vascular pattern, taking the macroscopic type and histological type in consideration.

(Tanaka, S., Hayashi, N.)

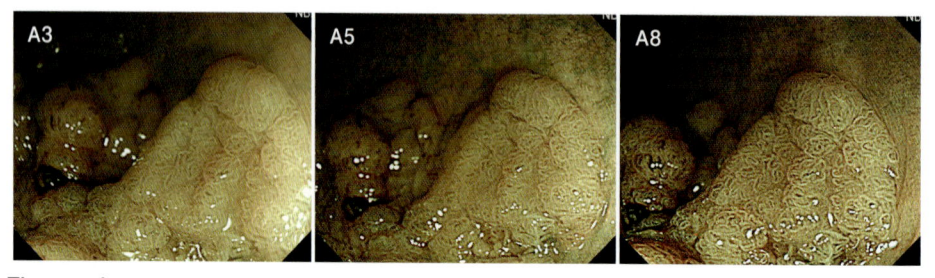

Figure Importance of System Condition Settings in NBI Magnifying observation

Structure enhancement can be set in eight steps of 1-8 in the A or B mode. The B mode enables detailed observation of vessels, but the A mode is suitable for balanced diagnosis based on both the vascular pattern and surface pattern. The images in this figure show NBI magnified images of the same part of the same lesion, captured under structure enhancement settings A3, A5 and A8 respectively. The surface pattern is clearest with A8 with color enhancement 3. The images show that the visibility of the surface pattern clearly differs depending on the structure enhancement settings. Although the structure enhancement for the NBI magnifying observation is best at A8, this setting can make images appear glittery under WLI, so a slightly lower setting is recommended for WLI. In any case, it should be noted that the images observed with the video endoscopy system vary greatly depending on the structure enhancement settings.

Index

(Page numbers in bold face indicate the presence of case images.)

A

AFI 176
ALDH-2 hetero deficiencies 37
Arima Classification 57
atypical vessel 41, 79
— proliferation 24, 38, 42, 75,123
avascular area (AVA) 58
— -large 58
— -middle 45, 58
— -small 58, 79, 80

B

B1 vessel 57, 58, 78, 80, 82, 84, 87
B2 vessel 44, 58, 76
B3 vessel 58, 76, 77
Barrett's esophageal adenocarcinoma
— : BLI **94**
— : NBI **92**
Barrett's esophagus 49
— : BLI **90**
— : NBI **88**
bile 99
biomarker of the pharyngeal carcinoma 37
black hood 85
Blue Laser Imaging (BLI) 16
— combined iodine staining 80
— laser 104
comparison between — and NBI 83, 85, 221
difference between — and FICE 19
NBI classification for — magnifying observation 168
principles of — 18
BLI-bright mode 18, 105, 168, 172
BLI mode 18, 105, 168, 172
usages of — and BLI-bright mode 105
BLI observation
— colon and rectum 168
— esophagus 56
— pharynx 26

— stomach and duodenum 104
brownish area 24, 26, 30, 34, 36, 38, 41, 42, 44, 50, 74, 78, 82, 84, 86, 104, 134, 186, 188
budding 183

C

capillary network 158
capillary pattern 162
— classification 207
chronic atrophic gastritis 113
chronic gastritis
— : BLI **112**
— : NBI **110**
collecting venules 111
color enhancement 19, 106
colorectal adenoma
— elevated serrated adenoma **182**
— elevated tubular adenoma **184**
— superficial tubular adenoma: NBI **186**
— tubulovillous adenoma: NBI **188**
— vascular pattern per macroscopic type 161
— villous adenoma **190**
columnar epithelium 91
contrast 12
corkscrew pattern 126, 130
crystal violet staining 174, 176, 182, 193, 195, 197, 201, 202, 205, 207, 208, 210, 215, 220, 223

D

demarcation line 116, 118, 138, 142, 154, 216
dense pattern 164
desmoplastic reaction 201
deep SM invasion not accompanied with — 199

differential diagnosis of erosion and early gastric carcinoma 120
differentiated gastric carcinoma 125, 129, 131, 135
atypical vessels of — 123
distal attachment 24, 39
distal hood 56
Dormicum 49
dot-shaped vessels 39, 40, 78
Dual Focus function 100, 230
duodenal adenoma
— : BLI **146**
— : NBI **144**
differentiation of — from carcinoid 145
differentiation of — from duodenal carcinoma 153
differentiation of — from ectopic gastric mucosa 145
duodenal carcinoma
— : BLI **150**, **152**
— : NBI **148**
differentiation of — from duodenal adenoma 153
duodenal normal mucosa 99, 101
NBI Near Focus observation of — 102
duodenal submucosal tumor 99
duodenal villus 101

E

early carcinoma in gastric remnant: NBI **138**
early colorectal carcinoma
— composite (Is+IIc) SM carcinoma: NBI **208**
— composite (IIa+IIc) SM carcinoma: BLI **202**, **204**
— composite (IIa+IIc) SM carcinoma: NBI **206**
— elevated M carcinoma: NBI 192
— elevated SM carcinoma: NBI

233

198
—— slightly depressed M carcinoma: NBI **196**
—— slightly depressed SM carcinoma: NBI **200**
—— slightly elevated M carcinoma: NBI **194**
early gastric carcinoma
　　—— : BLI **120**, **124**, **126**, **132**, **134**
　　—— : NBI **118**, **122**, **128**, **130**, **136**
　　—— extent diagnosis 122, 124, 135
　　differential diagnosis of —— from erosion 120
　　differentiated —— 125, 129, 131, 135
　　histological diagnosis of —— 130, 134
　　transnasal endoscopy of —— 136
　　undifferentiated —— 99, 127, 133
ectopic gastric mucosa 145
electronic zoom 100
elimination of saliva and mucus 48
endoscopy-pathology correlation 154
epiglottic vallecula 24, 29, 39
esophageal gland proper 93
esophageal hiatal hernia 65, 66
esophageal lavage 49, 57
esophageal papilloma: BLI **64**
esophageal superficial carcinoma
　　—— type 0-I: NBI **74**
　　—— type 0-Is: BLI **76**
　　—— type 0-IIa: BLI **78**
　　—— type 0-IIb: BLI **80**
　　—— type 0-IIc: BLI **82**, **84**, **86**
　　—— type 0-IIc: NBI **82**, **84**
　　differentiation of —— from Barrett's esophageal carcinoma 79
esophagogastric junction (EGJ) 49, 72, 79
　　—— identification 91

F
faint pattern 164
fine network pattern 95, 128
Flexible spectral Imaging Color Enhancement (FICE) 16, 168

flunitrazepam 49
fundic mucosa 111
fundic region 101
　　NBI Near Focus observation of normal mucosa in —— 102

G
Gascon 49, 57
gastric adenoma
　　—— : BLI **116**
　　—— : NBI **114**
　　differentiation of —— from gastric carcinoma 118
gastric MALT lymphoma 143
　　—— : BLI **142**
　　—— : NBI **140**
　　differentiation of —— from gastric carcinoma 141
gastric mucosa 101
gastroesophageal reflux disease (GERD) 65, 66, 70, 93
　　—— : BLI **72**
　　—— : NBI **70**
glycogenic acanthosis (GA): NBI **62**
　　differentiation of —— from papilloma 33
Grade B 70
Grade M 66, 68

H
H. pylori
　　—— negative/uninfected 110, 143
　　—— positive/infected 111, 112
hard palate 29
hemoglobin 13
heterotopic gastric mucosa 50
high-grade intraepithelial neoplasia (HGIN) 48
Hiroshima Classification 163, 171
human papilloma virus (HPV) infection 65
hyperplastic polyp (HP) 175
　　—— : NBI **174**
　　differentiation of —— from SSA/P 175
hypopharyngeal superficial carcinoma

　　—— 0-IIb: NBI **42**

I
illumination light 14, 17
inflammatory bowel disease 228
inflammatory pharyngeal lesion: NBI **30**
Inoue Classification 57
intervascular background coloration 40
intestinal metaplasia 111, 113, 135
intraepithelial papillary capillary loop (IPCL) 35, 50, 71, 83
invasive pattern 201, 208, 220
iodine staining 32, 39, 42, 60, 75, 76, 79, 80, 83, 85, 95
irregular pattern 162
irregularly branched (IB) vessels 58

J
Japan Esophageal Society Classification of Magnified Endoscopy (for the Diagnosis of Esophageal Superficial Carcinoma) 54, 57

L
laryngeal expansion under general anesthesia 33
laser illumination 17
laser light source 16, 104
laterally spreading tumor (LST) of colon and rectum
　　LST-G homogeneous type: NBI **210**
　　LST-G nodular mixed type: BLI **212**
　　LST-NG 162
　　LST-NG pseudo-depressed type: BLI **216**, **218**, **224**
　　LST-NG pseudo-depressed type: NBI **214**, **218**, **222**
light blue crest (LBC) 104, 111, 112, 113, 135
light wavelength 13
lingual surface of epiglottis 29
long-segment Barrett's esophagus

(LSBE) 92
Los Angeles Classification 68, 70, 71
— revised version 66
lower esophageal palisade vessel 66, 68, 69, 88, 89
low-oxygen imaging 109
lymphoepithelial lesion (LEL) 141

M

marginal crypt epithelium (MCE) 118, 125, 134
melanosis (pharyngeal)
— : BLI **36**
— : NBI **34**
differentiation of — from malignant melanoma 35
mesh pattern 123
midazolam 49
milk-white mucosa (MWM) 148
multi-layered (ML) vessels 58

N

Narrow Band Imaging (NBI) 12
brightness of — 14
comparison between — and BLI 83, 85, 221
principles of — 13
NBI magnifying observation under acetic acid spraying 199
NBI observation
— colon and rectum 158
— esophagus 48
— pharynx 24
— stomach and duodenum 98
— under acetic acid spraying 199
narrow-band light 13, 16
— imaging 104
Near Focus (mode) 53, 99, 100, 230
NBI — observation of normal duodenal mucosa 102
NBI — observation of normal mucosa in gastric pyloric gland region 102
network pattern 130, 149, 164
NICE Classification (NBI International Colorectal Endoscopic Classification) 164, 165
relationship between — and Sano, Hiroshima and Showa Classifications 165
non-erosive reflux disease (NERD)
— : BLI **68**
— : NBI **66**
non-lifting sign 197
Normal Focus mode 100, 230
normal gastric mucosa 101
NPG-type 208
NT tube 192

O

observation making use of speaking 24
omission of pit pattern observation 185
Opistan 49
optical zoom 100
oropharyngeal superficial carcinoma
— 0-IIa: NBI **38**
— 0-IIb: BLI **40**

P

palatine arch 29
palisade vessel 72, 91
lower esophageal — 66, 68, 69, 88, 89
pathological diagnosis 154
pethidine hydrochloride 49
pharyngeal papilloma: BLI **32**
differentiation of — from glycogenic acanthosis 33
pharyngeal reflex 24, 26, 33
pink color sign 83
pit
— -like structure 159, 162
enlargement of — openings 181
type II open-shape — 179
type III$_H$ — 183
type IV$_H$ — 183
pit pattern diagnosis 195, 197, 207
postcricoid area 26
precise observation of lesions 56
pseudopyloric gland metaplasia 111
pyloric gland mucosa 111
pyloric gland region 101
NBI Near Focus observation of normal mucosa in — 102
pyriform sinus 24, 26

R

remnant gastritis 138
Resect and Discard Trial 164
reticular (R) vessels 58
Rohypnol 49

S

Sano Classification 163
serrated adenoma **182**
sessile serrated adenoma/polyp (SSA/P) 166
— : BLI **178**, **180**
— : NBI **176**
differentiation of — from hyperplastic polyp 175, 179
differentiation of — from large hyperplastic polyp 177
short-segment Barrett's esophagus (SSBE) 88, 94
Showa Classification 164
signet-ring cell carcinoma 127
sniffing position 26
soft palate 29
sparse pattern 162
squamocolumnar junction (SCJ) 79, 94
squamous cell carcinoma (SCC) 43, 48
squamous epithelial island 90
structure enhancement 18, 105, 232
subepithelial capillary network (SECN) 143
surface pattern 159, 162, 170, 232

T

traditional serrated adenoma (TSA) 175
transnasal endoscope 32, 40, 78
NBI using — 136
tree-like appearance 141
tumor associated with inflammatory bowel diseases: NBI **228**

type II open-shape pit pattern 179

U
ulcerative colitis 228
　—— : BLI **226**
　—— associated early carcinoma 229
undifferentiated gastric carcinoma 99, 127, 133

uvula 29

V
Valsalva maneuver 28, 32
varicose microvascular vessel (VMV) 181
vascular pattern 158, 162, 170, 232
　—— per macroscopic type of colorectal adenoma 161
vomiting reflex 49

W
white light imaging (WLI) 12, 17
white mucosal disorder 72
white opaque substance (WOS) 115, 116, 124, 146, 204
white zone 111, 159